Fifth
Edition

The OTA's Guide to Documentation

Writing SOAP Notes

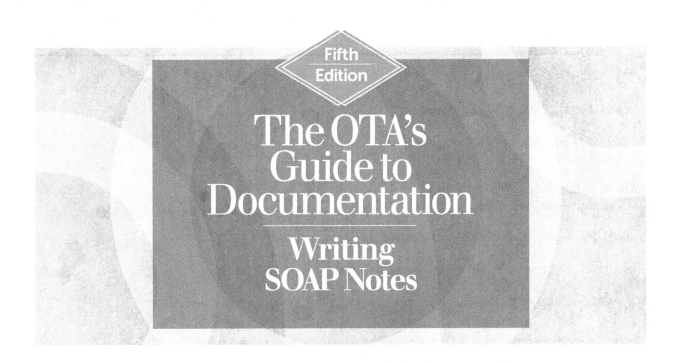

Fifth Edition

The OTA's Guide to Documentation

Writing SOAP Notes

Marie J. Morreale, OTR

Previously co-authored by:
Sherry Borcherding, MA, OTR/L

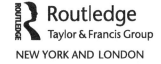

Routledge
Taylor & Francis Group

NEW YORK AND LONDON

Instructors: *The OTA's Guide to Documentation: Writing SOAP Notes, Fifth Edition* Instructor's Manual and videos are available. Don't miss this important companion to *The OTA's Guide to Documentation: Writing SOAP Notes, Fifth Edition*. To obtain these materials, please visit http://www.routledge.com/9781638220367

First published 2023 by SLACK Incorporated

Published 2024 by Routledge
605 Third Avenue, New York, NY 10158

and by Routledge
4 Park Square, Milton Park, Abingdon, Oxon OX14 4RN

Routledge is an imprint of the Taylor & Francis Group, an informa business

Copyright © 2023 Taylor & Francis Group.

Marie J. Morreale has no financial or proprietary interest in the materials presented herein.

Cover Artist: Tinhouse Design

Library of Congress Cataloging-in-Publication Data

Names: Morreale, Marie J., author.
Title: The OTA's guide to documentation : writing SOAP notes / Marie J.
   Morreale.
Other titles: Occupational therapy assistant's guide to documentation
Description: Fifth edition. | Thorofare, NJ : SLACK Incorporated, [2023] |
   Includes bibliographical references and index.
Identifiers: LCCN 2022025161 | ISBN 9781638220367 (paperback)
Subjects: MESH: Occupational Therapy--methods | Medical Records |
   Documentation--methods
Classification: LCC RM735.4 | NLM WB 555 | DDC 615.8/515--dc23/eng/20220708

ISBN: 9781638220367 (pbk)
ISBN: 9781003525523 (ebk)

DOI: 10.4324/9781003525523

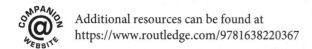

Additional resources can be found at
https://www.routledge.com/9781638220367

Dedication

This book is dedicated to OTA students everywhere. May you find joy and meaning in your work throughout your occupational therapy career.

Contents

Instructors: *The OTA's Guide to Documentation: Writing SOAP Notes, Fifth Edition* Instructor's Manual and videos are available. Don't miss this important companion to *The OTA's Guide to Documentation: Writing SOAP Notes, Fifth Edition*. To obtain these materials, please visit http:// www.routledge.com/9781638220367

Acknowledgments

Much appreciation goes to Sherry Borcherding, MA, OTR/L, for her vision in developing the initial materials for an occupational therapy documentation manual for therapist-level students. Following publication of her successful *Documentation Manual for Writing SOAP Notes in Occupational Therapy*, Sherry then partnered with Carol Kappel, COTA, to adapt this original material as a separate work to be more suitable for OTA students. As a result, Sherry and Carol co-authored *The OTA's Guide to Writing SOAP Notes*. After that first edition was published, I was honored to be able to collaborate with Sherry as co-author for the second, third, and fourth editions of that OTA documentation book. Along with an eventual title change, the initial OTA version has since morphed and expanded significantly over these subsequent editions to become what is now this current fifth edition text. I will always be truly grateful for Sherry's expertise and wisdom in the areas of mental health and documentation.

Thanks also go to University of Missouri occupational therapy students of the past who allowed some of their notes to be shared to teach others. Appreciation goes to Brien Cummings who is truly an asset at SLACK Incorporated. I am grateful for his kindness, help, and support with my multiple book projects throughout the past 15 years. Also, Jennifer Cahill and all the editorial team at SLACK have always been a pleasure to work with and they are dedicated professionals. Additionally, I will always be thankful to Ellen Spergel, past coordinator of the OTA Program at Rockland Community College, for giving me a start in academia that unexpectedly changed my path in life. Finally, special thanks to my husband, Richard. Without his love, patience, and support, this book would not have been possible.

About the Author

Marie J. Morreale, OTR, graduated Summa Cum Laude from Quinnipiac College (now Quinnipiac University) with a BS in occupational therapy. Throughout her professional career, Marie worked in a variety of practice settings, including inpatient and outpatient rehabilitation, cognitive rehabilitation, adult day care, skilled nursing facilities, home health, and hand therapy. She held the designation of Certified Hand Therapist for 25 years and served several years on a home health professional advisory committee, consulting on quality assurance issues.

For 17 years, Marie taught OTA students at Rockland Community College, State University of New York in Suffern as an adjunct faculty member. She taught a variety of courses there, which included Professional Issues and Documentation, Geriatric Principles, Occupational Therapy Skills, Advanced Occupational Therapy Skills, Therapeutic Activities, and Advanced Therapeutic Activities, in addition to serving briefly as interim coordinator of the OTA Program.

Marie co-authored the second, third, and fourth editions of *The OTA's Guide to Documentation: Writing SOAP Notes.* She also created the first and second editions of *Developing Clinical Competence: A Workbook for the OTA* and co-authored *The Occupational Therapist's Workbook for Ensuring Clinical Competence.* In addition, she wrote a chapter on documentation for *The Occupational Therapy Manager, Fifth Edition,* and published several occupational therapy articles. For the past several years Marie has been a test item writer for American Occupational Therapy Association continuing education products. She is active in her condo community and enjoys anything travel related.

Chapter 1

Documenting the
Occupational Therapy Process

An occupational therapy assistant (OTA) has many roles and responsibilities, including the essential task of documenting occupational therapy services. In addition to writing in the health record, documentation also encompasses accurate recordkeeping for school, community, or nontraditional settings. An OTA's professional documentation provides important information and feedback to the occupational therapist (OT) and other members of the health care or education team regarding clients. It also communicates the distinct value of occupational therapy to other audiences such as insurance companies and accrediting agencies. Initially, writing in the record might seem very intimidating to an OTA student or new practitioner. When you first see an experienced OT or OTA make an entry in a health, education, or early childhood record, you might be tempted to think you will never be able to do it. The technical language alone can be daunting, and then there is the amazing attention to detail in the client observation, the insightful assessment, and the documentation that just seems to flow from the pen, computer keyboard, or touch screen without apparent effort. You may wonder whether you will be able to organize all your client observations as effectively, predict what the next steps will be, and record interventions quickly and professionally. Perhaps you are also apprehensive about navigating the unfamiliar maze of templates and drop-down lists present in electronic health record (EHR) programs or being able to locate and decipher essential information in voluminous client charts. You might feel overwhelmed because the whole process seems a bit foreign to you. Rest assured that many occupational therapy practitioners felt the same way as you when they were students.

Professional documentation is a skill, and like any skill, it can be learned. Learning a skill, whether it is ice skating, playing the violin, or composing a progress note, requires three things of you: instruction, practice, and patience. This manual is designed to get you started with learning and practicing the process. Information is systematically provided on each part of the documentation process and the worksheets are designed to let you practice each step as you learn it. Use the manual as a workbook. Take time to integrate the information in each section, complete each exercise, and check it against the suggested answers in the Appendix. As you reflect and learn from your mistakes, you will develop more confidence in your documentation abilities.

Overview

This manual will help you to understand the purpose and standards of occupational therapy documentation for various practice settings and different stages of the occupational therapy process (evaluation, intervention, and targeting of outcomes; American Occupational Therapy Association [AOTA], 2018). Current occupational therapy practice is in many ways determined by which services are reimbursable, and documentation of skilled client care is the method by which that service is communicated. In the United States most hospitals and physician offices utilize

Morreale, M. J. *The OTA's Guide to Documentation:*
Writing SOAP Notes, Fifth Edition (pp. 1-15).
© 2023 Taylor & Francis Group.

EHRs (United States Department of Health and Human Services [USDHHS], n.d.). However, it is possible that you might encounter a facility or setting that continues to use a traditional paper-based charting system instead. It is also important to realize that even if a setting utilizes electronic medical records (EMR), some paper-based forms may still be necessary (e.g., a medical history questionnaire filled out by a client in the waiting room, or specific assessment forms used by an OTA in home care or a client's hospital room). These completed forms might then be scanned or the information manually transcribed into the EMR as appropriate. The fundamentals of both electronic documentation and traditional paper-based records are presented throughout this book.

This manual presents a thorough and systematic approach to one form of documentation, the **SOAP** note. SOAP is an acronym for the four parts of an entry into the record. The letters stand for *Subjective, Objective, Assessment*, and *Plan*. You will learn the origins and meanings of those terms in Chapter 2 along with an explanation of an alternate format, called a *narrative note*. The format this manual teaches for writing SOAP notes is one that is reimbursable by third-party payers, including Medicare, which has rigorous requirements. Not all funding sources require a SOAP note format and not all occupational therapy practitioners and facilities use SOAP notes. Practitioners using EHRs must conform professional documentation to specifications of the specific electronic documentation program in place. However, once you learn the basics for composing SOAP notes, you will then be able to adapt and apply those skilled observation and documentation skills to EHR formats and other methods of recording client care (e.g., flow sheets or narrative notes) required by your medical facility, school, or other practice setting. Also, if you learn to meet these strict standards, you are not likely to be denied reimbursement by any third-party payer.

Fundamentals of documentation, EHRs, billing, and reimbursement are explained in Chapters 2 and 3. These principles are also reflected in the many documentation examples presented throughout the manual. Each section of the SOAP note is also explained thoroughly in separate chapters for the S, O, A, and P. Other topics in this text include professional terminology, a review of grammar, an explanation of the initial evaluation process delineating the roles of the OT and OTA, a method for goal-writing, guidelines for selecting appropriate interventions, and an overview of the documentation requirements for different practice settings. A documentation checklist is also included at the end of this book to help ensure that your notes contain all the necessary elements. In addition, the Appendix in this book provides suggested "answers" for the worksheets. However, as there are many "right" ways to answer and compose therapy notes, these must be viewed as suggested best practice examples rather than the only "correct" answers. In actual clinical practice, you will see varied documentation styles among occupational therapy practitioners. Each OT and OTA develops individualized writing skills and a personal repertoire of professional language while complying with accepted legal and facility standards. Notes will also vary based on the type of practice setting and the specific documentation formats and systems used.

This manual reflects the collaboration of the OT and OTA and incorporates standards of AOTA and the Accreditation Council for Occupational Therapy Education (ACOTE) for education, documentation, and clinical practice. It reflects the scope of occupational therapy and emphasizes the basis of those services as described in the *Occupational Therapy Practice Framework: Domain and Process, Fourth Edition* (*OTPF-4*; AOTA, 2020d). This manual also incorporates educational standards delineated in the *2018 Accreditation Council for Occupational Therapy Education (ACOTE) Standards and Interpretive Guide* (ACOTE, 2018) along with concepts and guidelines delineated in AOTA official documents such as:

- *Guidelines for Documentation of Occupational Therapy* (AOTA, 2018)
- *Standards of Practice for Occupational Therapy* (AOTA, 2021b)
- *Occupational Therapy in the Promotion of Health and Well-Being* (AOTA, 2020c)
- *Guidelines for Supervision, Roles, and Responsibilities During the Delivery of Occupational Therapy Services* (AOTA, 2020b)
- *Scope of Practice* (AOTA, 2021a)
- *AOTA 2020 Occupational Therapy Code of Ethics* (AOTA, 2020a)
- *The Philosophical Base of Occupational Therapy* (AOTA, 2017)

The material presented in this book originally grew out of documentation courses taught to occupational therapy seniors at the University of Missouri–Columbia. The material was edited to be more appropriate for clinical practice of OTAs for the first edition of this book. Subsequent editions incorporated new material stemming from documentation courses taught to OTA students at Rockland Community College, State University of New York. The material has been field-tested to be sure it is practical, understandable, and effective in helping you learn both documentation and professional reasoning skills. This fifth edition reflects current guidelines for professional documentation, ethical occupational therapy practice, and includes updated billing and reimbursement information. Worksheets and learning activities have also been revised and new exercises added so that the reader can test attainment of knowledge and practice professional documentation skills. For new purchasers of this book, client intervention videos are available on the publisher's website for convenience and additional practice. An Instructor's Manual has been created for faculty as an online resource to accompany this book and includes client intervention videos, grading rubrics, and additional learning activities for documentation.

Occupational Therapy Professional Language and Focus

International Classification of Functioning, Disability and Health

The *International Classification of Functioning, Disability and Health (ICF)* is a health and disability framework established by the World Health Organization (WHO) and endorsed by WHO members in 2001 (WHO, 2002, 2021). *ICF* classifies, describes, and measures disability and health from the perspectives of not just physical health (pertaining to body structures and functions), but also a person's functional abilities (capacities) and actual performance levels for life tasks, while also considering the influence of social, personal, and environmental factors (WHO, 2002, 2021). The standard, universal language of *ICF* pertains to individuals, institutions, and society and influences public policy. *ICF* posits that most individuals will experience some level of disability through declining health as a result of illness, injury, or the normal aging process (WHO, 2002). Occupational therapy is a natural fit with the WHO viewpoint that health and disability are not based solely on a diagnosis but are impacted and intertwined with environmental factors, personal and social contexts, and actual abilities and limitations, all of which directly affect function, occupational participation, and performance of life tasks (AOTA, 2020d; WHO, 2002, 2021). It is useful to understand and incorporate terminology and concepts delineated in the *ICF* into your occupational therapy documentation.

Occupational Therapy Practice Framework

The *Occupational Therapy Practice Framework: Domain and Process, Fourth Edition* (AOTA, 2020d), also referred to as the *OTPF-4*, is an important document that embodies the focus and heart of occupational therapy and provides a foundational blueprint for the therapy process that occupational therapy practitioners reflect in professional documentation (Figure 1-1). The *OTPF-4* describes the domain and process of occupational therapy as "achieving health, well-being, and participation in life through engagement in occupation" (AOTA, 2020d, p. 5) and holistically delineates best practice for evaluation, intervention, and targeting of outcomes. This document includes taxonomy and standard definitions consistent with the *ICF* and presents a client-centered process that centers on enabling individuals to perform necessary and desired life activities for occupational participation and performance; the *OTPF-4* groups these broad and varied meaningful life tasks into **occupations** (AOTA, 2020d). The ability to engage in occupation is impacted by many interrelated factors: the client's **performance skills** (in the areas of motor, process, and social interaction), **performance patterns** (habits, routines, rituals, and roles), **client factors** (body structures and functions, spirituality, values, and beliefs), the influence of **contexts** (personal and environmental), as well as **activity and occupational demands** (AOTA, 2020b). Occupational therapy practitioners use professional reasoning, therapeutic use of self, empathy, activity analysis, and other specialized skills to plan and implement effective, evidence-informed interventions (AOTA, 2020d). An OTA's therapy notes should signify the skilled care provided and incorporate the professional language and underlying concepts set forth by the *OTPF-4*. The distinct value of occupational therapy should be evident to others reading your notes, such as payers and other disciplines.

By starting with an **occupational profile**, occupational therapy practitioners determine whether any personal or environmental features, activity demands, individual client factors or skills need to be addressed, depending on the occupational needs of the client (AOTA, 2020d). This allows appropriate goals and interventions to be determined for desired outcomes. The occupational profile is a client-centered approach to gathering information (occupational history, interests, experiences, habits, and patterns of daily living) as well as what the client values, needs, or hopes to gain from the present situation, allowing the client to set priorities for therapy (AOTA, 2020d). All this initial data, plus any subsequent changes in the client's status, priorities, interventions, goals, and targeted outcomes, will be recorded in the different types of notes that occupational therapy practitioners write throughout the intervention process.

OCCUPATIONS	CONTEXTS	PERFORMANCE PATTERNS	PERFORMANCE SKILLS	CLIENT FACTORS
Activities of daily living (ADLs) Instrumental activities of daily living (IADLs) Health management Rest and sleep Education Work Play Leisure Social participation	Environmental factors Personal factors	Habits Routines Roles Rituals	Motor skills Process skills Social interaction skills	Values, beliefs, and spirituality Body functions Body structures

Figure 1-1. Aspects of the occupational therapy domain. (Reproduced with permission from American Occupational Therapy Association. [2020d]. Occupational therapy practice framework: Domain and process [4th ed.]. *American Journal of Occupational Therapy, 74*[Suppl. 2], 7412410010. https://doi: 10.5014/ajot.2020.74S2001)

Engaging in Meaningful Occupation

Before documenting the occupational therapy process, OTs and OTAs must differentiate occupational therapy from other health care disciplines. Occupational therapy practitioners provide interventions for people who have problems engaging in *occupation*. This distinction is essential to convey in an OT or OTA's notes. In documentation, a focus on ability to engage in occupation is critical for demonstrating the necessity for occupational therapy and for preventing any question of duplication of services (Youngstrom, 2002). Occupational therapy practitioners in *all* service delivery settings have this common goal of facilitating occupational engagement (AOTA, 2020d; Youngstrom, 2002). Targeted outcomes can include occupational participation, health and well-being, occupational justice, quality of life, and role competence (AOTA, 2020d). It is also important to understand that each funding source has an interest in different outcomes or areas of occupation, meaning that payers have specific guidelines for what services they allow or consider necessary and will reimburse. This includes the specific type of occupational therapy interventions, frequency and duration of therapy services, or any special equipment clients may need (e.g., hospital beds, orthotic devices, adaptive equipment, assistive technology, customized wheelchairs). Your documentation should reflect those payer interests and requirements as they pertain to the client's condition and needs, physical environment, personal factors, and realistic expected outcomes. For example, Worker's Compensation will be interested in a client's ability to return to work, Medicare may be concerned about a home care client's ability to perform ADLs safely at home, whereas a school district will be focused on a child's ability to perform educationally related tasks as per the Individualized Education Program (IEP). The *OTPF-4* describes the following nine occupations (AOTA, 2020d):

Activities of Daily Living

ADLs are necessary tasks for self-care and personal independence. These are tasks such as bathing, grooming, hygiene, dressing, eating, toileting, sexual activity, and functional mobility (AOTA, 2020d). It is important to consider not just the physical ability to care for self, but also other components, such as cognitive deficits or mental health conditions that might cause limitations in performance. For example, rather than being unable to perform grooming skills due to a physical factor, a client might fail to notice that their poor hygiene is problematic or, perhaps, might have depression and lack of motivation to perform self-care. If your services are being reimbursed by Medicare, you will often find yourself writing goals for ADLs. For children, you will address ADLs as developmentally appropriate.

Instrumental Activities of Daily Living

IADLs require more complex problem-solving and social skills in addition to the physical aspects involved. IADLs include such tasks as money management, cleaning, laundry, childcare, driving, shopping, and meal preparation (AOTA, 2020d). While these are necessary skills in adulthood, IADLs are also important developmental milestones for children and teenagers and can include tasks such as caring for a pet, managing an allowance, babysitting, and using a microwave or stove. Occupational therapy practitioners who work with persons with brain injuries also consider executive functions that are an issue in frontal lobe damage. Executive functions involve planning, goal setting, and organizational tasks, which impact the ability to perform IADLs effectively and safely. If your client population has cognitive impairment, intellectual disability, or mental health problems, you may find that your goals include multiple IADLs.

Health Management

This area includes activities to improve or manage one's health to support occupational participation (AOTA, 2020d). In addition to looking at the motor skills needed to perform specific health management activities such as; opening pill containers to take prescribed medication, using birth control, handling and caring for personal care devices (i.e., glucometer, contact lenses, orthotics, hearing aids), OTs and OTAs also consider the mental functions, process skills, and performance patterns involved with procuring and using these items safely, effectively, and as directed by the person's health providers. Occupational therapy documentation includes relevant factors that hinder or support the individual's ability to self-monitor and manage symptoms of a specific condition or disease (i.e., rheumatoid arthritis, gluten/peanut allergy, diabetes), have emotional well-being, or maintain a healthy weight or lifestyle (AOTA, 2020d). OTs and OTAs collaborate with other health team members and document the skilled interventions working toward improving or maintaining the client's health and wellness. Examples of these interventions can include establishing individualized exercise programs, adapting personal care devices/methods to enable use, recommending stress-reduction activities, and teaching strategies to help maintain sobriety or adhere to a prescribed diet.

Work

Work includes successfully seeking and carrying out paid employment, as well as participating in volunteer experiences and planning for retirement (AOTA, 2020d). Work is a primary area of occupation for adults, forms a part of adult identity, and helps to structure one's day. If your services are being reimbursed by Workers' Compensation, you will generally find that the client's goals and interventions center around the return to work. Other work goals might include injury prevention, implementing interventions such as ergonomic education, occupational adaptations, safety training, and the elimination of hazards. If vocational rehabilitation is your funding source, you might find instead that your work goals involve helping prepare a client for work that is both meaningful and within the client's capabilities.

Leisure

Leisure activities are those intrinsically rewarding things one does when not obligated to do anything else. Leisure is a very important area of occupation, particularly for older people. Leisure is generally considered as activities that enhance one's quality of life and is not usually regarded as being a reimbursable goal. However, the performance skills and patterns required to perform leisure activities are transferable to a variety of occupations that are reimbursable. Therefore, leisure is usually approached indirectly in documentation, with a focus on functional performance skills and patterns. However, in some practice settings, such as mental health, it could be appropriate to have leisure-related goals addressing certain areas such as the appropriate use of leisure time, application of recommended coping strategies, and intrapersonal, interpersonal, or social components.

Play

In a young child, play can be solitary or social and may consist of organized tasks, such as games with rules or spontaneous activities such as exploratory play. One of the primary occupations for a child is acquiring those skills necessary to progress through age-appropriate developmental milestones, and these skills are acquired through play. When providing occupational therapy to young children, you will often find yourself talking about play in your documentation.

Education

Education is another of the primary occupations of a child. Those activities and skills needed to perform well in formal or informal educational settings are unique. Occupational therapy services to children in the educational system are for the purpose of the child performing school-related activities successfully. If you are working in school-based practice, your goals and interventions must relate to behaviors and skills needed in the classroom or school environment to be reimbursable. You should also consider the child's ability to engage in extracurricular activities such as music, clubs, and sports. Education for adults encompasses college classes and formal, informal, or personal educational situations such as attending a continuing education seminar for professional needs or personal enrichment (AOTA, 2020d).

Social Participation

People, as social beings, need to be able to interact successfully with others, have friendships and intimate partner relationships, and to keep one's behavior within the contextual norms of the community, the family, and peer groups (AOTA, 2020d). If you are working with clients who have a brain injury, intellectual disability, or mental health conditions, you might find yourself documenting goals and interventions for social participation.

Rest and Sleep

Proper rest, relaxation, and sleep are essential for physical and emotional health, stamina, and safety. Clients who have pain, illness, incontinence, or who are caregivers of young children or a parent with Alzheimer's disease may have interrupted sleep patterns or limited opportunities to rest or relax. Mental health conditions such as depression or anxiety can result in excessive or inadequate sleep. Other factors such as a noisy environment or working the night shift or multiple jobs may also adversely impact attainment of proper rest and sleep. Your documentation should include any concerns related to sleep preparedness or inadequate rest and sleep patterns.

Influencing Contexts

The *OTPF-4* also describes the variety of internal and external **contexts** that influence one's ability to engage in meaningful occupations (AOTA, 2020d). Contexts include **personal factors** unique to the individual such as, age, gender, culture, socioeconomic status, character traits, life experiences, and so forth (AOTA, 2020d). Contexts also encompass **environmental factors** which are the person's surroundings such as, the physical setting, geography, climate, available systems, products and technology, types of relationships and support, etc. (AOTA, 2020d). If your client is being seen in an environment such as a hospital or clinic that is not usual for that person, it is important to determine whether the skills you are teaching are transferable to that client's own environment. It is especially important to document how specific contextual factors relate to the client's condition and may be barriers to occupational participation. For example, a client who has good functional mobility in the hospital may be completely stopped by three steps into a mobile home, an old-fashioned bathtub on legs, or lack of an elevator at the jobsite. A client who lives in a rural area and can no longer drive may not have availability of public transportation or ride-sharing service for grocery shopping or getting to work. Due to peer pressure, a teenager may refuse to wear leg braces, orthotic devices, or might avoid use of adaptive equipment or assistive technology in public. A recently retired executive or empty nester might have difficulty adjusting to an abundance of leisure time or, perhaps, a nursing home resident may have difficulty getting adequate sleep due to a roommate crying out frequently during the night. Your documentation should always include relevant personal and/or environmental contextual factors that support or hinder occupational participation along with any interventions or occupational adaptations to address problematic situations.

Underlying Factors

Occupational therapy practitioners document the pertinent underlying factors that impact a client's abilities, limitations, and occupational participation. **Client factors** consist of **body structures and functions**, which refer to the client's anatomy and physiology, along with internal **spirituality, values, and beliefs,** which influence a client's meaning of life and motivation (AOTA, 2020d). For example, an amputation of a limb, a hysterectomy, or a dental extraction would be considered loss of a body structure. An adult with hip joint degeneration, scoliosis, aneurysm, or a child born with cleft palate, spina bifida, or club foot have impairment in a particular body structure. Body structures provide a physical framework to enable all the body's systems to function, just like a water heater requires a metal container, pipes, nuts, and bolts before it can begin to work.

Some deficits in body structures can be "fixed" permanently or semi-permanently (total joint replacement, organ transplant, corrective surgery) or temporarily (dentures, prosthesis, wig). As some of these underlying deficits and surgical/medical "corrections" could affect body functions and limit performance skills, a referral to occupational therapy might be indicated to help manage the condition and improve occupational participation. For example, intervention may include teaching compensatory dressing and bathing techniques following a total hip replacement, improving activity tolerance using a prosthesis, teaching energy conservation and occupational adaptations following a heart transplant, or improving body image and upper limb function after a mastectomy.

The term *body functions* refers to making the body systems perform their physiological and psychological duties, just like a water heater getting turned on and heating the water. Body functions include the vital processes of basic life and movement functions, such as breathing, righting reactions, reflexes, wound healing, digestion, cardiovascular functions, and immunology (AOTA, 2020d). More overt body functions include areas such as strength, the senses, and joint motion. Mental functions encompass cognitive and perceptual aspects and also include intrapersonal characteristics such as personality, self-image, and emotions (AOTA, 2020d). If any of these client factors do not limit the client's ability to engage in desired activities and occupations, they do not necessarily need to be assessed or addressed in treatment. However, if a client has problems that do impact occupational participation such as poor memory, a non-healing wound, dyspraxia, orthostatic hypotension, low vision, impaired sensory processing, decreased strength, spasticity, low vital capacity, poor self-esteem, hallucinations, or anxiety, then these might be relevant client factors or conditions to document and target in your interventions.

Performance Skills

Occupational therapy practitioners use knowledge and professional reasoning to assess the demands or requirements of activities/occupations in addition to observing and analyzing **performance skills**; these are client behaviors and actions grouped into three primary areas: **motor, process,** and **social interaction skills** (AOTA, 2020d). As your client is performing activities and occupations, you will examine and document how these task skills are performed and consider what factors may impede or support occupational participation (AOTA, 2020d). For example, you can note specific motor capabilities as a client tries to carry dishes to the table; reach to get clothes out of the dryer; brush teeth; draw a picture with crayons; push a toy shopping cart; manipulate knitting needles and yarn; bend to pick boxes up from the floor; grip pliers; or stand at a workstation for a specific time-period. Process skills levels become apparent when you observe a client try to sort laundry; put away clean utensils; play checkers; choose proper coins for the vending machine; attend to the math teacher; organize a locker; pay bills and so forth. You can note social interaction skills by observing, for example, whether the client has ability to initiate casual conversation; request a pain pill appropriately; handle a frustrating situation; ask for help with homework; share a toy; sustain eye contact; or maintain personal boundaries. You will be recording your professional observations and skilled analysis of client behaviors, actions, skills, and underlying client factors in your clinical (SOAP) notes.

Activity Demands

Occupation and activity demands are interactive. They are most easily thought of in terms of task analysis. The demands of an occupation/activity include both what is needed for successful performance (specific materials, methods, skills, sequence of steps) and how that influences or relates to the client's stated goals. Occupational therapy documentation should specify the occupation and activity demands that are challenging for a particular client along with any interventions, grading methods, and adaptations needed for occupational performance.

Interventions

Occupational therapy practitioners record the varied interventions that are planned and implemented for the attainment of desired client outcomes such as managing chronic conditions, enabling occupational participation, and improving quality of life. According to the *OTPF-4* (AOTA, 2020d) types of occupational therapy interventions include the following: occupations and activities; interventions to support occupations (skilled methods and tasks); group interventions; advocacy; education and training. Documentation should delineate the specific methods used, the client's response to intervention, progress made toward goals, and any changes to the intervention plan.

Roles of the OT and OTA

When communicating about occupational therapy, it is important to understand that the terms *therapist* and *clinician* are used to refer only to the OT, *not* an OTA (AOTA, 2020b; Centers for Medicare & Medicaid Services [CMS], 2019). An OTA, of course, uses the term *occupational therapy assistant* and should never be referred to as a therapist. OTs and OTAs are also identified as *occupational therapy practitioners*. In documenting the occupational therapy process, OTs and OTAs have different roles and responsibilities. AOTA's *Guidelines for Supervision, Roles, and Responsibilities During the Delivery of Occupational Therapy Services* (AOTA, 2020b) and *Standards of Practice for Occupational Therapy* (AOTA, 2021b) delineate specifically the roles and responsibilities of both OTs and OTAs regarding documentation and clinical practice. In partnership with the supervising OT, the OTA performs delegated aspects of client care and can assist in designing, implementing, and assessing occupational therapy services (AOTA, 2020b, 2021b). The OTA may also contribute to documentation at all stages of treatment under the supervision of the OT and concurring with relevant laws and regulations (AOTA, 2018, 2020b, 2021b).

Although these guidelines are considered "best practice," state statutes and licensure laws may differ from the guidelines. The guidelines may also differ from federal laws that delineate mandatory documentation requirements. In addition, funding sources may specify who would be an approved documenter or service provider for reimbursement purposes. You, as an occupational therapy professional, are accountable for adhering to the mandatory policies and procedures adopted by state and federal regulatory agencies. However, you will find the standards established by the AOTA very useful in interpreting and following regulations.

Types of Notes

Different kinds of notes are written at different stages of the occupational therapy process. Notes also vary according to the type of practice setting. From the first notation in the chart that a referral has been received to the closing lines of the discharge report, occupational therapy practitioners document the many varied activities of the intervention process. The specific content of the note, format and organization of the note, and the timelines required all vary greatly according to type of setting, accrediting and regulatory agencies involved, and requirements of the funding source. The contents required for the following types of notes are described in *Guidelines for Documentation of Occupational Therapy* (AOTA, 2018) and will be addressed in this manual.

Initial Evaluation Reports

Before beginning intervention, the client is evaluated to determine whether occupational therapy is appropriate, and if so, what kind of therapeutic intervention will be most useful. The OT directs the evaluation process, documents the results, and establishes the intervention plan; although, the OTA can contribute to this process (AOTA, 2018, 2020b, 2021b). Each practice setting or facility has its own way of evaluating a client. A behavioral or mental health center, for example, may not do the same kind of an evaluation as a public school or a skilled nursing facility. Evaluations are usually documented by completing a specific form provided by the setting or using a particular software program linked to the facility's EHR system. Sometimes, even if an EHR system is in place, the therapist might utilize a paper-based form or take handwritten notes during the actual evaluation session (for convenience or portability), then formally enter that information into an electronic format afterward. In some instances, an evaluation may also be done in a SOAP format for entry into the record.

Contact Notes (Treatment Notes)

Each time an intervention is provided by the occupational therapy practitioner, a notation is made of what occurred (AOTA, 2018). Documentation might also include relevant information obtained from communications with the client, family/significant others, health professionals, or service providers such as from telephone conversations or meetings. Depending on the setting, each intervention session is documented in the health or school record using a formal contact note or, perhaps, the occupational therapy practitioner might fill out a simple flow sheet or checklist of services provided instead. In other settings where no formal contact notes are required, the occupational therapy practitioner might only keep an attendance sheet, informal log, or perhaps just jot down some observations to refer to later when writing progress notes. Contact notes can be written in many different formats, but in this manual the SOAP format will primarily be taught.

Progress Report

At the end of a certain time period, a progress note is written. The occupational therapy practitioner records the client's progress toward goals and details any changes made in the intervention plan. Different practice settings vary regarding time periods for reporting, but progress notes are usually written in specified time frames such as weekly, every 2 weeks, monthly, or after a particular number of intervention sessions have been implemented. Progress notes may also be written in different formats but will be taught in a SOAP format in this manual. Regulatory and payer mandates often delineate the required frequency of progress notes (or benchmark reporting in school settings) and specify whether an OTA is allowed to write a progress note for clients in that setting or not.

Reevaluation Report

The OT directs and documents the reevaluation that is part of the occupational therapy intervention process and modifies the intervention plan according to the client's needs and changes in status. The OTA may contribute to this reevaluation process (AOTA, 2018, 2020b, 2021b). Some settings and payers require a formal reevaluation report. For example, in a practice setting where managed care is involved, a client may need to be reevaluated in order to be recertified for treatment after the number of initially allocated visits are completed. EHR programs may use a reevaluation format similar to the evaluation, making it easy to compare results.

Transition Plan

Transition notes are written when a client is transferring from one service setting to another (e.g., from early intervention to preschool or from special education to vocational services) within the same system of service delivery (AOTA, 2018). Transition notes ensure that the client's intervention plan remains intact through the move and that services that have already been provided are not duplicated. The transition plan is the responsibility of the OT, but the OTA may contribute to this process (AOTA, 2018, 2020b, 2021b).

Discharge or Discontinuation Report

At the end of the intervention process, a discharge or discontinuation report is written to describe changes in the client's ability to engage in meaningful occupation as a result of occupational therapy intervention (AOTA, 2018). The discontinuation plan is directed and documented by the OT, but the OTA may contribute to this process (AOTA, 2018, 2020b, 2021b). Discharge notes summarize the course of intervention; progress toward goals; status at the time of discharge; provision or recommendation of any durable medical equipment, orthotic devices, assistive technology, adaptive equipment, home programs, and any other referrals or follow-up required. Some settings will provide a specific form for the discharge note, whereas other facilities might use a similar form that was used for the client's evaluation. Some EHR programs might use a format that automatically pulls up the initial evaluation data, making it easy to compare and record discharge results side by side.

Conclusion

Professional documentation pulls together all of your observation skills, clinical reasoning, and knowledge of occupational therapy. It communicates important information to the health, education, or early childhood team and substantiates the need for occupational therapy services to third-party payers. The content and style of notes will vary according to the type of practice setting and the specific systems and formats in place.

Due to space limitations in this book, some required contents of various notes have been purposely left out. Understand that if you were writing an actual note in a client's health or education record, you would always use the client's whole name and identification information along with any other required demographic data and insurance information. For clients already established in an EHR system, this information is usually incorporated when the record is opened again. A "real" note might also include additional pertinent background facts and assessment findings. All notes must be signed with the occupational therapy practitioner's full name and credentials and an OTA's notes cosigned by the OT when required by law, facility policy, or payer requirements (AOTA, 2018).

It is important to understand that each client has unique circumstances and needs. Although this manual provides sound guidelines and examples of best practice, occupational therapy practitioners must always use professional reasoning when interacting with clients and documenting in the record. For the many notes and examples presented throughout this manual, fictitious names have been used and any specific resemblance to a real person is coincidental. The following worksheets will test your knowledge of documentation basics and help you understand and practice using the *OTPF-4* terminology to record your observations and interventions. Then, in the next chapters, you will be introduced to important aspects of the health record, billing and reimbursement fundamentals, and the specifics of your documentation in the record. There will be ample explanation and opportunity for practice so that you will systematically acquire the appropriate documentation skills. Eventually, **you** will be the OTA we talked about in the beginning paragraph whose documentation was so amazing to the beginning student.

Worksheet 1-1
Documentation Basics

Indicate whether each of the following statements is true (T) or false (F).

1. _____ OTs and OTAs can be referred to as occupational therapy practitioners or therapists.

2. _____ When skilled therapy is no longer needed, the OTA has responsibility for writing the discharge report if they treated the client for the final therapy session.

3. _____ Most hospitals and physician offices in the U.S. utilize EHRs.

4. _____ The acronym SOAP stands for Subjective, Objective, Appraisal, and Plan.

5. _____ An occupational therapy note is only written when the OT or OTA has physical contact with the client.

6. _____ An alternate format to a SOAP note is a narrative note.

7. _____ A transition note might be written when a client is transferring from special education to vocational services within the same system of service delivery.

8. _____ It may be necessary for an OT or OTA to utilize various paper-based health forms in a setting that has an EHR system in place.

9. _____ The *OTPF-4* incorporates terminology and concepts compatible with the WHO health and disability framework *International Classification of Diseases* (*ICD*).

10. _____ In educational settings, benchmark reporting refers to documenting a student's progress for specific time periods during the school year.

11. _____ To differentiate occupational therapy from other disciplines, OTs and OTAs should focus their documentation on the client's ability to engage in occupation.

12. _____ An occupational profile is established once appropriate client goals are established.

13. _____ ADL occupations include activities to improve or manage one's health, such as wearing an orthotic device, taking prescribed medication, or using a glucometer.

14. _____ An OTA should expect that a client's ability to perform an activity/occupation in the clinic will always be transferable to the client's home setting.

15. _____ OTAs document performance skills such as reflexes and range of motion.

16. _____ Occupational therapy notes tend to be very consistent in content and style across different types of practice settings.

17. _____ The OT cannot change an established occupational therapy intervention plan once treatment has been initiated.

18. _____ Third-party payers always approve reimbursement for durable medical equipment or assistive technology if the client would benefit from it.

19. _____ Activity demand refers to a task the client insists on doing during an intervention session rather than what the OT or OTA is recommending.

20. _____ Because leisure tends to improve one's quality of life, it is usually regarded by third-party payers as a reimbursable goal in physical rehabilitation settings.

Worksheet 1-2
The *Occupational Therapy Practice Framework: Domain and Process, Fourth Edition (OTPF-4)*

Refer to the *OTPF-4* (AOTA, 2020d) to answer the following multiple-choice questions. Questions may have more than one correct answer. For each question, indicate all the answer choices that are correct.

1. Which of the following are examples of a performance pattern?
   a. Tracing a client's hand during orthotic device fabrication
   b. One's family or work role
   c. Bilateral coordination
   d. A religious ritual
   e. Bedtime routine
   f. Two-point gait

2. Which of the following are examples of a performance skill?
   a. Bending far enough to retrieve clothing from dryer
   b. Muscle strength of Good (4/5) for shoulder flexion
   c. Standing for 10 minutes
   d. Reciting a prayer from memory
   e. Normal muscle tone
   f. Gag reflex

3. Which of the following are considered occupations?
   a. Spirituality
   b. Social participation
   c. Range of motion
   d. Sleep
   e. Rest
   f. Play

4. Which of the following are client factors?
   a. Values
   b. Sleep
   c. Mental functions
   d. Roles
   e. Blood pressure
   f. Age

5. Which of the following are examples of contextual factors?
   a. Gender
   b. Completing high school or college
   c. Internet access
   d. Lack of public transportation for a client who is unable to drive
   e. Presence of lead or pesticides in client's home
   f. Income below poverty level

Morreale, M. J. (2023). *The OTA's guide to documentation: Writing SOAP notes* (5th ed.). SLACK Incorporated.

6. A client is recovering from a stroke and has deficits in upper extremity function and difficulty performing ADLs/IADLs. Which of the following are examples of possible interventions to support occupations?
   a. Using pulleys to increase range of motion
   b. Squeezing therapy putty to improve grip strength
   c. Practicing buttoning a shirt
   d. Measuring ingredients to make a cake
   e. Passive range of motion to increase elbow flexion
   f. Fabricating and issuing an orthotic device

7. Which of the following are activities?
   a. Practicing writing one's name in cursive
   b. Preparing a meal after shopping for ingredients
   c. Peeling potatoes
   d. A 50-year-old client stacking cones to improve upper limb function
   e. Maintaining balance while sitting on a therapy ball
   f. Completing morning grooming routine

8. Which of the following are examples of interventions to support occupations?
   a. Rolling out pie dough
   b. Performing wound care on a client
   c. Application of hot pack
   d. Using hand weights to increase upper extremity strength
   e. Teaching client strategies to reduce stress
   f. Washing lettuce for a salad

9. Which of the following are delineated as the primary performance skills categories in the *OTPF-4*?
   a. Motor skills
   b. Emotional regulation skills
   c. Social interaction skills
   d. Sensory integration skills
   e. Preparatory skills
   f. Process skills

10. Which of the following are rituals?
   a. Biting one's fingernails when feeling anxious
   b. Lighting candles on the Sabbath
   c. Wearing a seatbelt when driving
   d. Showering, dressing, and buying coffee at Starbucks prior to work every day
   e. Always making Irish soda bread for St. Patrick's Day
   f. Making the sign of the cross when entering a church

Worksheet 1-3
Using the *Occupational Therapy Practice Framework*

Observe someone make an object out of clay or another craft project. Use terminology from the *Occupational Therapy Practice Framework: Domain and Process, 4th Edition* (AOTA, 2020d) and list 10 specific client factors or performance skills that you observe happening during this activity. Try to describe, qualify, or quantify levels of performance.

Activity observed: _____

Examples:

Process skill: Attends well to task

Client factor: Has good range of motion in both hands

1.

2.

3.

4.

5.

6.

7.

8.

9.

10.

Morreale, M. J. (2023). *The OTA's guide to documentation: Writing SOAP notes* (5th ed.). SLACK Incorporated.

Worksheet 1-4
Occupational Therapy Practice Framework—More Practice

Observe someone perform a simple cooking task such as making tea, a sandwich, or a can of soup. Use terminology from the *Occupational Therapy Practice Framework: Domain and Process, 4th Edition* (AOTA, 2020d) and list 10 specific client factors or performance skills that you observe happening during this activity. Try to describe, qualify, or quantify levels of performance.

Activity observed: _____

Example:

   Motor skill: Coordinates use of both hands well when using can opener

   Client factor: Able to hear whistling tea kettle

1.

2.

3.

4.

5.

6.

7.

8.

9.

10.

Morreale, M. J. (2023). *The OTA's guide to documentation: Writing SOAP notes* (5th ed.). SLACK Incorporated.

References

Accreditation Council for Occupational Therapy Education. (2018). 2018 Accreditation Council for Occupational Therapy Education (ACOTE) standards and interpretative guide (effective July 31, 2020). *American Journal of Occupational Therapy, 72*(Suppl. 2), 721241005. https://doi.org:10.5014/ajot.2018.72S217

American Occupational Therapy Association. (2017). The philosophical base of occupational therapy. *American Journal of Occupational Therapy, 71*(Suppl. 2), 7112410045. https://doi.org: 10.5014/ajot.2017.716S06

American Occupational Therapy Association. (2018). Guidelines for documentation of occupational therapy. *American Journal of Occupational Therapy, 72*(Suppl. 2), 7212410010. https://doi.org :10.5014/ajot.2018.72S203

American Occupational Therapy Association. (2020a). AOTA 2020 occupational therapy code of ethics. *American Journal of Occupational Therapy, 74*(Suppl. 3), 7413410005. https://doi.org: 10.5014/ajot.2020.74S3006

American Occupational Therapy Association. (2020b). Guidelines for supervision, roles, and responsibilities during the delivery of occupational therapy services. *American Journal of Occupational Therapy, 74*(Suppl. 3), 7413410020. https://doi.org/10.5014/ajot.2020.74S3004

American Occupational Therapy Association. (2020c). Occupational therapy in the promotion of health and well-being. *American Journal of Occupational Therapy, 74*, 7403420010. https://doi.org/10.5014/ajot.2020.743003

American Occupational Therapy Association. (2020d). Occupational therapy practice framework: Domain and process (4th ed.). *American Journal of Occupational Therapy, 74*(Suppl. 2), 7412410010. https://doi.org: 10.5014/ajot.2020.74S2001

American Occupational Therapy Association. (2021a). Occupational therapy scope of practice. *American Journal of Occupational Therapy, 75*(Suppl. 3), 7513410020. https://doi.org/10.5014/ajot.2021.75S3005

American Occupational Therapy Association. (2021b). Standards of practice for occupational therapy. *American Journal of Occupational Therapy, 75*(Suppl. 3), 7513410030. https://doi.org/10.5014/ajot.2021.75S3004

Centers for Medicare & Medicaid Services. (2019). *Medicare benefit policy manual* (Pub. 100-02: Ch. 15, Section 220). Retrieved October 11, 2021 from https://www.cms.gov/Regulations-and-Guidance/Guidance/Manuals/Downloads/bp102c15.pdf

U.S. Department of Health and Human Services. The office of the national coordinator for health information technology. (n.d.) *Health IT Dashboard: Quick Stats.* Retrieved May 25, 2022 from https://healthit.gov/data/quickstats

World Health Organization. (2002). *Towards a common language for functioning, disability and health: ICF.* Author. https://cdn.who.int/media/docs/default-source/classification/icf/icfbeginnersguide.pdf?sfvrsn=eead63d3_4

World Health Organization. (2021). *Classifications: International classification of functioning, disability and health (ICF).* Author. Retrieved October 11, 2021 from https://www.who.int/standards/classifications/international-classification-of-functioning-disability-and-health

Youngstrom, M. J. (2002). The occupational therapy practice framework: The evolution of our professional language. *American Journal of Occupational Therapy, 56*(6), 607-608.

Chapter 2

The Health Record

Definition, Types, and Purpose

The medical record is also referred to as the *health record*. It is a ***legal document*** that provides an electronic or written history of a client's past and present health, substantiates care, and creates proof of advance directives, vital statistics, course of treatment, and related correspondence (Fremgen, 2020; Scott, 2013). The primary purpose of the health record is the exchange of information among health care providers in order to determine a client's problems and strengths, establish an appropriate plan of care, record treatment, facilitate continuity of care upon discharge (or in the future), and fulfill legal documentation requirements (Fremgen, 2020; Scott, 2013). In addition to an individual's health care information, records typically contain standard content such as the person's identifying information, demographic data, insurance and physician information, assignment of benefits, privacy notices, and consent forms. Any ***advance health care directives*** (e.g., health care proxy, living will, organ donor, "do not hospitalize" or "do not resuscitate" [DNR] orders) should also be contained in the record and kept updated as appropriate. Occupational therapy practitioners working in inpatient, outpatient, or community settings utilize the health record to obtain and record client data, document planned and implemented interventions, and validate services for reimbursement. An OTA provides valuable communication in the health record to support intraprofessional and interprofessional collaboration.

As medicine advanced, so did the complexity and detail of the health record. A profession called *health information management* was created to oversee the health record. Useful resources regarding various aspects of the record are offered by The American Health Information Management Association (AHIMA) at www.ahima.org. As of 2019, 96% of non-federal acute care hospitals and nearly 75% of office-based physicians in the United States have now shifted from the use of traditional paper-based records to a certified computerized format, called an ***electronic health record*** (EHR) or ***electronic medical record*** (EMR; Office of the National Coordinator for Health Information Technology [ONC], n.d.b). The ONC, part of the United States Department of Health and Human Services (USDHSS), differentiates between these two terms using the following descriptions:

Morreale, M. J. *The OTA's Guide to Documentation: Writing SOAP Notes, Fifth Edition* (pp. 17-45).
© 2023 Taylor & Francis Group.

> "<u>Electronic medical records</u> (EMRs) are **digital versions of the paper charts** in clinician offices, clinics, and hospitals. EMRs contain notes and information collected by and for the clinicians in that office, clinic, or hospital and are mostly used by providers for diagnosis and treatment. EMRs are more valuable than paper records because they enable providers to track data over time, identify patients for preventive visits and screenings, monitor patients, and improve health care quality."
>
> "<u>Electronic health records</u> (EHRs) are built to go beyond standard clinical data collected in a provider's office and are inclusive of a broader view of a patient's care. EHRs contain information from **all the clinicians involved in a patient's care** and all authorized clinicians involved in a patient's care can access the information to provide care to that patient. EHRs also share information with other health care providers, such as laboratories and specialists. EHRs follow patients – to the specialist, the hospital, the nursing home, or even across the country."
>
> Reproduced from Office of the National Coordinator for Health Information Technology. (2019c). What are the differences between electronic medical records, electronic health records, and personal health records. Retrieved October 11, 2021 from https://www.healthit.gov/faq/what-are-differences-between-electronic-medical-records-electronic-health-records-and-personal

Providers can choose from a variety of available EHR software programs and systems but must use **certified EHR** technology to meet specific Centers for Medicare & Medicaid Services (CMS) requirements for security and functionality (CMS, 2021b).

Another type of computerized record, called a ***personal health record* (PHR)** is an EHR used and controlled by the individual to track and maintain their own health information for personal use. It also allows the individual to select information to be shared with family/caregivers or health providers (ONC, 2019c). PHRs may include data that the individual enters, such as allergies and medication history, along with information obtained from home monitoring devices and various health providers (ONC, 2019c). Health providers may provide a ***patient portal***, which is a website through which individuals can access their personal health information (e.g., lab test results, medications, discharge summaries) anytime. These portals might also allow patients to exchange email securely with their health providers, request refills for prescriptions, schedule appointments, pay bills, fill out forms, and perform other related tasks (ONC, 2017b). Besides enhancing communication between the patient and health care team, portals help to empower clients, save time, and support clinical care (ONC, 2017b).

OTs and OTAs working in school-based settings provide interventions and documentation that focus primarily on the educational needs of children requiring special services. It is important to understand that a student's **education records** (including any occupational therapy documentation) also require accurate recordkeeping, confidentiality, and adherence to established protocols. Education records provide a means of communication among professionals in the child's school and district concerning the child's academic abilities and pertinent health or social concerns. If you are an OTA working in a school-related setting, understand that it is also very likely that a parent or guardian will eventually read what you and the OT have written about a child receiving services (Sames, 2015). In addition, education records are used to obtain aggregate data for local, state, and federal reports. While this manual often refers to the *health record*, many of the documentation "rules" also apply to education records. Specific information regarding occupational therapy documentation in school-based settings is presented in Chapter 17.

Legislation Impacting Health Care and Documentation

Education and health care in the United States are regulated by numerous federal and state laws that impact access to care, costs, reimbursement, professional roles, and types of services available in various communities. Government mandates influence how health and education services, including occupational therapy, are delivered, paid for, communicated, and valued. Some legislation specifically applicable to the documentation, management, and meaningful use of health information include the following:

Health Insurance Portability and Accountability Act

In 1996 Congress passed the Health Insurance Portability and Accountability Act (HIPAA), which established national standards to manage and protect the privacy and security of an individual's health information (USDHHS, 2003a). HIPAA delineates an individual's right to understand and control the use of one's own health information and to be informed about a provider's privacy practices, including how one's information will be used and shared (USDHHS, 2003a, 2003b).

The Privacy Rule required compliance by April 14, 2003 (with a 1-year extension for small health plans; USDHHS, 2003a). It specified regulations for the use and disclosure of **protected health information (PHI)**, which is defined as "individually identifiable health information" (USDHHS, 2003a, p. 3). Facilities and individuals providing health or medical services and transmitting health information electronically (i.e., claims, referral authorization requests, payment) are considered a **covered entity** (USDHHS, 2003a). Occupational therapy practitioners come under this category and must adhere to the HIPAA regulations.

A written **Notice of Privacy Practices (NPP)**, which must be given to each patient, delineates the provider's privacy practices regarding PHI. The patient signs this document which grants permission for their PHI to be disclosed for treatment, reimbursement, and certain other health care reasons. The signed document is maintained in the patient's medical record. A major part of the Privacy Rule is the **minimum necessary** standard, which states that only the minimum amount of PHI must be requested or disclosed to accomplish the intended purpose (USDHHS, 2002, 2003a, 2003b). In addition, the covered entity must establish reasonable safeguards, workplace policies, and procedures protecting PHI, such as allowing access only to the personnel requiring that information for their job duties and locking up records when not in use (USDHHS, 2002, 2003b, 2007). Some instances in which PHI disclosure is permitted without express written authorization include public health activities (e.g., tracking certain communicable diseases or adverse effects of products), various law enforcement situations, organ and tissue donation, reports of child abuse or neglect, and national security (USDHHS, 2003a).

In practical terms, as an OTA, you typically cannot provide information about the client's condition with the client's family, friends, or employer without the client's permission. However, you can usually communicate with the referring physician and other team members involved in the client's care. Also, although you might be very curious and concerned, these are not acceptable reasons to look up information on a friend, colleague, family member, or public figure admitted to the facility if you are not authorized to be involved in that individual's care. Most importantly, you must always try to protect client privacy and safeguard information. If you happen to have a client in your facility or on your caseload that is famous, such as a movie star, musician, high-profile athlete, or politician, you are still *not allowed* to divulge this to your friends or family, or provide information to any news outlet, even though you might be very tempted to do so. Understand that these public figures also have the right to privacy. They should not have to worry that their PHI will be plastered across the front page of a newspaper or supermarket tabloid. Any information released to the public must be expressly authorized through the proper channels and personnel, such as the facility's legal department or public relations staff, and only with the client's permission. As this is only a brief overview of HIPAA, **it is essential that you do not disclose or give out any health records or client information without fully understanding the law and knowing your facility's policies and procedures**.

Family Educational Rights and Privacy Act

The Family Educational Rights and Privacy Act (FERPA) outlines a student's rights and privacy regarding their education records. FERPA applies to all schools receiving U.S. Department of Education funding for pertinent programs (U.S. Department of Education, 2021). This federal law allows the parent or eligible student (e.g., students 18 or older or who attend schools beyond high school) to fully review the student's education record and to formally request correction of any inaccuracies, including what is written in occupational therapy (U.S. Department of Education, 2021). FERPA also mandates that, in order for a school to release a student's protected information, written permission from a parent or eligible student is needed. There are some exceptions for the consent requirement, such as for emergencies, a student's financial aid or school transfer, judicial orders, legitimate functions of school officials, accreditation, and certain types of studies (U.S. Department of Education, 2021). Schools are also allowed to release basic directory information (e.g., names, awards, honors) provided that parents are notified of this general practice and can opt out (U.S. Department of Education, 2021). At schools, a student's health information (including Individualized Education Program [IEP] designated special services) is typically contained in education records and, as such, would be subject to FERPA privacy requirements rather than the HIPAA Privacy Rule (USDHHS, 2008). However, HIPAA rules for transactions would still apply if third-party payers such as Medicaid are billed for a student's health services such as occupational therapy (USDHHS, 2008). It is essential that you do not disclose student information or give out any records without fully understanding the law and adhering to your school district's or facility's policies and procedures.

Box 2-1
MANDATES INCLUDED IN THE AFFORDABLE CARE ACT

- Affordable quality health care and health insurance coverage for all Americans
- Requirement for individuals to maintain minimum essential coverage
- Ensuring that consumers get value for their dollars
- Essential health benefits requirements
- Health information technology enrollment standards and protocols
- Development of quality outcome measures
- Data collection and public reporting
- Quality reporting for long-term care hospitals, inpatient rehabilitation hospitals, and hospice programs
- Hospital readmissions reduction program
- Improving Medicare and Medicaid for patients and providers
- Ensuring beneficiary access to physician care and other services
- Linking Medicare payment to quality outcomes
- Medicare shared savings program
- National pilot program on payment bundling
- Hospital readmissions reduction program
- Payment adjustment for health care–acquired conditions
- Clinical and community preventive services
- Increasing access to clinical and community preventative services
- School-based health centers
- Removing barriers and improving access to wellness for individuals with disabilities

Adapted from United States Department of Health and Human Services. (2010). Compilation of Patient Protection and Affordable Care Act. Retrieved May 20, 2022 from: https://www.hhs.gov/sites/default/files/ppacacon.pdf

Health Information Technology for Economic and Clinical Health Act

To promote EHR infrastructure and use across the United States, the Health Information Technology for Economic and Clinical Health (HITECH) Act of 2009 was enacted (ONC, 2021). HITECH set technology standards to improve health information quality, safety, and efficiency through the promotion of health information technology, creation of a nationwide health infrastructure with funding, and authorized CMS to initiate incentive programs for implementation (ONC, 2021). HITECH established an Office of National Coordinator for Health Information Technology and created committees for policies and standards to make recommendations and create standards for establishment of individual EHRs, ensure health information privacy and security protections, create certification criteria, improve coordination of care between facilities, increase care quality, develop telemedicine technologies, and collect health information data for public reporting, public health, and research (ONC, 2021).

The Patient Protection and Affordable Care Act

The Patient Protection and Affordable Care Act (ACA) was passed in 2010 to establish reforms for health care insurance. Aims of the ACA include increasing health care access, lowering costs, providing new protections for consumers, and improving health care quality and efficiency (USDHHS, 2010, 2021a). The ACA has led to various changes regarding the purchase and cost of health insurance. It also influences the coverage of various services and impacts how health care is delivered and paid for. Some of the numerous provisions in this legislation that may directly or indirectly impact occupational therapy are listed in Box 2-1 (USDHHS, 2010).

Food and Drug Administration Safety and Innovation Act

The Food and Drug Administration Safety and Innovation Act (FDASIA) of 2012 requires collaboration among the FDA and several other governmental agencies to propose strategies and recommendations for a health IT regulatory framework that is appropriate, risk-based, and includes medical mobile applications. Aims of FDASIA include protecting patient safety, avoiding regulatory duplication, and promoting innovation (ONC, 2015; 2021).

Improving Medicare Post-Acute Care Transformation Act of 2014

The Improving Medicare Post-Acute Care Transformation Act of 2014 (the IMPACT Act) is legislation that requires long-term care hospitals, inpatient rehabilitation facilities, home health agencies, and skilled nursing facilities to submit standardized client assessment data and report on specific quality measure domains and resource use, such as: total Medicare spending per beneficiary; changes in functional status and cognitive function; major falls incidence; skin integrity status and changes; whether the client was discharged to community; risk-adjusted hospital readmission rates that were potentially preventable; and various other measures (CMS, 2021d). This legislation aims to enhance care coordination, improve client outcomes, provide overall comparisons of quality, and reduce costs through more efficient care (CMS, 2021d). The IMPACT Act and the ACA are requiring providers to be more accountable for the care they provide and are a fit with CMS quality initiatives. As a result, health care has been trending toward *value-based care*, which includes different payment models such as episode-based management and bundled (consolidated) payments over the traditional fee-for-service model (DeJong, 2016). DeJong (2016) posits that OTs need to be "smart" clinicians who use the available data to improve client care, outcomes and provide more value for consumers and payers.

Medicare Access and CHIP Reauthorization Act of 2015 (MACRA)

This legislation created the **Quality Payment Program (QPP)** that changes how Medicare "rewards clinicians for value over volume"; provides bonus payments to providers participating in eligible alternative payment models (APMs), and implements a new Merit Based Incentive Payments System (MIPS) which streamlines multiple quality programs under it (CMS, 2019a). Providers can choose from these two tracks; those involved with Advanced APMs can earn incentive payments from Medicare for participating sufficiently in an "innovative payment model" while clinicians eligible for MIPS are subject to a performance-based payment adjustment (CMS, 2020c; ONC, 2021).

21st Century Cures Act

Aims of the 21st Century Cures Act (Cures Act) include improving flow and interoperability of electronic health information, enhancing privacy and security, increasing accessibility and usability, and ensuring individuals, families and health providers have suitable access to EHRs to enable overall improvement of health in the United States (ONC, 2021). The Cures Act also strives for development of innovative software and smartphone apps for both individuals and providers to allow for easier records access, more transparency, and competitive care options (ONC, n.d.a.)

Individuals with Disabilities Education Act

The Education for All Handicapped Children Act (PL 94-142) Section 504 was enacted in 1975 to address the individual needs (i.e., development, education) of infants and children with disabilities and their families (U.S. Department of Education, n.d.a). The law was reauthorized in 1990 (PL 110-476) and renamed the Individuals with Disabilities Education Act (IDEA). This reauthorization now included autism and traumatic brain injury as new disability categories and mandated that post high school transition plans be established for individuals (U.S. Department of Education, 2020). A 1997 reauthorization (PL-105-17) included emphasis on general curriculum access and expanded the definition of "developmental delay" in students up to age 9 years (U.S. Department of Education, 2020). IDEA was again reauthorized in 2004 as the Individuals with Disabilities Improvement Act to provide services to students needing academic and behavioral support but who are not classified as requiring special education. Additional aims of the 2004 reauthorization included improved standards, better educational outcomes, greater accountability, plus alignment with requirements of the No Child Left Behind Act (U.S. Department of Education, 2020). Subsequently, periodic new regulations for IDEA have also been issued to revise definitions and address various areas such as parental consent, due process, state monitoring, and others (U.S. Department of Education, 2020).

IDEA Part C mandates the provision of **early intervention** services to children less than 3 years of age who are experiencing or are at risk for developmental delay (due to a diagnosed condition) in one or more areas. The five areas of development delineated in IDEA include physical, cognitive, communication, adaptive (e.g., daily living skills), and social/emotional (Center for Parent Information and Resources, 2017; U.S. Department of Education, n.d.b). States have discretion to expand the definition of various factors that put a child at risk for needing early intervention services and the law mandates that early intervention services must be provided in the child's "*natural* *environment*," which can include the home or a community setting with nondisabled children, such as a daycare center or preschool (Center for Parent Information and Resources, 2017). Specific documentation for each child is required, including an **Individualized Family Service Plan (IFSP)** that describes the child's development, family situation, and identifies specific services needed.

IDEA Part B applies to children ages 3 to 21 years old with a disability or qualifying health condition, mandating that schools provide an appropriate free public education in the "*least restrictive environment*" (LRE). The LRE regulation requires that children be educated (and perform other typical school activities) in settings alongside non-disabled peers to the maximum extent possible (Center for Parent Information and Resources, 2021). As appropriate, special education, related services (e.g., skilled services, which can include occupational therapy), and supplementary aids and services may be provided to help the child succeed in school. Supplementary aids and services can include student accommodations and modifications, such as an aide, extra time to take tests, physical adaptations, slower-paced instruction, communication aids, etc. (Center for Parent Information and Resources, 2021). The law requires that an **Individualized Education Program [IEP]** be established for each child requiring special education and related services. The specific documentation requirements for early childhood and school settings will be described further in Chapter 17 of this manual.

Electronic Documentation Systems

The switch from traditional paper-based charts to electronic documentation systems has changed how occupational therapy practitioners approach the documentation process, obtain data, use specific formats to enter information, communicate with others, and obtain reimbursement for services. Health information can now be entered and obtained from different locations and means, such as handheld wireless devices, computers, and smart phones. As an authorized user you will be given a user name and password, and the facility will provide training for whatever electronic systems are in place there.

Digital Technology in Health Care

Facilities may utilize digital technology such as electronic client wristbands with memory chips or barcodes that link to a client's identifying data, medications, or other health information (Scott, 2013). Barcode scanning helps to reduce errors by ensuring that the correct patient is getting the intended medication, diagnostic tests, or treatment.

Health practitioners are also able to obtain client information from a variety of **remote patient monitoring (RPM) devices** that can be used to track patients' vital signs and deliver alerts if suboptimal results occur. Some examples of RPM devices include wearable heart monitors, digital scale, thermometer, pulse oximeter, blood pressure device, etc. These devices might provide data in real-time remotely to the medical practitioner or, perhaps, track data that the client enters through an app or phone call at scheduled intervals. In some situations, clients may be instructed to keep a handwritten log or bring a particular device's memory chip to appointments.

Electronic Health Record Systems

Electronic documentation requires computer *hardware*, which is the actual physical equipment, such as a computer hard drive, server, printer, monitor, handheld devices, etc. *Software* are specific programs that run on a computer. They include the basic operating system, anti-virus software, and other installed programs that perform various functions. EMR systems are generally classified into two types: on-site (e.g., local) and web-based systems, which must meet legal requirements (i.e., HIPAA, HITECH) for privacy, security, and functionality (Cohen, 2013; CMS, 2021a). Systems must have proper firewalls and be able to effectively back up data.

Local/on-site systems have their own server to run an EMR program on *local* networks and store the data privately in-house whereas, web-based systems use a program that runs on an *internet-based system* (Cohen, 2013). Data centers are used to store information from web-based systems (e.g., cloud), enabling authorized personnel to access certain records via the internet from any location such as a client's residence or the practitioner's home (Utzman, 2020). Web-based systems typically entail a subscription model with recurring monthly costs that can vary according to the number of users or amount of data and claims processed, but the subscription price usually includes training, upgrades, and technical support (Cohen, 2013). Depending on the setting, the OTA might share a computer in the occupational therapy office, enter data in a more central area (such as a mobile computer station on a hospital unit), or have a personal laptop or hand-held device to access and record information. Some clinics also have designated tablets or kiosks for clients to enter information, such as to complete a questionnaire or check in for a scheduled appointment.

Advantages of Electronic Health Records

Electronic records are legible and organized, which benefits the different audiences that might be reading them, such as the client, family/caregiver, other health care providers, attorneys, etc. EHR systems may include various short-cuts or organizational functions, such as schedule management; automated patient appointment reminders (e.g., emails, phone calls); application of proper code sets for billing claims; comparing prior test results to the present assessment; and ability to track and analyze various data in the facility/agency for productivity, resource use, quality measures, clinical outcomes, etc. (ONC, 2018, 2019b). EHRs can also improve efficiency by centralizing chart management, eliminating duplicate paperwork, requiring less storage space for cumbersome charts, decreasing time to pull and file information, etc. (ONC, 2018). Also, EHRs typically have integrated program prompts to help ensure that necessary paperwork and information are all in place such as privacy and consent forms, insurance information, medication history, diagnosis and billing codes, plan of care, and so forth, along with possible links to public health systems for required reporting of communicable diseases, CMS quality measures, etc. (ONC, 2017a, 2018). Authorized users also have easy, immediate access to comprehensive patient information from multiple sources and locations. Several people can collaborate and review a client's data simultaneously which can help to coordinate care and reduce unnecessary services such as duplication of tests or procedures. Secure patient portals allow for convenient electronic communication between the client and provider, such as for prescription requests, questions, or client's access to test results.

Documentation completed using paper and pen often necessitates that health care providers fill out duplicate information (particularly client identifiers and demographic data) on facility and regulatory forms; this redundancy is minimized with EHRs (ONC, 2017a; Herbold, 2016; Utzman, 2020). Another benefit of electronic documentation is that it typically includes the use of prompts or templates for the information necessary to meet requirements for the setting or funding sources (ONC, 2017a; Herbold, 2016). For example, rehabilitation software might have templates guiding the therapist through all required aspects of an evaluation report and the specific factors that must be addressed and documented in that setting, for example, living situation, functional cognition, pain level, ADL abilities, and so forth. Also, electronic documentation systems often allow for entered data to be routed into regulatory systems to facilitate reporting of mandated CMS outcome measures used in various settings, such as the *Minimum Data Set (MDS)* in nursing homes, *Outcomes Assessment Information Set (OASIS)* in home care, and the *Inpatient Rehabilitation Facility-Patient Assessment Instrument* (*IRF-PAI*; Herbold, 2016). These standard quality measures will be explained further in Chapter 17. Practitioners can also save time by selecting from standard menus of problems, goals, and possible intervention strategies specific to a particular practice setting, such as hand therapy, mental health, or pediatrics. Programs might also include established clinical pathways for specific diagnoses commonly treated at that setting, for example, total knee or hip replacement. Additionally, medical errors can be reduced by built-in safeguards to alert the provider to possible drug interactions, allergies, or other potential adverse events (ONC, 2019a). Other helpful EHR features can include electronic reminders or alerts telling health providers when code modifiers are needed, therapy is reaching a therapy cap (requiring an Advanced Beneficiary Notice), or that a certification or report is due. EHR programs may provide links to evidence-based information and articles that the health provider can use to help with clinical decision-making, in addition to linking to patient education materials (Swigert, 2018).

EHR systems designed for use by rehabilitation professionals might include various tools such as balance or pain scales, cognitive or behavioral assessments, and functional questionnaires. Optional compatible accessories may be available for integration into the system such as grip and pinch meters or a goniometer. These allow assessment results to be scored and incorporated automatically into the treatment note as tests are administered. Also, as a timesaving measure, there might be an option for specific types of data or standard phrases to be copied and pasted into subsequent notes and reports, as appropriate, without having to retype the same information over and over. Of course, practitioners must ensure that any information copied and pasted must be completely accurate for the current client and not substituted for critical thinking in a note. Some standard phrases that might be used as shortcuts are presented in the following examples, although additional clarification still needs to be included in the note such as, listing the exact exercises shown; identifying specific resistance level of therapy putty/exercise bands used or kind of orthotic device issued; noting right or left hand; indicating purpose of exercises/adaptive equipment/orthosis for that individual, and so forth.

"Client was instructed in home program of therapy putty exercises and precautions. Client provided with written instructions and demonstrated good understanding by performing all exercises accurately."

or, perhaps,

"Client was instructed in use and care of orthotic device. Written copy of instructions provided. Client demonstrated ability to don/doff orthosis independently and verbalized understanding of wearing schedule and precautions.

Client was advised to contact OT Dept. if any problems/questions re: orthosis and to bring orthosis next session for follow-up assessment of use/wearing tolerance."

Disadvantages of Electronic Health Records

There can be significant costs related to setting up an electronic documentation system such as purchasing equipment/software, technical support services, plus subscription costs if using an EHR cloud service (Utzman, 2020). A specific data backup plan must also be in place (USDHHS, 2007). Although staff training might be included in the purchase or subscription price of an EHR system, costs are still incurred for the *time* needed to train staff in the use of a particular software program or system. Training could be time consuming or meet resistance from persons who are inexperienced with technology or are opposed to switching over from a different system because they prefer "doing things the old way." Practitioners used to paper-based records may also experience an adjustment period with additional documentation time needed to merge their own organizational style with a more structured format that "flows" quite differently. It may also take extra time to shift through a maze of various menus and pages to find and enter information in the appropriate places.

There can be challenges with interoperability due to providers using different networks and systems. Other concerns regarding electronic documentation include security, privacy, computer downtime, and crashing. Information could possibly be destroyed accidentally or entered inaccurately due to errors in typing or using a touch screen, misdirected pointing and clicking, or mistakes in digital cutting, copying, and pasting. Additionally, devices containing sensitive information on hard drives or portable memory storage items could be stolen, lost, or hacked into.

When accessing or entering computer data at point of service, health practitioners can have tendency to focus on the computer screen, keyboard, and mouse but must ensure that their attention is also directed toward the client. An OTA should display a caring approach, make eye contact with the client, and not cut off the person's conversation just because it doesn't fit with the present data entry page. Practitioners should have awareness of one's nonverbal communication (e.g., frowning, sighing, having a too casual sitting/standing posture), and remain patient if the computer happens to be temperamental or very slow at inopportune times.

Use Professional Reasoning and a Client-Centered Approach in Documentation

Occupational therapy practitioners must always use professional reasoning and a client-centered approach throughout the occupational therapy process, such as when gathering information, creating goals, selecting and implementing interventions, developing home programs, and documenting in the record. Although there are a variety of EHR vendors and products that facilities, agencies, and private practices can choose from, the terminology or methods for a specific program may not be fully compatible with occupational therapy language, process, or departmental needs. Therefore, occupational therapy practitioners must be careful to avoid a rote or cookbook approach when selecting problems, goals, interventions, and other clinical options from a program menu. Some software programs are very structured and rigid while others offer flexibility in terms of customizing formats to the specifications of a facility or department (such as for evaluations, contact notes, and intervention plans). Some software programs allow for greater individualized detail by providing places for comments or allowing users to mix-and-match programs or menus. Practitioners must not lose sight of a client's individual needs or compromise quality of care by making the client conform to the specifications of a particular software package. One resource, AOTA PERFORM, consists of a variety of templates created as a layout for inclusion in EMR systems to aid in documenting the occupational therapy three-part evaluation process: Occupational Profile, Analysis of Occupation, and Intervention/Plan of Care (AOTA, 2018a, 2021c). Aim of this tool is to integrate the evaluation process into EMRs efficiently and effectively by incorporating, at that time, the *Occupational Therapy Practice Framework: Domain and Process, 3rd Edition* (AOTA, 2014b) terminology, concepts, and detailed elements (AOTA, 2018a, 2021c).

Storing, Managing, and Disposing of Health Records

There are federal and state guidelines for storing, managing, and retaining health records, such as the types of safeguards that must be put in place to protect client privacy and the length of time records must be kept. Each facility/agency establishes policies and procedures to comply with established laws, and the OTA must follow these protocols.

Privacy Protocols

To safeguard protected health information, workers must be trained regarding proper privacy practices and appropriate disposal of client files (USDHHS, 2002, 2007, 2015). One typical security measure is for health care workers to have *password-protected* computer access to the patient information necessary to perform their job functions. This helps to ensure that unauthorized users cannot view that information (USDHHS, 2002, 2007). Systems can track who accessed patient data and when. Items containing protected health information such as traditional paper-based charts, computers, tablets, and portable memory storage devices should be kept in a secure location such as a locked cabinet or office. Never leave records where others can see them, such as open on a desk or treatment table. Ensure that the computer screen is not in view of others when entering or accessing information and always remember to log out and close the computer screen when you are done. Volunteers, visitors, other clients, or staff (i.e., housekeeping, maintenance, secretaries, rehab disciplines) may have valid reasons to enter the treatment area or your office, so you should always manage records in a way that protects client confidentiality. In addition, be very careful if you must have conversations about a client with relevant health team members, third-party payers, family/significant others, etc. in public areas such as an elevator or cafeteria. You must try to ensure that other people cannot inappropriately see or hear the confidential information.

Paperwork should normally remain and be completed on-site and not taken home to review or complete documentation. However, it might be necessary for an occupational therapy practitioner working in home care or traveling among several sites to have secure access to electronic record systems off-site or be allowed to keep a temporary working copy of paper records while the original stays within the agency. Do not leave briefcases, laptop computers, or other equipment on the seat of a parked car where it might be tempting for someone to steal them. Again, it is essential to always follow HIPAA guidelines and facility policies.

Storage of records depends on federal and state regulations and the type of practice setting, but methods include keeping the original paper format, microfilm, hard drives, or computer media. Individual states mandate the specific minimum time periods (usually 10 years) for retaining medical records for minors and adults, including occupational therapy documentation (Fremgen, 2020). Most states also require that the health records of minors be kept until a certain number of years after the child reaches the age of majority in that state (Fremgen, 2020). Providers may choose to keep records longer than what the state requires, such as for potential future legal issues or client care.

Disposal of Records

If records containing PHI are no longer needed, they must be disposed of properly according to legal guidelines (USDHHS, 2007, 2015). Your facility will have specific policies and procedures in place to comply with this. Paper records with PHI must *never* just be put in a dumpster or ripped up in a few pieces and thrown in a garbage pail because someone might find them and possibly reconstruct and read the confidential information. Instead, paper records must be destroyed completely by incinerating, pulverizing, or shredding (USDHHS, 2007, 2015). Disposal of electronic records must be done by specified methods of clearing or purging data or destroying the computer media through shredding, disintegrating, incinerating, etc. (USDHHS, 2007, 2015). Realize that any other paperwork or electronic files containing confidential client information not yet entered in the chart (such as any attendance logs, working copies used for day-to-day occupational therapy intervention, or temporary drafts), must be properly secured and destroyed when no longer needed. Your department or facility should have a shredding machine or designated locked bin (to contain items for later shredding) readily available for proper disposal of confidential records.

Health Record Access

The medical record is the physical property of the health care facility that furnishes the client's care, but clients normally have a legal right to obtain and review copies of their billing records and health information, including what you have written in occupational therapy (Fremgen, 2020; USDHHS, 2020). However, this right excludes psychotherapy notes (e.g., personal notes of the mental health provider kept separate from the record) and information that will be used in a criminal, civil, or administrative action/proceeding (USDHHS, 2020). Additionally, there are certain instances when a patient or their representative can be denied access to medical records upon the review of a licensed medical professional who determines access would endanger that patient or others (USDHHS, 2020).

To obtain their records, clients may have to submit a formal signed request and can also be charged for copying, postage, and certain labor costs. Fees cannot be charged to a client just for the opportunity to inspect their records but not get a personal, physical copy (USDHHS, 2020). Individual states usually determine the maximum reasonable fees that may be charged for copies of reports, X-rays, etc.; and your facility or agency will have specific policies regarding this process. In addition, third-party payers may require health record documentation to substantiate claims for reimbursement. In these situations, only the *minimum necessary* is sent. Some occupational therapy documentation, such as for outpatient Medicare Part B services, might require physician review and certification (requiring a hand-written or electronic signature) to certify the patient requires skilled services and the physician approves the plan of care, even if an initial order is in place (CMS, 2021f). As previously mentioned, **privacy laws regulate the disclosure of medical information, so never, ever give out or send any health records or client information without knowing the exact policies and procedures in your facility**. To comply with legislative and payer requirements regarding the exchange of health information, each setting establishes policies and procedures delineating which departments or personnel (such as the Health Information Services Department, outpatient department secretary, private practice owner, etc.) are responsible for the sending of specific records or reports to clients, physicians, other professionals, or funding sources, depending on the situation. All staff must be very careful when using electronic communication, fax machines, and copiers to avoid breaches of confidentiality to unintended recipients. Paperwork must always be removed after using the copier, printer, or fax machine and it is prudent for the sender to always double check fax numbers, email addresses, and phone numbers for accuracy. A copy of pertinent correspondence, including letters, home exercise programs, or instructions given to the client, should be maintained in the record.

Organization of the Health Record

How information is entered and organized in the record depends largely on the specific format used by the facility or the specifications of the electronic documentation program used. Software programs display various templates, menus, and comment areas in a particular order for various functions. This structures how data is entered and organized into notes and presented as reports, with the amount of flexibility dependent on the specific program.

Medical records have traditionally utilized formats such as a **source-oriented medical record** or **integrated medical record** to organize all of the client's health information in the chart. A source-oriented record is divided into sections for each discipline (i.e., nursing, lab results, occupational therapy). Within each section, the discipline's information is presented in chronological order using SOAP notes (or another format) to record that discipline's care and the client's status. This type of organization makes it easy to locate information or track progress for a particular discipline such as occupational therapy. This is especially beneficial when contributing to an occupational therapy progress report or discharge report. A disadvantage is that one has to search through many sections to determine the client's overall status at a given time. With an integrated medical record format, all disciplines record information in chronological order, one right after the other. For example, an occupational therapy note might come directly after a nursing note, followed by a physical therapy or respiratory therapy note. If using paper-based records, this format makes it easy to find client information pertaining to a particular time period but it is harder to find or track information for a particular discipline. For example, the OTA might have to search through all of the shift changes of nursing notes to find out what was done in the client's occupational therapy session yesterday. It is also more difficult to locate and gather information for the occupational therapy discharge report, such as the number of sessions provided. However, the use of EMRs can help eliminate such unnecessary steps by being able to click on a menu to pull up a particular discipline's notes or automatically tracking how many occupational therapy sessions have been provided.

SOAP Note History

In the 1960s, Dr. Lawrence Weed advocated the problem-oriented medical record (POMR) in order to provide more meaning and organization to the client's record through a structured, objective, and client-centered approach to documentation (Weed, 1971, Erikson, 2020).

Weed recommended that the client information (i.e., history, physical findings, lab results) be structured and organized according to a list of the patient's problems with planned interventions for each problem (Erickson, 2020). Weed also suggested a specific progress note format of four distinct sections which addressed the identified problems and evolved into a SOAP note (Erickson, 2020).

The acronym SOAP stands for subjective, objective, assessment, and plan and consists of the following:

- **S (Subjective):** The *client's perception* of the treatment being received, progress, limitations, needs, and problems. Normally the subjective section of a treatment note is brief. However, in an occupational therapy initial evaluation note, the "S" might be longer because it contains the information obtained by occupational therapy practitioners in the initial interview (i.e., occupational profile).

- **O (Objective):** The *health professional's observations* of the treatment being provided, such as the specific interventions implemented, the client's performance, and levels of assistance needed. In an occupational therapy initial evaluation note, this section also contains all of the measurable, quantifiable, and observable data that the OT determines should be collected. In an evaluation, the first two sections form the data base from which the OT, with contributions from the OTA, develops a problem list and treatment plan.

- **A (Assessment):** The *health professional's clinical judgment and interpretation* of the statements and events reported in the subjective and objective sections. This section includes the client's progress, functional limitations, problems, and expectations of the client's ability to benefit from therapy (sometimes called *rehabilitation potential*). In an initial evaluation, the OT, with feedback from the OTA, will determine and include the problem list, which is one of the key elements of the POMR method of charting.

- **P (Plan):** *What the health professional plans to do next* to help meet the goals and objectives in the intervention plan. In an occupational therapy initial evaluation, this section contains the OT's intervention plan, including the anticipated frequency and duration of treatment.

SOAP is simply a format—an outline for organizing information. Any note can be written in this format, although some notes lend themselves to it better than others, such as contact (treatment) notes and progress notes. Of course, electronic documentation programs may delineate how specific information needs to be entered and organized in the record. However, OTs and OTAs can still incorporate important aspects of SOAP criteria when recording data and documenting progress toward goals in a standard, organized way. Also, some practitioners still include all or part of a SOAP note in the comments section of an EMR note to ensure that no important client details have been missed and to further substantiate the care provided in case claims are later audited. A more detailed discussion of each section of the SOAP note will follow in Chapters 6 through 10.

Narrative Notes

An alternative to the structured SOAP format is the **narrative note**. Narrative notes are typically written in a less restricted paragraph format; although the information may still be organized into various pertinent categories such as client factors or occupations. As narrative notes are not divided into standard sections like the SOAP note, the occupational therapy practitioner must be very careful to ensure that all of the necessary information is still organized and included. A good narrative note will contain all the components of the SOAP note but just not have the information divided into separate categories for the S, O, A, and P. The general documentation rules in this manual still apply to narrative notes. However, you might find that the information typically entered in the S and O sections of the SOAP note is sometimes ordered a little differently in a narrative note. For example, a SOAP note might begin with something like the following:

S: *Client reported having a "constant dull ache" in his right shoulder for the past 2 days which he described as 3/10.*

O: *Client participated in 30-minute session in rehab gym to work on decreasing pain and increasing strength/ function of right upper extremity to enable return to work...*

Whereas, a narrative note might begin like this:

Client participated in 30-minute session in rehab gym to work on decreasing pain and increasing strength/function of right upper extremity to enable return to work. When client arrived at therapy today, he reported having a "constant dull ache" in his right shoulder for the past 2 days which he described as 3/10...

If you first learn the SOAP note format presented in this manual, you can easily convert your client information into a proper narrative note if that is the format your facility uses. An example of a narrative discharge report is provided in Chapter 16 and several examples of narrative contact notes are provided in Chapter 18.

Users and Uses of Health Records

The health record is a communication tool, and thus has many different uses and users. As an OTA, it is important to consider all of your different audiences when you make an entry in the client's record.

Client Care Management

The record is one method the health care team uses to communicate with each other about the day-to-day aspects of a client's condition and treatment. Other occupational therapy practitioners in your department or other members of the health care team will read your notes in order to coordinate appropriate care. The OT, with contributions from the OTA, will document the results of the occupational therapy evaluation in the health record and establish the intervention plan. The OT and OTA will then collaborate to implement interventions, record the client's progress toward established goals, and advise other team members of the occupational therapy plan for continuing care. This communication is extremely important to the health care team. One occupational therapy practitioner may not be providing all of the client's care and may depend upon the treatment notes to find out what interventions were provided in their absence. A particular advantage of electronic documentation is that it organizes information and makes it easy to generate multiple written patient reports for various audiences as needed (Herbold, 2016).

The Client

Of course, another significant user is the client. When you are writing in the record, always remember that clients (or parents/guardians as appropriate) have access to information in the health or education record and may choose to exercise their right to read what you have written.

Reimbursement

The record is the source document for what services were provided, and thus for what occupational therapy services may be billed. It is used in billing to substantiate reimbursement claims. For example, if a question arises about the duration and frequency of interventions provided, the record would be the source document used to answer that question. Often in managed care, initial evaluation data and periodic progress reports must be submitted to obtain authorization for additional therapy sessions.

The Legal System

The health record is a legal document that substantiates what occurred during a client's illness or condition and course of treatment. If you are an OTA having to appear in court to testify, you will be very glad that your documentation is clear and thorough. Sometimes court cases will occur years after the event or intervention that is being contested and you may not even remember the client or the event. What you have written in the record should provide you with the information you need to testify. Therapy records may be subpoenaed for many reasons, including cases involving Workers' Compensation; malpractice; personal injury lawsuits; child, spousal, or elder abuse.

Research and Evidence-Based Practice

The record is also used to provide data for medical research and evidence-based practice. Researchers might use individual data specific to that client or aggregate data where no client name is attached to the data. In either case, the source document is often the health record, under the security regulations of HIPAA.

Accreditation

Accrediting organizations, such as the Joint Commission and the Commission on Accreditation of Rehabilitation Facilities (CARF), review medical records (including your occupational therapy notes) to help ascertain whether the extent and quality of services provided by your facility and/or your department meet the standards of care set by the accrediting agency. If the facility is found not in compliance, accreditation may be withdrawn. Accreditation from specific national accrediting organizations, including the Joint Commission, Accreditation Commission for Health Care, Inc. (ACHC), Community Health Accreditation Program (CHAP), and several others, can be used to meet Medicare certification requirements for facilities and providers that bill Medicare (CMS, 2021b). If the facility or equipment provider does not meet CMS standards, claims made by that facility for Medicare services (including occupational therapy) will be denied. The health record is one of the primary sources used during a visit from an accrediting organization or a CMS State Survey Agency.

Education

The record may be used as a teaching tool. A fieldwork student uses the health record to gain information about clients and learn about quality of care, other disciplines, occupational therapy intervention and best practices, in accordance with HIPAA guidelines.

Public Health

The health record is used to identify and to document the incidence of certain diseases, such as tuberculosis, COVID-19, HIV, and outbreaks of contagious illness within a facility. In addition, the health record is used to report vital statistics (births, deaths); substantiate and report child, spousal, or elder abuse; and provide statistics for epidemiology.

Business Development

Management teams use the information contained in the record to review what kinds of clients are being seen and how services in the facility or agency are being utilized. This information is used to help plan and market the services provided and to determine appropriate levels of personnel. For example, are enough cases of clients with cardiac conditions being admitted to justify developing a specialized cardiac rehabilitation program? Would this necessitate hiring more staff in the occupational or physical therapy departments?

Clinical Quality Measures

Legislation such as the ACA and IMPACT Act require that health providers report on various patient quality measures to improve efficiency and quality of care, reduce costs, and provide better client outcomes. Some of these measures may involve monetary incentives to providers for implementation or outcomes. Individual client data (such as level of function) is recorded according to specific required measures for certain settings, such as a skilled nursing facility, inpatient rehabilitation facility, or home health agency. Aggregate data, such as hospital readmission rates and overall incidence of falls or pressure injuries, is used to determine and compare a provider's quality of service and whether care there is value-based.

Documentation for Quality Improvement

The health record is one of the primary sources of information used in the quality assurance (QA) process, which provides accountability, assesses the quality of care provided, and compares it to established standards (Fremgen, 2020). Clinical data is gathered (such as mandatory clinical quality measures, incidents, outcomes, etc.) and analyzed. Various mandatory and/or voluntary quality measures reported to Medicare and Medicaid can impact the payment amounts facilities and providers receive.

Quality Improvement Committees

Most facilities have a QA or Quality Improvement (QI) committee whose duty it is to oversee the appropriateness and adequacy of the care that is being provided. These committees are charged with finding and solving problems in client care. Employees are normally encouraged to help make positive changes in their facility to reduce medical errors, improve safety, increase efficiency, and ensure high standards of care. For example, the occupational therapy staff might determine that one problem they are seeing is that a certain percentage of outpatients are not complying with their orthosis-wearing schedule, which impedes the clients' recovery. The QI team might collaborate with the occupational therapy department to brainstorm possible solutions, determine appropriate outcome measures, and implement new procedures (e.g., develop a checklist for proper fitting, provide clients with additional training and written instructions, implement reminder emails/phone calls and timely follow-up appointments) to address this problem. The occupational therapy practitioners will then document and track whether these new methods increase compliance and meet desired outcomes.

Facilities also use other kinds of quality measures to determine if policies and procedures are being followed and to help ensure proper standards. One method that may be utilized is periodic **peer review**. Health professionals may be assigned various client records to review peer documentation and look for any deficiencies in notes or care implemented. For example, you might review another OTA's notes or another occupational therapy practitioner might review your notes for a client who has been discharged from therapy. Typically, the reviewer fills out a facility checklist or form as the chart is examined for predetermined criteria, such as if verbal orders have been followed up with a written order, all goals in the intervention plan have been addressed, or all the OTA's notes have been cosigned by the OT (if required).

LEARNING ACTIVITY 2-1: QUALITY IMPROVEMENT

Imagine you are working in a skilled nursing facility as an OTA. One problem the occupational therapy staff is seeing is that residents' adaptive equipment and orthotic devices often go missing. Sometimes these items get mixed up in the sheets and inadvertently get sent to the laundry department when linens are changed. In other instances, devices may be left on a meal tray and arrive in the dietary department when the used tray is sent back. The dietary and laundry departments often do not know who these items belong too or might throw items out because they do not even know what they are. Describe the negative effects of this situation. Brainstorm a list of ideas to help minimize this problem of lost devices and determine the pros and cons of each. Determine which ideas you think will work best and explain how you will implement your plan. Include specific procedures, costs that will be incurred, and personnel needed. Discuss if your plan is actually feasible to achieve the outcome you want.

Client Satisfaction Surveys

Following discharge from therapy or from the facility or agency, clients may be asked to fill out a **client satisfaction survey,** which is a feedback form asking for the client's perspective about the care that was received from the facility, rehabilitation department as a whole, or single discipline such as occupational therapy. These questionnaires are a useful tool to help improve client care through identification of recurring areas of concern or specific problems. In addition, positive reviews could be a consideration used in incentive programs honoring deserving staff members for exceptional care. Some feedback forms are very detailed and lengthy to allow for a wide variety of areas to be addressed, whereas others can be much shorter and consist only of a few basic questions (Morreale, 2022). An internet search engine can be used to find and compare various health care feedback forms. An example of an occupational therapy client satisfaction survey is presented in Figure 2-1.

LEARNING ACTIVITY 2-2: CLIENT SATISFACTION SURVEY

Instructions: Recall your last visit to a health provider (e.g., doctor, dentist, physical therapist, nurse practitioner, chiropractor). Complete the client satisfaction survey in Figure 2-1 based on your experience, adapting the form to reflect the discipline you chose. After completing the questionnaire, create a list of five additional questions that you feel would be beneficial to include on this survey.

Additional questions to add to this survey:

1.

2.

3.

4.

5.

We Really Care Rehabilitation Facility

Occupational Therapy Department

Thank you for choosing to receive rehabilitation services at our facility. Please answer the following questions based on your experience here and return this survey in the postage-paid envelope provided. We appreciate your feedback.

	Strongly Agree	Agree	Neither Agree nor Disagree	Disagree	Strongly Disagree
I was able to schedule my initial appointment in a timely manner.	O	O	O	O	O
Parking was convenient.	O	O	O	O	O
I was seen on time for scheduled appointments.	O	O	O	O	O
The facility was clean/sanitary.	O	O	O	O	O
I was treated with courtesy/respect.	O	O	O	O	O
My privacy and confidentiality were well protected.	O	O	O	O	O
My concerns were listened to and addressed satisfactorily.	O	O	O	O	O
My OT/OTA spent sufficient time with me.	O	O	O	O	O
Treatment was clearly explained.	O	O	O	O	O
Therapy helped the problem(s) I was being treated for.	O	O	O	O	O
I would not have gotten better without therapy.	O	O	O	O	O
I would recommend this facility.	O	O	O	O	O

How did you hear about us?   Physician ☐   Family member/friend ☐   Internet ☐

Newspaper ☐   Other ☐

Comments/suggestions:

Name and contact information (optional):

Figure 2-1. Client satisfaction survey. (Reproduced with permission from Morreale, M. J. [2022]. *Developing clinical competence: A workbook for the OTA* [2nd ed.]. SLACK Incorporated.)

LEARNING ACTIVITY 2-3: DEVELOPING A CLIENT SATISFACTION SURVEY

Imagine you are responsible for developing a client satisfaction survey for the occupational therapy department either in an elementary school or home care agency. List 10 aspects of care that you would include on this survey. Would these aspects of care be the same for inpatient clients?

CMS Quality Initiatives

Meaningful Measures is a CMS initiative that determines the top priorities for quality measures, improvement, and looks at the issues integral for assessing high care quality and improving individual outcomes (CMS, 2021e). It links CMS Strategic Goals with individual initiatives/measures, and addresses concrete areas such as hospital admission and readmission rates; prevention and treatment of opioid and substance use disorders; health care–associated infections; end-of-life care; and others (CMS, 2021e).

Care-Compare

CMS has also created an online tool, called *Care-Compare*, that allows health care consumers to find and compare information about health providers and their ratings of various quality measures (CMS, 2021c).

Writing in the Record

As health and education records are not only a communication tool during the client's course of treatment, but also the source document for financial, legal, and clinical accountability, the record should indicate the following:

- What services were provided, where and when they occurred.
- What happened and what was said.
- How the client responded to the services provided.
- Why skilled occupational therapy services were needed rather than what an aide, teacher, or family member could do.
- How skilled occupational therapy is different from the services being provided from another discipline.

AOTA's *Guidelines for Documentation of Occupational Therapy* (2018b) includes a list of fundamental elements that should be incorporated into all occupational therapy documentation (Box 2-2).

Before you write anything in the record, make the following assumptions:

- Someone else will have to read and understand what I write because I may be sick or have the day off the next time this client needs to be treated.
- This entry I am about to make will be the one scrutinized by a CMS review team, Child Study Team, or managed care representative. If I were a funding source, would I want to pay for the occupational therapy services I am about to record?
- This entry I am about to make will be subpoenaed and scrutinized by attorneys. If I am called upon to testify, will I be able to recall pertinent client information based on this record?
- My client (or the client's parent/guardian) will exercise their right to read this record.
- When using an EMR, my name will be attached to any information I enter and save (Swigert, 2018).
- Once I have entered information in the record it needs to remain there. Proper protocols must be followed to correct any mistakes.

It is critical to know your payment sources when documenting. Payers have different requirements and time frames, and some look for quite different outcomes than others. With a client who has Medicare, you will normally discuss and write goals for specific occupations such as self-care, functional mobility, and home management, as CMS generally looks for **functional** improvement. It is not enough to simply indicate that the client is working toward a goal of increasing elbow range of motion or attaining a better grip score with a dynamometer. You must indicate what this increased motion or improved strength will enable the client to do, such as get food out of the refrigerator, open a jar, or put on a shirt. There are certain exceptions for skilled maintenance care, which will be explained in Chapter 3. With a Workers' Compensation case, your documentation will likely be oriented toward the client's return to work or prevention of a costly injury. For example, a software engineer who has carpal tunnel

---

Box 2-2
FUNDAMENTALS OF DOCUMENTATION

- Documentation practices and storage and disposal of documentation must meet all state and federal regulations and guidelines, payer and facility requirements, practice guidelines, and confidentiality requirements.
- Client's full name, date of birth, gender, and case number, if applicable, are included on each page of the documentation.
- Identification of type of documentation and the date service is provided and documentation is completed are included in the documentation.
- Acceptable terminology, acronyms, and abbreviations are defined and used within the boundaries of the setting.
- Clear rationale for the purpose, value, and necessity of skilled occupational therapy services is provided. The client's diagnosis or prognosis is not the sole rationale for occupational therapy services.
- Professional signature (first name or initial, last name) and credential; cosignature and credential when required for documentation of supervision; and, when necessary, signature of the recorder are included with each documentation entry.
- All errors are noted and initialed or signed.

Reproduced with permission from American Occupational Therapy Association. (2018b). Guidelines for documentation of occupational therapy. *American Journal of Occupational Therapy, 72*(Suppl. 2),7212410010. https://doi.org/10.5014/ajot.2018.72S203

---

syndrome might benefit from skilled interventions such as ergonomic education, occupational adaptations, and use of an orthotic device to help alleviate symptoms for work tasks and avoid surgery. When working in home care, your documentation might focus on your client being homebound and the reasons why the client is unable to leave home to receive services at this time. Additionally, you will document the skilled occupational therapy services implemented in the home such as ADL retraining, adaptations for safety, functional mobility for IADLs, and client/family education. If your documentation states that your client is shopping at the mall or routinely driving to the local coffee shop, then payment for home care services will likely be denied, as these activities suggest the client is not truly homebound (CMS, 2020a). For a child receiving early intervention services, occupational therapy notes will be oriented toward the developmental needs and concerns identified in the IFSP and describe the skilled interventions and family/caregiver education provided. In school settings, documentation addresses the specific skills or occupational adaptations the student needs to achieve success in that educational setting. Also described in documentation are the related services, supplementary aids and services provided as per the IEP. Documentation for children in pediatric medical settings or outpatient clinics describes occupational therapy interventions that focus on managing/improving the child's health condition or circumstances to support occupational participation, performance, and quality of life.

Additionally, you must **always follow established facility, payer, and legal time frames for entering client information into the record**. Some settings or payers may require that contact notes be entered right at the time the client is being seen (point of service). Other settings might allow you to complete your daily notes by the end of that workday or other established time frame. Electronic records typically track the date and time each note is entered into the record or altered. If you are unable to compose and enter a formal note into the record as you are working with a client but planning to do it later in the day (if allowed), it is helpful to at least jot down some observations/information for yourself to avoid forgetting pertinent facts when you finally write the note. Realize that you must properly secure and dispose of any informal notes or drafts containing PHI as per HIPAA guidelines. Consider the following recommendations when planning to write in the health record:

- Accuracy is your best protection against problems. You cannot be accurate if you wait too long to record what happened.
- A note in the health or education record is a reflection of your professional identity and abilities as well as that of your department and occupational therapy as a profession.
- No activity or contact is ever considered a service that has been provided until a clinical entry is in the record. In terms of legal and fiscal accountability, as the saying goes, "If it is not written, it did not happen."

The following are some helpful hints on writing notes:
- Avoid generalities.
- Be as concise as possible without leaving out pertinent data.

- Report behavior objectively and avoid judgments except in assessing your data.
- Be sparse with technical jargon, which may be unfamiliar to the reader.
- To help avoid errors, be *extremely careful* when entering or transposing data; typing; tapping touch screens; pointing and clicking on drop-down menus or check-off boxes; copying, cutting, and pasting digital information.
- Ensure that autocorrect functions have not changed any words or phrases to unintended entries.
- Proofread your work before hitting the submit button.

Use Respectful Language

Use appropriate terminology for the recipients of services. When referring to the persons who use occupational therapy services, terms such as *client, patient, consumer, resident, veteran, participant, individual, student, infant, child, caregiver,* and *family* may be used. Please use these or other terms that are considered most respectful and appropriate for your practice setting.

Use people-first language. Emphasize the person rather than the disability. Do not refer to an individual *as a* diagnosis. Avoid referring to clients as *victims* or stating that an individual is "afflicted with" or "suffers from" a condition (American Psychological Association [APA], 2020; Quinn & Gordon, 2016).

For example:

Rather than saying *"the para …"*
It is better to say *"the person with paraplegia."*

Rather than saying *"total hip patient …"*
It is better to say *"patient who had total hip replacement surgery."*

Rather than saying *"suffers from Alzheimer's …"*
It is better to say *"diagnosed with Alzheimer's."*

Rather than saying *"wheelchair bound …"*
It is better to say *"wheelchair user."*

Keep current with new trends and changes in acceptable terminology. Certain terms such as "crippled" are no longer appropriate and have been replaced with more respectful words such as "wheelchair user" or "non-ambulatory." Rosa's law resulted in changes to IDEA in 2017 that replaced the term "mental retardation" with "intellectual disability" in Federal law (U.S. Department of Education, 2017). Terms such as "addict" and "alcoholic" are also considered stigmatizing and should be replaced with more suitable phrases such as "person with substance use disorder" or "has problem with unhealthy use of alcohol on weekends." Also, the 11th version of the *International Classification of Diseases (ICD-11)* includes various new diagnostic categories (e.g., gaming disorder) plus redefines and recategorizes other conditions, and replaces stigmatizing terms such as mental retardation (Reed, et.al, 2019).

Use culturally sensitive language when referring to individuals, groups, and populations. Avoid words with negative connotations such as crazy person, fat, lazy, difficult, or old people. Do not use slang terms for a person's culture, ethnicity, gender, or sexual orientation. Using an appropriate term, you might say something like, "The person identifies as _____." Do not refer to an individual as *"the Italian guy in room 246."* It is better to say, *"Mr. Rigatoni in room 246"* or *"the patient in room 246."* Complete Worksheets 2-1, 2-2, and 2-3 at the end of this Chapter to test your knowledge of professional language, practice using people-first language and more culturally sensitive terminology.

The Mechanics of Documentation

There are certain "rules" that must be followed when writing in the health record:

1. **Use black ink that is waterproof and nonerasable for handwritten notes.** For any paper-based documentation, do not use a pencil or marker for notes entered into the record. Indelible ink will help ensure that notations are not altered or smeared accidentally (Gateley & Borcherding, 2017).

2. **Never use correction fluid/correction tape.** For handwritten or printed health records, using correction fluid or correction tape to alter entries or copies is not allowed. Health records are legal documents that must always stand as originally written.

3. **Correct errors properly.** Corrections/alterations for an EMR must follow the established standards in place for that particular facility and software program, such as "*correction*," "*late entry*," "*entered in error*," "*addition*," "*deletion*" (Fairchild et al., 2018, p. 8). The program will indicate when and who altered the record and only certain personnel may be authorized to make corrections, such as the original author of the note (Fairchild et al., 2018). If you make an error in a handwritten record, draw a single line through it, then date and initial your correction (CMS, 2020b; Fairchild et al., 2018; Fremgen, 2020; Quinn & Gordon, 2016). Do not attempt to change a word or phrase by writing over it or squeezing in additional words.

mm 4/15/22
Pt. able to dress lower body with ~~verbal cues~~ min Ⓐ using a reacher.
Pt. able to dress lower body with ~~mod~~ (mm 4/15/22) min Ⓐ using a reacher.

If you are using traditional paper-based records and inadvertently write your note in the wrong client's chart, draw a single line through the entire entry and write "wrong chart" beside it with your signature and date.

4. **Adding information.** For handwritten records, if you need to add something immediately after you have written and signed your note, write "addendum" with the current date and time. For an EMR, follow the established standards in place for that specific software program and your facility.

5. **Do not erase or delete previously entered data.** This is also considered illegally altering the record and is another reason that indelible ink should be used. Electronic records normally indicate the date and time that previously entered information is modified, deleted, or new information added.

6. **Do not leave blank spaces or lines when using traditional paper-based forms/records.** Draw a horizontal line through the center of blank spaces in handwritten notes. If completing a form, do not leave any questions blank. Write an appropriate answer such as, "N/A," "not applicable," "to further assess," etc. This prevents the record from being altered at a later time or date.

7. **Be sure all required data are present.** The *Guidelines for Documentation of Occupational Therapy* (AOTA, 2018b) specify requirements for each type of occupational therapy note such as an evaluation report, contact note, or discharge report. This information will be addressed in other chapters of this manual. Make certain that each page of your documentation contains the necessary basic information such as the facility name, department name, and specific type of note. If paper-based forms are being used, this information is usually preprinted as a heading at the top of each page (Figures 2-2 and 2-3). Your facility or agency might utilize different forms depending on the specific type of note. The following are some examples of headings:

Best Rehabilitation Center
Occupational Therapy Department
Progress Note

ABC Therapy for Children
Occupational Therapy Department
____Contact Note   ____Progress Note   ____Discharge Note

WeCare Home Health Care Agency
☐OT ☐PT ☐SLP Department
Progress Note

8. **Ensure names are spelled correctly.** The full name of your client must be included on each piece of documentation along with any applicable health record number or identification number (AOTA, 2018b). This will ensure that you are looking at the correct EMR or that documentation is placed in the correct chart if paper-based forms/reports/notes accidentally get misplaced, mixed-up, or if loose papers fall out of charts. Identifying and other demographic information will generally come up in an EMR system automatically if you click on a particular individual who is already entered in the system. Always check with your facility and the specific software program template, but the client's name is generally written as last name, comma, then first name (Doe, Jane). Be especially careful to avoid clerical errors with case numbers or complicated ethnic names you are unfamiliar with. It is prudent to clarify if a name is a nickname or not, such as Jen vs. Jennifer or Alex vs. Alexander. It is also important to avoid clerical errors with names that might differ by only one or two letters (i.e., Marie/Maria, Brian/Brien) and/or sound similar, for example:

- *Steven/Stephen*
- *Riley/Rylee*
- *Jayden/Jaden vs. Jaylin or Zayden*
- *Kobe/Coby/Koby vs. Kody/Cody*
- *Jean/Gene/Jeanne*
- *Caitlin/Kaitlyn*
- *Kylee vs. Kaylee*

9. **Sign and date every note.** Remember, it is absolutely essential that you date and sign all of your notes with your legal signature and credentials. **Do not** sign or enter information in the health record for someone else and do not ask another OTA or rehabilitation discipline to write or sign a note for you. CMS (2021f) requires that health providers sign their documentation with a handwritten or electronic signature but does *not* allow for stamped signatures as a substitute (except in very limited special circumstances). Notes written by an OTA and students may need a co-signature by a supervising OT when the agency, state, or federal regulations require this (AOTA, 2018b). In addition, some facilities require that practitioners also document the exact time of day that occupational therapy services were provided or phone calls were made.

10. **Be sure to save information in an electronic record (Scott, 2013).** When you have completed an entry be sure to save it. EMR programs may provide prompts or save information automatically if you accidentally log out.

11. **Be concise.** In today's health care system, busy professionals are often pressed for time. They will appreciate being able to read what you have written in the shortest time possible, and your own time for documentation will also be limited under today's productivity standards.

12. **Be prudent in using abbreviations.** While you might use slang abbreviations in social emails and text messages to friends and family, many of these casual abbreviations such as *SLAP* (sounds like a plan) and *IDK* (I don't know) are not appropriate for use in professional documentation. Use **only** the abbreviations that are approved by your facility and do not make up abbreviations. This will be further addressed in Chapter 4.

13. **The use of emoticons and emojis do not give a professional appearance.** These should not be used in professional documentation.

14. **Refer to yourself, the OTA, in the third person (Sames, 2015).** Avoid referring to yourself with the words "I" or "me." For example, instead of recording, *"Child attempted to kick me,"* write, *"Child attempted to kick OTA."* As another example, instead of writing, *"I instructed the client in dressing skills,"* you could write, *"OTA instructed the client in dressing skills."* However, in this instance, it is even better to use a more formal style and focus on the client rather than the health care practitioner in your note such as, *"Client was instructed in dressing skills"* (Sames, 2015).

15. **Use proper spelling and grammar.** To demonstrate professionalism, use proper spelling and grammar when communicating with faculty, fieldwork educators, and other professionals. Facilities have different styles of organizing and writing information. Some facilities will allow you to use sentence fragments or incomplete sentences, and you will notice this in some of the examples in this book. Other facilities may have a more formal style and may insist on complete sentences (Sames, 2015). Follow the style used in your facility or agency and always use proper spelling and grammar. This will be addressed further in Chapter 5.

16. **Notes continued.** When using a paper-based record, if your note for a particular entry does not fit on one page, at the end write "*(cont.)*." Then, on the next page that you resume writing the same note, write the date and "*(OT note cont.)*" on the first line.

17. **Always adhere to ethical and legal guidelines.** Keep abreast of laws, regulatory guidelines, facility policies, and AOTA's guidance and documents concerning both the delivery of occupational therapy services and documentation. This includes anti-discrimination and privacy laws; current billing and reimbursement requirements; avoiding fraud and abuse; maintaining certification, licensure and continuing competency requirements; ensuring appropriate supervision; and so forth. OTs and OTAs should *never compromise ethics* even if nursing home or school administrators are applying pressure to keep clients on program longer than medically necessary to maintain clients in a higher payment category. It is unethical to falsify documentation or submit claims for extra sessions of therapy that are not reasonable and necessary (AOTA, 2014a, 2020b). Services should reflect interventions within the scope of occupational therapy practice (AOTA, 2020c, 2021a).

18. **Always be truthful and objective.** The information you record should never be misleading, fabricated, or falsified (AOTA, 2020a; Fremgen, 2020). Don't guess at or embellish information; be careful to avoid personal complaints; and do not judge, criticize, or blame other employees in your note. Defamatory statements could potentially be considered libel (Fremgen, 2020; Sames, 2015; Scott, 2013).

19. **Enter all information accurately.** Write legibly, type carefully, and point and click accurately. Remember that other professionals and insurance company personnel will be reading and reviewing your occupational therapy notes. You will also be providing written home programs for clients and caregivers. Sloppy handwriting or data entry errors using a keyboard, touch screen, or misdirected pointing and clicking of a mouse may result in serious inaccuracies, substandard work, or could lead to possible client harm. In addition, ensure that you are always identifying right and left accurately (e.g., parts of the body) as documentation of your interventions must match the identified condition (Fairchild, et.al, 2018). Your notes must be understandable and accurate in order to present client information truthfully and effectively, minimize denial of claims, and help avoid medical errors.

20. **The OTA should not be referred to as *therapist*.** There is a clear distinction between an OT and an OTA regarding roles and responsibilities (AOTA, 2020b, 2021b). The OTA should be referred to as an *occupational therapy assistant* or an *occupational therapy practitioner* rather than a *therapist*. CMS regulations regarding occupational therapy also state that the words *therapist* and *clinician* apply only to the OT and are not appropriate terms for the OTA (CMS, 2019b).

21. **Do not include other clients' names in your note.** There are times when it is important to note that your client is interacting with other clients but, for confidentiality reasons, their names should not be listed in another client's notes. You can state something like:

    - *Client reports that his roommate's yelling kept him from getting a good night's sleep.*
    - *During activity group, client initiated conversation with three other group members.*
    - *Student reports that a classmate helps her with opening containers for lunch.*
    - *Resident played checkers with another resident.*

22. **Always review the client's chart and communicate with the client and team members as appropriate before beginning intervention.** It is important to determine if there have been any changes in the client's status, discharge plan, or if new medical orders are in place. For example, the client may have developed complications recently or may be undergoing testing that necessitates fasting, bed rest, or measuring fluid intake and output.

23. **Don't assume you will find all the information you need in the chart.** You must always use professional reasoning and good communication skills to decipher and clarify information present in the chart and determine what data or medical orders could be missing or incomplete. If you are unsure of something regarding a client, discuss it with your supervising OT or other team members as appropriate. When in doubt, always err on the side of caution.

Conclusion

Federal regulations have influenced greatly how health information is managed and communicated. Mandates at the federal, state, and local levels also impact significantly how health care and educational services are prioritized, delivered, paid for, and evaluated for quality and accountability. The use of EHRs in the United States is widespread and has many advantages, but also presents some disadvantages. Occupational therapy documentation serves many purposes and has various audiences. Therapy notes can be organized into different formats and must meet third-party payer requirements for reimbursement. When writing in the health or education record, all occupational therapy practitioners and students are obliged to follow professional, legal, and ethical standards (AOTA, 2018b, 2020a). The Advocacy and Policy section of the AOTA website (www.aota.org) contains helpful resources for OTs and OTAs regarding reimbursement, value-based occupational therapy practice, and documentation.

XYZ Home Health Care Agency
☐ OT   ☐ PT   ☐ ST Department
Progress Note

Name: _____   Record #: _____

Dx: _____   SOC: _____

Date	

Figure 2-2. Example of a facility paper-based form.

Healthy Hospital
Occupational Therapy Department
Contact Note

Name: _____   Record #: _____

Date/Time	

Figure 2-3. Example of a facility paper-based form.

Worksheet 2-1
Internet and Chat Slang

Consider the following messages intended for a fieldwork educator, supervisor, or other members of the health care and education team. Rewrite each of the sentences to make them more professional and determine what abbreviations could be appropriate to leave in place. A list of commonly used acceptable abbreviations is included in Chapter 4. Slang abbreviations are identified in the worksheet answers in the Appendix. *Remember that HIPAA guidelines and facility policy must be followed regarding electronic communication pertaining to a client's protected health information, such as using a secure portal.*

1.   TX, SLAP. Pt's DH and DD will be instructed in use of the equipment you suggested.

2.   Client AWOL today. Could not reach her by phone 2X.

3.   K, I will call parents. FWIW the student did not hurt herself when she fell. TTYL.

4.   OMG, the client's wound stinks and has bad yellow drainage. Please TMB ASAP.

5.   IDK why the adaptive equipment was not ordered. Sorry, G2G.

6.   Resident negative for TB and AFAIK will be discharged in am.

7.   Got ur message. IMHO client is unsafe transferring by herself and needs SBA.

8.   The MS pt. tires easily when AMB short distances and needs a w/c eval before discharge. TIA.

9.   Transporting the CA victim to his room now. BRB.

10. Doc, WDYT about US and TENS to pt's wrist?

Morreale, M. J. (2023). *The OTA's guide to documentation: Writing SOAP notes* (5th ed.). SLACK Incorporated.

Worksheet 2-2
People-First and Culturally Sensitive Language

Rewrite the following sentences using more appropriate people-first and culturally sensitive language.

1. The TBI was alert and oriented to person but not place or time.

2. The cerebral palsy child demonstrated difficulty fastening ½" buttons on her shirt because she is spastic.

3. The first grader is fat and mentally retarded. She seems lazy.

4. The resident diagnosed with polio is crippled and wheelchair bound.

5. The three Mexicans were teaching their classmates some Spanish phrases.

6. The client had a sex change.

7. The OTA led an activity group consisting of two schizophrenics and two borderlines.

8. The Haitian stroke victim speaks only Creole.

9. The client suffers from amyotrophic lateral sclerosis and lives in an old folks home.

10. The quad has an upper respiratory infection. He is being very difficult and won't come to therapy.

Morreale, M. J. (2023). *The OTA's guide to documentation: Writing SOAP notes* (5th ed.). SLACK Incorporated.

Worksheet 2-3
Written Communication

Critique the following email message that an OTA student sent to a professor. List 10 suggestions to improve this note.

Prof,
OMG, my activity analysis grade is HORIBLE!!!!! 🙁 *I DON'T WANT TO FAIL UR CLASS. Lets meet ASAP. Tell me when. TTYL.*
Stewart

Suggestions to improve this note:

1.

2.

3.

4.

5.

6.

7.

8.

9.

10.

Adapted from Morreale, M. J. (2022). *Developing clinical competence: A workbook for the OTA* (2nd ed.). SLACK Incorporated.

References

American Occupational Therapy Association. (2014a). Consensus statement on clinical judgment in health care settings AOTA, APTA, ASHA. Retrieved May 25, 2022 from http://www.aota.org/~/media/Corporate/Files/Practice/Ethics/APTA-AOTA-ASHA-Concensus-Statement.pdf?la=en

American Occupational Therapy Association. (2014b). Occupational therapy practice framework: Domain and process (3rd ed.). *American Journal of Occupational Therapy, 68*(Suppl. 1), S1-S48. doi.org: 10.5014/ajot.2014.682006

American Occupational Therapy Association. (2018a). AOTA PERFORM Documentation Templates. *American Journal of Occupational Therapy, 72*(Suppl. 2), 7212420023p1–7212420023p31. https://doi.org/10.5014/ajot.2018.72S213

American Occupational Therapy Association. (2018b). Guidelines for documentation of occupational therapy. *American Journal of Occupational Therapy, 72*(Suppl. 2), 7212410010. https://doi.org:10.5014/ajot.2018.72S203

American Occupational Therapy Association. (2020a). AOTA 2020 occupational therapy code of ethics. *American Journal of Occupational Therapy, 74*(Suppl. 3), 7413410005. https://doi.org: 10.5014/ajot.2020.74S3006

American Occupational Therapy Association. (2020b). Guidelines for supervision, roles, and responsibilities during the delivery of occupational therapy services. *American Journal of Occupational Therapy, 74*(Suppl. 3), 7413410020. https://doi.org/10.5014/ajot.2020.74S3004

American Occupational Therapy Association. (2020c). Occupational therapy practice framework: Domain and process (4th ed.). *American Journal of Occupational Therapy, 74*(Suppl. 2), 7412410010. https://doi.org: 10.5014/ajot.2020.74S2001

American Occupational Therapy Association. (2021a). Occupational therapy scope of practice. *American Journal of Occupational Therapy, 75*(Suppl. 3), 7513410020. https://doi.org/10.5014/ajot.2021.75S3005

American Occupational Therapy Association. (2021b). Standards of practice for occupational therapy. *American Journal of Occupational Therapy, 75*(Suppl. 3), 7513410030. https://doi.org/10.5014/ajot.2021.75S3004

American Occupational Therapy Association. (2021c). Use "AOTA PERFORM" to add OT-specific fields to your electronic health record system. Retrieved September 19, 2021 from https://www.aota.org/Practice/Manage/Reimb/perform-template.aspx

American Psychological Association. (2020). *Publication manual of the American Psychological Association* (7th ed.). Author.

Center for Parent Information and Resources. (2017). Key terms to know in early intervention. Retrieved September 18, 2021 from https://www.parentcenterhub.org/keyterms-ei/

Center for Parent Information and Resources. (2021). Considering LRE in Placement Decisions. Retrieved October 29, 2021 from https://www.parentcenterhub.org/placement-lre/

Centers for Medicare & Medicaid Services. (2019a). MACRA. Retrieved October 1, 2021 from https://www.cms.gov/Medicare/Quality-Initiatives-Patient-Assessment-Instruments/Value-Based-Programs/MACRA-MIPS-and-APMs/MACRA-MIPS-and-APMs

Centers for Medicare & Medicaid Services. (2019b). *Medicare benefit policy manual* (Pub. 100-02: Ch. 15, Section 220). Retrieved October 1, 2021 from https://www.cms.gov/Regulations-and-Guidance/Guidance/Manuals/Downloads/bp102c15.pdf

Centers for Medicare & Medicaid Services. (2020a). *Medicare benefit policy manual* (Pub. 100-02: Ch. 7, Section 30.1.1). Retrieved October 1, 2021 from https://www.cms.gov/Regulations-and-Guidance/Guidance/Manuals/Downloads/bp102c07.pdf

Centers for Medicare & Medicaid Services. (2020b). *Medicare program integrity manual* (Pub. 100-08: Ch. 3, Section 3.3.2.5). Retrieved May 26, 2022 from https://www.cms.gov/Regulations-and-Guidance/Guidance/Manuals/Downloads/pim83c03.pdf

Centers for Medicare & Medicaid Services. (2020c). Quality payment program. Retrieved October 1, 2021 from https://www.cms.gov/Medicare/Quality-Payment-Program/Quality-Payment-Program

Centers for Medicare & Medicaid Services. (2021a). Certified EHR technology. Retrieved October 29, 2021 from https://www.cms.gov/Regulations-and-Guidance/Legislation/EHRIncentivePrograms/Certification

Centers for Medicare & Medicaid Services. (2021b). CMS-approved accrediting organizations. Retrieved October 1, 2021 from https://www.cms.gov/Medicare/Provider-Enrollment-and-Certification/SurveyCertificationGenInfo/Downloads/Accrediting-Organization-Contacts-for-Prospective-Clients-.pdf

Centers for Medicare & Medicaid Services, (2021c). Find & compare nursing homes, hospitals and other providers near you. Retrieved October 1, 2021 from https://www.medicare.gov/care-compare/

Centers for Medicare & Medicaid Services. (2021d). IMPACT Act of 2014 Data standardization & cross setting measures. Retrieved September 15, 2021 from https://www.cms.gov/Medicare/Quality-Initiatives-Patient-Assessment-Instruments/Post-Acute-Care-Quality-Initiatives/IMPACT-Act-of-2014/IMPACT-Act-of-2014-Data-Standardization-and-Cross-Setting-Measures

Centers for Medicare & Medicaid Services. (2021e). Meaningful measures hub. Retrieved October 1, 2021 from https://www.cms.gov/Medicare/Quality-Initiatives-Patient-Assessment-Instruments/QualityInitiativesGenInfo/MMF/General-info-Sub-Page

Centers for Medicare & Medicaid Services. (2021f). *Medicare program integrity manual* (Pub 100-08: Ch 3, Section 3.3.2.4). Retrieved May 26, 2022 from https://cms.gov/Regulations-and-Guidance/Guidance/Manuals/Downloads/pim83c03.pdf

Cohen, J. (2013). Which way to go? Comparing the advantages of web-based vs. on-site EMR systems. *Advance for Occupational Therapy Practitioners, 29*(15), 7-9.

DeJong, G. (2016). Coming to terms with the IMPACT Act of 2014. *American Journal of Occupational Therapy, 70*(3), 7003090010p1-7003090010p6. doi.org: 10.5014/ajot.2016.703003

Erickson, M. L. (2020). Documentation formats. In M. L. Erickson, R. R. Utzman, & R. S. McKnight (Eds.), *Physical therapy documentation: From examination to outcome* (3rd ed., pp. 33-52). SLACK Incorporated.

Fairchild, S. L., O'Shea, R. K., & Washington, R. D. (2018). *Pierson and Fairchild's principles & techniques of patient care* (6th ed.). Elsevier.

Fremgen, B. F. (2020). *Medical law and ethics* (6th ed.). Pearson Education, Inc.

Gateley, C. A., & Borcherding, S. (2017). *Documentation manual for occupational therapy: Writing SOAP notes* (4th ed.). SLACK Incorporated.

Herbold, J. (2016). Electronic medical record. In L. Quinn & J. Gordon (Eds.), *Documentation for rehabilitation: A guide to clinical decision making in physical therapy* (3rd ed., pp. 56-68). Elsevier.

Morreale, M. J. (2022). *Developing clinical competence: A workbook for the OTA* (2nd ed.). SLACK Incorporated.

Office of the National Coordinator for Health Information Technology. (n.d.a). About ONC's Cures Act final rule. Retrieved October 1, 2021 from https://www.healthit.gov/curesrule/overview/about-oncs-cures-act-final-rule

Office of the National Coordinator for Health Information Technology. (n.d.b). Health IT dashboard: Quick stats. Retrieved May 26, 2022 from https://dashboard.healthit.gov/quickstats/quickstats.php

Office of the National Coordinator for Health Information Technology. (2015). FDSAIA. Retrieved September 16, 2021 from https://www.healthit.gov/hitac/committees/fdasia

Office of the National Coordinator for Health Information Technology. (2017a). Improved patient care using EHRs. Retrieved September 15, 2021 from https://www.healthit.gov/topic/health-it-and-health-information-exchange-basics/improved-patient-care-using-ehrs

Office of the National Coordinator for Health Information Technology. (2017b). What is a patient portal? Retrieved September 16, 2021 from https://www.healthit.gov/faq/what-patient-portal

Office of the National Coordinator for Health Information Technology. (2018). Medical practice efficiencies & cost savings. Retrieved September 16, 2021 from https://www.healthit.gov/topic/health-it-and-health-information-exchange-basics/medical-practice-efficiencies-cost-savings

Office of the National Coordinator for Health Information Technology. (2019a). Benefits of EHRs: Improved diagnostics and patient outcomes. Retrieved October 29, 2021 from https://www.healthit.gov/topic/health-it-and-health-information-exchange-basics/improved-diagnostics-patient-outcomes

Office of the National Coordinator for Health Information Technology. (2019b). What are the advantages of electronic health records? Retrieved October 11, 2021 from https://www.healthit.gov/faq/what-are-advantages-electronic-health-records

Office of the National Coordinator for Health Information Technology. (2019c). What are the differences between electronic medical records, electronic health records, and personal health records. Retrieved October 11, 2021 from https://www.healthit.gov/faq/what-are-differences-between-electronic-medical-records-electronic-health-records-and-personal

Office of the National Coordinator for Health Information Technology. (2021). Health IT legislation. Retrieved October 29, 2021 from https://www.healthit.gov/topic/laws-regulation-and-policy/health-it-legislation

Quinn, L., & Gordon, J. (2016). *Documentation for rehabilitation: A guide to clinical decision making in physical therapy* (3rd ed.). Elsevier.

Reed, G. M., First, M. B., Kogan, C. S., Hyman, S. E., Gureje, O., Gaebel, W., Maj, M., Stein, D. J., Maercker, A., Tyrer, P., Claudino, A., Garralda, E., Salvador-Carulla, L., Ray, R., Saunders, J. B., Dua, T., Poznyak, V., Medina-Mora, M. E., Pike, K. M., Ayuso-Mateos, J. L., … Saxena, S. (2019). Innovations and changes in the ICD-11 classification of mental, behavioural and neurodevelopmental disorders. *World psychiatry: official journal of the World Psychiatric Association (WPA), 18*(1), 3-19. https://www.ncbi.nlm.nih.gov/pmc/articles/PMC6313247/

Sames, K. M. (2015). *Documenting occupational therapy practice* (3rd ed.). Pearson Education, Inc.

Scott, R. W. (2013). *Legal, ethical, and practical aspects of patient care documentation: A guide for rehabilitation professionals* (4th ed.). Jones & Bartlett Learning.

Swigert, N.B. (2018). *Documentation and reimbursement for speech-language pathologists: Principles and practice.* SLACK Incorporated.

U.S. Department of Education. (n.d.a) About IDEA. Retrieved September 18, 2021 from https://sites.ed.gov/idea/about-idea/#IDEA-Purpose

U.S. Department of Education. (n.d.b). IDEA: Statute and Regulations. Retrieved September 18, 2021 from https://sites.ed.gov/idea/statuteregulations/

U.S. Department of Education. (2017). July11, 2017 (82 FR 31910). https://sites.ed.gov/idea/idea-files/july-11-2017-82-fr-31910/

U.S. Department of Education. (2020). A History of the Individuals with Disabilities Education Act. Retrieved September 28, 2021 from https://sites.ed.gov/idea/IDEA-History

U.S. Department of Education. (2021). Family Educational Rights and Privacy Act (FERPA). Retrieved October 29, 2021 from https://www2.ed.gov/policy/gen/guid/fpco/ferpa/index.html

U.S. Department of Health & Human Services. (2002). Incidental uses and disclosures. https://www.hhs.gov/hipaa/for-professionals/privacy/guidance/incidental-uses-and-disclosures/index.html

U.S. Department of Health & Human Services. (2003a). OCR privacy brief: Summary of the HIPAA Privacy Rule. Author. https://www.hhs.gov/sites/default/files/privacysummary.pdf

U.S. Department of Health & Human Services. (2003b). Uses and disclosures for treatment, payment, and health care operations [45 CFR 164.506]. Retrieved October 29, 2021 from https://www.hhs.gov/hipaa/for-professionals/privacy/guidance/disclosures-treatment-payment-health-care-operations/index.html

U.S. Department of Health & Human Services. (2007). HIPAA security series 3: Security standards: Physical safeguards. Retrieved September 20, 2021 from https://www.hhs.gov/sites/default/files/ocr/privacy/hipaa/administrative/securityrule/physsafeguards.pdf?language=es

U.S. Department of Health & Human Services. (2008). Does the HIPAA Privacy Rule apply to an elementary or secondary school? Retrieved October 29, 2021 from https://www.hhs.gov/hipaa/for-professionals/faq/513/does-hipaa-apply-to-an-elementary-school/index.html

U.S. Department of Health & Human Services. (2010). Compilation of Patient Protection and Affordable Care Act. Retrieved May 20, 2022 from https://www.hhs.gov/sites/default/files/ppacacon.pdf

U.S. Department of Health & Human Services. (2015). What do the HIPAA Privacy and Security Rules require of covered entities when they dispose of protected health information? Retrieved September 20, 2021 from https://www.hhs.gov/hipaa/for-professionals/faq/575/what-does-hipaa-require-of-covered-entities-when-they-dispose-information/index.html

U.S. Department of Health & Human Services. (2020). Individuals' rights under HIPAA to access their health information 45 CFR 164.524. Retrieved October 11, 2021 from https://www.hhs.gov/hipaa/for-professionals/privacy/guidance/access/index.html

U.S. Department of Health & Human Services. (2021a). About the Affordable Care Act. Retrieved September 16, 2021 from https://www.hhs.gov/healthcare/about-the-aca/index.html

Utzman, R. R. (2020). Health informatics and electronic health records. In M. L. Erickson, R. R. Utzman, & R. S. McKnight (Eds.), *Physical therapy documentation: From examination to outcome* (3rd ed., pp. 53-60). SLACK Incorporated.

Weed, L. L. (1971). Editorial: The problem oriented record as a basic tool in medical education, patient care and clinical research. *Annals of Clinical Research*, 3(3). 131-134. https://pubmed.ncbi.nlm.nih.gov/4934176/

Chapter 3

Billing and Reimbursement

Health care spending in the United States reached $4.1 trillion in 2020 and accounted for 19.7% of the Gross Domestic Product (GDP), with sharp increases due primarily to the COVID-19 pandemic (Centers for Medicare & Medicaid Services [CMS], 2021c). This chapter describes various funding sources for health care and presents an overview of the billing and reimbursement process. This includes the necessity of documenting occupational therapy services as *skilled* in accordance with established legal and ethical standards. Although this manual contains information based on current practice guidelines and legislation at time of publication, it is important to realize that reimbursement criteria and documentation requirements could change as new laws are enacted and health care systems evolve.

Health Care Funding Sources

Although individuals can pay providers directly for health care services received, the majority of health care is funded through a wide range of public and private health insurance programs and managed care plans. Primary funding sources in 2020 included Medicare (20% share), Medicaid (16% share), private health insurance (28% share), out-of-pocket (9% share), with the remainder consisting of various other public and private programs (CMS, 2021c). Hospital costs in 2020 accounted for the biggest share of health care spending at 31% ($1.3 trillion), followed by physician and clinical services with a 20% share (CMS, 2021c). Payers have been moving toward reimbursement aligned to outcomes that justify treatment over the traditional fee-for-service model (DeJong, 2016). Various attempts at more cost-effective ways of improving client outcomes and providing value-based care have been implemented, such as quality measures, bundled payments, and episode-based management, influencing how occupational therapy and other health services are managed, delivered, and paid for (DeJong, 2016).

Third-party payers (e.g., private insurance companies, managed care plans, governmental programs) vary greatly regarding program eligibility, premiums, out-of-pocket expenses, provider networks, and plan benefits such as types of coverage for prescriptions, mental health services, catastrophic care, rehabilitation services, medical equipment/supplies, and so forth. Health providers and suppliers (e.g., institutions, agencies, medical equipment vendors, pharmacies, and individuals such as physicians and therapists in private practice) contract with various third-party payers to be an approved health care provider for patients with that insurance. For reimbursement, these contracted providers agree to accept **assignment** which are the predetermined amounts the insurer will pay for each covered service or medical equipment/supplies if certain criteria are met. Although this allowable amount is considered payment in full, the consumer could be responsible for paying a portion of this preset cost if the insurance plan stipulates copayments, deductibles, and/or coinsurance. Thus, if a health care consumer uses a practitioner or equipment

Morreale, M. J. *The OTA's Guide to Documentation: Writing SOAP Notes, Fifth Edition* (pp. 47-69).
© 2023 Taylor & Francis Group.

vendor that accepts their insurance plan, all sides agree to the plan terms regarding what is or is not covered as a benefit and the maximum amount the consumer and third-party payer will each owe the provider. The billing and reimbursement process will be explained in more detail a little later in this chapter.

The Affordable Care Act (ACA) mandates that insurers must offer certain standard benefits, such as specific health screenings, immunizations, and other services (U.S. Department of Health and Human Services [USDHHS], 2021). These requirements include specific evidence-based preventative services (e.g., cancer screenings, flu shots, well-baby visits, tests for diabetes and cholesterol) that must be covered at no cost to the consumer (CMS, 2010). The Shared Responsibility Payment (which required individuals without qualifying health coverage to pay a fee) is no longer applicable for Federal tax returns as of 2019, but such fees are still allowable at the state level (HealthCare.gov, n.d.).

An individual may purchase a private policy directly from an insurance company or might obtain insurance through a group plan from one's own employer or an employer of a parent or spouse (Gateley & Borcherding, 2017). **Premiums** are the yearly costs to purchase the plan, usually paid in monthly intervals. A person who is covered by an insurance plan is called the plan **beneficiary**. In certain circumstances, private organizations and foundations may provide some charitable assistance or special grants to needy individuals to help pay for certain out-of-pocket health care expenses such as rehabilitation therapy, medical equipment, or other services.

A government-funded program called **TRICARE** provides health care benefits for active and retired military personnel and their families. Another funding source is **Workers' Compensation**, which is a mandatory insurance paid by businesses to cover employees who are injured on the job. Workers' Compensation pays for an injured employee's wages, medical care, and rehabilitation; although programs and benefits do vary from state to state. Medicare and Medicaid are major public programs that provide health care benefits to eligible populations, as described briefly in the following sections. Chapter 17 provides further explanation of the Medicare and Medicaid documentation requirements for rehabilitation therapy in specific practice settings, such as home care, hospitals, rehabilitation facilities, outpatient clinics, and skilled nursing facilities.

Coordination of Benefits

Individuals could be covered by two kinds of health insurance (payers) simultaneously or, in rare instances, three different insurances. For example, a person might have Medicare plus a Medigap insurance or, perhaps, Medicare along with Medicaid. The "coordination of benefits" rules determines which insurer is the primary payer that pays first up to coverage limits, then sends the remaining costs to the secondary (supplemental) payer (CMS, n.d.a). However, depending on the specific plans' designated benefits, not all costs may be fully covered.

Medicare (www.Medicare.gov)

Medicare is a federal insurance program for people ages 65 years and older, individuals with end-stage renal disease or amyotrophic lateral sclerosis (ALS), and eligible people younger than 65 who have permanent disabilities. In 2020, Medicare spent more than $829 billion, which accounted for 20% of total health care spending in the United States (CMS, 2021c). Individuals may choose either Original Medicare (Parts A and B) managed by the federal government (through regional contractors) or a Medicare Advantage Plan (Medicare C), which is a plan managed by a private insurance company. The Medicare program obtains revenue through a designated Medicare payroll tax and consists of the following four parts:

1. **Medicare Part A (Hospital Insurance):** This covers inpatient hospital care (including inpatient rehabilitation facilities and psychiatric care), limited skilled nursing facility stays, hospice, and medically necessary home health services. Premiums are generally free for individuals (and spouses) if they paid enough Medicare taxes while working, but the beneficiary must pay deductibles and some other expenses for care received.

2. **Medicare Part B (Medical Insurance):** For persons with Part A, this is an optional, supplemental insurance that covers medically necessary outpatient care (such as occupational therapy), medical supplies, doctor visits, and preventative services (such as health screenings and immunizations). Part B also provides benefits for some therapy services in skilled nursing facilities and home health. In 2022 the Part B standard monthly premium cost is $170.10 (typically subtracted from Social Security benefits automatically, if applicable) and there are also some additional out-of-pocket expenses for care received.

3. **Medicare Part C (Medicare Advantage Plans):** This is a type of Medicare plan contracted with private insurance companies such as a Health Maintenance Organization (HMO) or Preferred Provider Organization (PPO) to provide Medicare Parts A and B benefits. There are a variety of plans the beneficiary can compare and choose from so the cost of premiums will vary depending on the specific plan. Medicare Advantage Plans usually include some coverage for prescription drugs and may provide dental, vision, and hearing benefits.

4. **Medicare Part D (Prescription Drug Coverage)**: This provides prescription drug coverage through Medicare-approved companies. The costs of premiums and out-of-pocket expenses vary depending on the specific plan. Individuals who have Medicare Parts A and B can purchase a Medicare Part D prescription plan.

Further information about Medicare eligibility, benefits, out-of-pocket costs, and plan limits can be found at www.medicare.gov.

Medigap Insurance

There are supplemental plans offered by private insurance companies to "bridge the gap" and help pay for out-of-pocket medical expenses (e.g., deductibles, copayments, and coinsurance) incurred by individuals with Original Medicare (CMS, n.d.b). There is a yearly cost for premiums that individuals pay to the private insurer, usually in installments. Medicare does not cover health services when an individual is traveling outside of the United States so an individual might select a particular Medigap plan that provides foreign travel benefits. Also, as Medigap plans sold after 2006 can no longer provide prescription benefits, Medicare beneficiaries can choose to additionally purchase a Medicare D prescription plan if desired (CMS, n.d.b). Purchasing a separate plan might not be needed if supplemental benefits are already provided as secondary insurance through an individual's employer retiree health plan or covered by a working spouse's group health plan.

Medicaid (www.Medicaid.gov)

Medicaid is a joint federal and state program that funds health care for eligible low-income people in the United States and its territories. In 2020, total Medicaid spending cost $671.2 billion and accounted for 16% of total national health care costs (CMS, 2021c). In the United States, Medicaid mandates coverage of specific health services (such as inpatient/outpatient hospital services, physician visits, lab tests, transportation to medical care, etc.) but allows individual states flexibility to administer programs, process claims, and determine other optional benefits (such as prescriptions, rehabilitation therapy, dental services, eyeglasses, and so forth). Therefore, income eligibility, types of services covered, and reimbursement rates will vary from state to state. Within a particular state, the scope of covered health services may be different for children than for adults. States often contract with managed care organizations to administer their Medicaid programs more effectively. Children (up to age 19 years) who are uninsured and in families with incomes exceeding Medicaid eligibility could receive free or low-cost health benefits through the **Children's Health Insurance Program** (CHIP). OTs and OTAs must follow documentation and reimbursement guidelines for the specific state in which occupational therapy services are provided (Gateley & Borcherding, 2017). Further information about Medicaid and links to state programs can be found at www.medicaid.gov.

Early Intervention and Schools

As described in Chapter 2, children under 3 years old who are experiencing a developmental delay (or are at risk for developmental delay due to a diagnosed condition) are eligible for **early intervention** services under Part C of the Individuals with Disabilities Education Act (IDEA; U.S. Department of Education, n.d.; Center for Parent Information and Resources, 2017). Early intervention services are reimbursed through private insurance plans or public programs such as Medicaid. Part B of IDEA pertains to children ages 3 to 21 years and mandates that schools provide an appropriate free public education in the least restrictive environment for students with a disability or qualifying health condition. A state's Medicaid program will reimburse schools for medically necessary direct services (including occupational therapy) provided under IDEA for qualifying health conditions if the child is Medicaid eligible in that state, services are delineated in the IEP, and documentation substantiates the services (AOTA, 2021a; Frolek-Clark & Holahan, 2015). However, if Medicaid is the payer, it usually only pays for direct contact with the student present, not consultation (Frolek-Clark & Holahan, 2015). In certain states, services implemented by an OTA might not be Medicaid reimbursable (Frolek-Clark & Holahan, 2015). The unique documentation requirements for school-based settings are described in Chapter 17.

Skilled Occupational Therapy

Throughout this documentation manual, occupational therapy service is described as *skilled occupational therapy*. This term originated in Medicare regulations, which define the difference between skilled and nonskilled services (CMS, 2014a, 2019b, 2020a). Because Medicare requirements are quite stringent, these guidelines are being followed in this manual to help ensure that your services will not be denied payment by any payer. *Skilled* services have specific criteria and are performed by **qualified professionals**, including OTs and OTAs under the OT's supervision (CMS, 2014a, 2019a, 2020a). They require professional education, decision making, and highly complex competencies that have a well-defined knowledge base of human functioning and occupational performance. Skilled occupational therapy is also considered a service that can only be safely and effectively performed by an OT or an OTA under the OT's supervision (CMS, 2014a, 2019b). *Nonskilled* services are defined as those that are routine or maintenance types of therapy, both of which could be carried out by nonprofessional personnel, caregivers, or family members (CMS, 2019b, 2020a). This manual emphasizes the necessity of documenting your intervention as *skilled occupational therapy*. However, **the mere fact that an OT or OTA provided a service does not necessarily make that service billable**, as the intervention must still meet the qualification criteria for *skilled, reasonable, and medically necessary* care (CMS, 2019b). This means you must demonstrate the client's potential for functional improvement and safety, or that professional intervention is necessary for equipment recommendations, family/caregiver training, establishment of an effective and safe maintenance program, or to address a specific medical need requiring the expertise of an occupational therapy practitioner (CMS, 2019b, 2020a). These criteria justify the services of an OT or OTA.

Reasonable and Necessary Care

The frequency, duration, type, and amount of therapy services must be **reasonable and necessary** based on the client's condition, rehabilitation potential, complexity of the situation, and accepted standard practices (CMS, 2019b). Various payers, including Medicare, also require that the individual receiving reimbursable services be under a physician's (or approved non-physician practitioner) care who then certifies the therapy plan of care. Medicare and other payers do **not** reimburse for services considered unskilled or unnecessary for the client's condition, or if there is no expectation that treatment will be effective (CMS, 2019b, 2020a). Billing for extra services the client does not really need or keeping a client on a program longer than medically necessary (or educationally necessary in schools) for additional reimbursement is unethical and can potentially lead to severe legal and professional consequences.

Rehabilitative Therapy

CMS defines rehabilitative therapy as "*services designed to address recovery or improvement in function and, when possible, restoration to a previous level of health and well-being*" (CMS, 2019b). A diagnosis of a chronic condition or terminal illness does not automatically negate the need for skilled rehabilitative services if the potential exists for that client's functional abilities to reasonably improve in areas such as self-care, mobility, or safety (CMS, 2019b). CMS considers the deciding factor to be whether *the skills of a therapist are truly needed* (i.e., to design, implement, or supervise treatment) rather than nonskilled individuals (such as a family member or aide) being able to implement those same tasks effectively and safely instead (CMS, 2019b). It is essential to document in a way that differentiates your skill as an occupational therapy practitioner from that of nursing or other rehabilitation disciplines. It is also very important to document objective, measurable information; describe the skilled interventions implemented; and clearly indicate any progress the client is making toward minimizing the impairment and restoring the prior level of function (CMS, 2019b). In addition, as the training of clients and family/significant others is an integral aspect of care that enhances recovery, this should be carried out and documented throughout the course of treatment (CMS, 2019b).

Maintenance Programs

Maintenance programs are not considered rehabilitative but are created instead to help clients maintain present function or slow down/prevent further functional deterioration (CMS, 2019b). CMS covers skilled therapy services to **design and establish** maintenance programs only if the specialized judgment, knowledge, and skill of a qualified therapist are needed to do this (CMS, 2019b). Client/family instruction for the maintenance program is also a reimbursable service. In certain instances, periodic reevaluations/assessments are also covered (such as for progressive or degenerative conditions) so long as these services meet the criteria for skilled therapy and require a qualified therapist to perform (CMS, 2019b). Understand that payers might only reimburse one or two sessions for client and family/caregiver training for basic positioning or routine exercise programs. It is generally expected that these established maintenance programs will then be able to be carried out safely by nonskilled personnel or a family member. However, under certain circumstances, the actual **delivery** of maintenance programs is a covered service if the **safe and effective performance** of the maintenance program requires the specialized judgment, knowledge, and skills of a qualified therapist (CMS, 2019b). For example, the skill of a therapist is needed if the client requires range of motion but presently has an unhealed, unstable fracture in that area (CMS, 2019b). CMS delineates the following criteria for **delivery of maintenance programs** as a skilled service (CMS, 2019b):

> a) The therapy procedures required to maintain the patient's current function or to prevent or slow further deterioration are of such complexity and sophistication that the skills of a qualified therapist are required to furnish the therapy procedure
>
> or
>
> b) The particular patient's special medical complications require the skills of a qualified therapist to furnish a therapy service required to maintain the patient's current function or to prevent or slow further deterioration, even if the skills of a therapist are not ordinarily needed to perform such therapy procedures. Unlike coverage for rehabilitation therapy, coverage of therapy to carry out a maintenance program does not depend on the presence or absence of the patient's potential for improvement from the therapy.
>
> Reproduced from Centers for Medicare & Medicaid Services. (2019b). *Medicare benefit policy manual* (Pub. 100-02: Ch. 15, Section 220.2). Author. Retrieved Sept. 28, 2021 from https://www.cms.gov/Regulations-and-Guidance/Guidance/Manuals/downloads/bp102c15.pdf

Safety Concerns

The ability to perform a task must include the ability to do it safely. Intervention strategies targeting safety are usually considered cost-effective services by third-party payers because they prevent costly re-injury. Safety concerns include situations such as a high probability of falling; lack of environmental awareness; severe pain; absent skin sensation; abnormal, aggressive, or maladaptive behaviors; or suicide risk. These all fall within the scope of skilled occupational therapy, but practitioners must follow the guidelines for reasonable and necessary care in order to be reimbursed by third-party payers.

Prevention of Secondary Complications

Preventative interventions are within the scope of skilled occupational therapy if it can be shown that the client has a high risk of developing complications and therapy is justified as medically necessary and reasonable. Secondary complications might include prevention of repetitive strain injuries, progressive joint contractures, fracture nonunion, skin breakdown, or pressure injuries. Other kinds of prevention programs and strategies might include early intervention programs, drug/alcohol relapse prevention programs, assessment of ergonomics in the workplace, instruction in joint protection, energy conservation, programs for at-risk youth, provision of health and wellness programs, and so forth. To meet third-party payer requirements, the skill of a therapist must be needed to design, implement, and supervise (an OTA, if applicable) the occupational therapy intervention.

Justification for Skilled Therapy

Proper wording is critical to justify continuation of skilled occupational therapy and to demonstrate the level of complexity or sophistication of the services you are providing. **Never embellish or fabricate information to substantiate treatment**. Documentation must also reflect intervention appropriate to the individual's condition and rehabilitation potential. It is very important to describe the occupational therapy practitioner's **skilled services** provided to clients rather than simply noting the client was *assisted* or *helped* with specific occupations such as ADLs. For example, an aide or family member can *help* a client diagnosed with chronic obstructive pulmonary disease (COPD) to perform difficult or strenuous tasks such as bathing, laundry, or rising from a chair. However, an occupational therapy practitioner might provide **skilled ADL or IADL training** such as *equipment recommendations* for safety and *education* regarding proper pacing and breathing. Additional occupational therapy services for that client might include skilled instruction in *compensatory methods* such as energy conservation and work simplification to *improve* occupational performance and safety.

OTs and OTAs collaborate to ***design*** and provide *skilled instruction* and *training* in home programs, which will then be carried out by aides, caregivers, and family members. Why should third-party payers reimburse you to watch clients carry out a home exercise program or do a self-care task, such as dressing, that they perform daily on their own? However, if you are *assessing* a client's ability to perform all the components of it correctly and safely, *modifying* it to compensate for recent progress or changes, or *teaching* certain strategies, then your professional skill as an OTA is clearly required, under the supervision of the OT. Consider the following list of specialized skills and services that occupational therapy practitioners provide. While not an all-inclusive list, it will give you an idea of the various types of skilled interventions and professional wording that might be used in occupational therapy documentation:

- **OTs, with contributions from the OTA, provide the following services** (AOTA, 2020d, 2021b, 2021c):
  - Evaluate and reevaluate clients; create occupational profiles; identify problems; establish goals; and develop intervention, transition, and discontinuation plans
  - Assess or reassess the effectiveness of adaptive equipment, compensatory techniques, occupational adaptations, methods/tasks to support occupations, activities, occupations and modify the intervention plan for desirable client outcomes (e.g., occupational participation, quality of life, health, wellness)
- **OTs and OTAs provide an array of skilled services such as the following** (AOTA, 2020c, 2020d, 2021b):
  - Modify and adapt activities, occupations, and environmental contexts such as workstations, classrooms, and homes to enable safe occupational performance
  - Enhance performance of activities/occupations through the provision, instruction, training, and use of adaptive equipment and assistive technology
  - Promote physical and psychosocial health and well-being
  - Intervene to address safety hazards and unsafe or at-risk behaviors
  - Teach adaptive and compensatory techniques to minimize barriers for occupational participation
  - Improve and enhance acquisition of developmental and educational skills
  - Fabricate/fit/customize/select/recommend and provide training in use of orthotic devices, durable medical equipment (DME), seating and positioning, adaptive devices, and assistive technology
  - Design individualized exercise and home programs
  - Provide skilled instruction and training to the client/family/caregiver
  - Determine safety and effectiveness of performance skills, task procedures, and equipment
  - Improve/restore performance skills and client factors through remediation approaches
  - Administer various methods and tasks (e.g., physical agent modalities, therapeutic exercises, sensory strategies) to support occupational performance
  - Implement skilled group interventions to enhance occupational role performance
  - Provide skilled coordination of care, case management, and consultation
  - Advocacy and consultation
- **Examples of skilled occupational therapy instruction, training, and education that may be provided to a client, family, or caregiver to enhance occupational participation include the following** (AOTA, 2020c, 2020d, 2021b):
  - Instruction in the development, acquisition, or remediation of specific life skills for occupational roles and contexts
  - Training in social skills, such as communication and interpersonal behaviors, to fit within social and cultural norms
  - Education to enhance health, wellness, safety, and life satisfaction
  - Education to help manage chronic diseases/conditions for occupational participation
  - Instruction in individualized therapeutic exercise programs
  - Instruction in home, school, community, and workplace safety
  - Fall prevention
  - Training in use of adaptive equipment, DME, assistive technology, wheelchairs/mobility aids, and orthotic/prosthetic devices
  - Training in strategies to manage stress, anger, anxiety, or prevent relapse of substance use
  - Instruction in specific leisure or play skills
  - Education to improve parenting skills
  - Education regarding community services and support systems
  - Driver rehabilitation and education
  - Teaching methods of energy conservation and work simplification

- o Instruction in joint protection
- o Teaching compensatory techniques to minimize challenges in functional cognition
- o Instruction in strategies to enhance sensory processing for occupational participation
- o Teaching of strategies to enhance educational and work performance (such as organizational skills and time management)
- o Instruction in body mechanics, ergonomics, functional mobility in home/community for safe occupational performance
- o Instruction in specific prevocational and vocational task skills
- o Instruction in positioning of the limbs, trunk, and head to improve client factors (e.g., managing tone, improving lymph drainage, safe swallowing) for occupational participation
- o Self-advocacy
- **Skilled occupational therapy is NOT evident when an OT or OTA provides the following services** (CMS, 2019b, 2020b, 2021c):
  - o Provides unnecessary or unreasonable services for a client who cannot tolerate interventions, has poor potential to meet rehabilitation goals, or is expected to spontaneously recover a transient loss of function, such as after a general surgery
  - o Carries out diversionary activities or groups not appropriate or relevant to the intervention plan
  - o Duplicates services with another discipline or provides services that nonskilled personnel can do
  - o Continues routine interventions or maintenance programs, such as self-care activities; passive range of motion; or monitoring of exercise programs after the adapted procedures are in place, outcomes are reached, no further significant progress or changes are expected, and the skills of a therapist are not needed
  - o Provides services that are not part of an occupational therapy intervention plan
  - o Has a patient watch a video or read a handout regarding total hip or cardiac precautions, home safety, ergonomics, body mechanics, etc. without providing skilled instruction or practice of the skills
  - o Administers routine physical agent modalities without relating them to the performance of occupational tasks (AOTA, 2018)

Use of Aides

Occupational therapy settings often have support staff such as rehabilitation aides (or technicians) to assist with various departmental tasks and improve productivity. It is important to realize that these positions are not licensed roles requiring professional education. Aides typically only receive on-the-job training specific to their roles in that setting. Even if an aide is attending college and working toward a degree in a rehabilitation discipline, this factor alone does not qualify that person to perform skilled therapy services. AOTA's *Guidelines for Supervision, Roles, and Responsibilities During the Delivery of Occupational Therapy Services* (AOTA, 2020b) also asserts that **aides cannot provide skilled therapy**. They may be assigned client-related tasks only when the client outcome and environment are stable and predictable, professional judgment is not needed, and the task routine has already been established and performed by the client (AOTA, 2020b). Additionally, the aide must be under the supervision of the occupational therapy practitioner and properly trained in the delegated tasks (AOTA, 2020b). CMS regulations also clearly state that services provided by an aide are considered unskilled and, as such, are not a billable covered service, even under the supervision of an OT (CMS, 2009a, 2019b, 2020a). Billing for services rendered by an aide as skilled client care is unethical and could create legal and professional ramifications.

Although not an all-inclusive list, some acceptable functions of an aide might include clerical tasks (e.g., scheduling, photocopying, filing paperwork); routine maintenance (e.g., laundry, sanitizing equipment, keeping temperature logs and maintaining proper volume levels for hydrocollator and paraffin units); and other unskilled departmental tasks (e.g., servicing wheelchairs, organizing work areas, maintaining inventory/ordering supplies, prepping areas/ gathering intervention materials for the OT/OTA, transporting clients, assisting the OT/OTA with a client in a group or during a transfer). It is crucial to know your facility's exact policies regarding specific roles and responsibilities of occupational therapy support staff and volunteers. Complete Worksheet 3-1 to test your knowledge of skilled and unskilled services as they relate to delegating tasks to an aide.

Worksheet 3-1
Delegating Tasks to Aides

Indicate which of the following tasks can be delegated to an occupational therapy aide by putting a Yes (Y) or No (N) beside each item.

1. _____ Help maintain inventory of adaptive equipment and supplies.
2. _____ File OT department paperwork.
3. _____ Instruct the client in new therapy putty exercises.
4. _____ Perform retrograde massage to decrease edema.
5. _____ Assist the OT practitioner with a client transfer by stabilizing chair or walker.
6. _____ Upgrade a client's exercise program.
7. _____ Photocopy a home exercise program for the client's chart.
8. _____ Transport a stable client in a wheelchair from their hospital room to the OT room.
9. _____ While the OTA is leading a sensory group, encourage a client in that group to handle and share the tactile objects.
10. _____ Assist client in filling out routine client information forms.
11. _____ Teach a client how to use lower extremity adaptive equipment following a total hip replacement.
12. _____ Determine what adaptive feeding equipment is needed for a client who has a CVA with right hemiparesis.
13. _____ Schedule OT appointments.
14. _____ Select activities for a client's fine motor exercises.
15. _____ Assist the OTA with client wound care by opening packages of bandages and instruments without touching sterile materials inside.
16. _____ Adjust settings on a TENS unit when client reports not feeling the treatment modality work.
17. _____ Sit and talk with a client while client is receiving a hot pack or other modality.
18. _____ Assist a child with scissors skills when more practice is needed after child learns the task and condition is stable.
19. _____ Obtain therapeutic equipment that the OTA will be using with the client.
20. _____ Cut out Velcro tabs and straps for an orthosis that the OTA is fabricating.
21. _____ Administer part of a standardized assessment.
22. _____ Add more paraffin to unit when paraffin levels are low.
23. _____ Maintain temperature log of hydrocollator.
24. _____ Determine if a client should have a paraffin treatment rather than a hot pack that day.
25. _____ Set up client's meal tray in preparation for an occupational therapy feeding session.
26. _____ Clean equipment and treatment tables/mats.
27. _____ Place reality orientation calendar in client's room.
28. _____ Determine if a client is adhering to weight-bearing precautions during morning ADLs.
29. _____ Call a client as a reminder to bring orthosis to tomorrow's therapy appointment.
30. _____ To work on a client's dynamic balance, play catch with the client as the OTA is providing contact guard assist.

Morreale, M. J. (2023). *The OTA's guide to documentation: Writing SOAP notes* (5th ed.). SLACK Incorporated.

Billing Procedures and Codes

More than 5 billion claims for health services are processed every year in the United States (CMS, 2022a). Diagnosis and billing codes are used by physicians and other health care providers when submitting claims for reimbursement. The appropriate codes need to be assigned to the client's condition and specific interventions provided. Billing codes identify specific health services rendered, provision of any DME (purchase or rental), orthotic/prosthetic devices, and certain supplies deemed medically necessary for the client and are covered by the specific plan. Skilled services provided by an OTA are normally billed through an enrolled occupational therapist or another approved therapy provider (CMS, 2009a). Facilities establish specific procedures for the billing process to meet payer requirements and will provide you with the necessary resources. Some electronic documentation programs assign the proper codes automatically as interventions are recorded. Code books can be purchased from various sources and codes are also published on the CMS website.

Billing Forms and Procedures

Providers submit **claim forms** to third-party payers, usually electronically, when payment is being requested for covered health services and equipment/supplies. Medicare use alone accounted for more than 1.1 billion claims in fiscal year 2020 (CMS, 2022b). A claim form called the CMS-1450 (also called the UB-04) is a uniform billing form used by institutional providers such as hospitals and skilled nursing facilities (CMS, 2014b). It can be used to enter standard billing codes and bill multiple third-party payers (CMS, 2014b). Another type of claim form called the CMS-1500 is used by health providers who are exempt from submitting claims electronically and must use this paper form to bill CMS for services covered by Medicare (CMS, 2014c). These two forms can be viewed on the CMS website at www.cms.gov.

To process and manage claims (medical care, orthotics, prosthetics, and DME) for beneficiaries with Medicare Parts A and B, CMS uses regional **Medicare Administrative Contractors (MACs)**. These are private health care insurers, chosen through a competitive process, for a particular geographic area or jurisdiction (CMS, 2022b). These MACs are the *operational contact* between fee-for-service Medicare and enrolled health providers. In addition to processing claims and making payments, MACs enroll providers, handle first stage appeals, review medical records for specific claims, and provide cost audits (CMS, 2022b; Fearon & Levine, 2016). MACs also make **local coverage determinations (LCDs)** to justify payments and determine if a particular item or service is reasonable and necessary (CMS, 2022b; Fearon & Levine, 2016). Claims that are rejected due to clerical errors may be resubmitted with corrections. However, for fully denied claims or those reimbursed with reduced amounts, the provider might choose to go through an **appeals process**. The appeals process entails the provider trying to substantiate the claim to the insurer and overturn the denial. This could potentially turn into a time-consuming and lengthy multi-step process and there is no guarantee that the claim will ultimately be approved for reimbursement.

ICD-10 and ICD-11 Codes

The World Health Organization (WHO) is responsible for the *International Classification of Diseases (ICD)* which is a large set of codes used to define and classify the spectrum of health-related conditions, injuries, disorders, and diseases worldwide (WHO, 2021). These are usually referred to as *diagnosis codes*. ICD is used by more than 150 countries, enabling nations to track diseases and deaths (morbidity and mortality), manage health, allocate resources, and is the standard diagnostic classification system used for all research and clinical purposes (WHO, 2021). ICD-10 refers to the 10th version of the ICD codes, which the USDHHS mandated be used in the United States for electronic health care transactions as of October 1, 2015 (Centers for Disease Control and Prevention [CDC], 2015). ICD-10 codes have three to seven alphanumeric characters and are used for multiple purposes in the United States, such as health care statistics; epidemiology research; measuring patient outcomes; billing and claims processing; and identifying fraud/abuse (CDC, 2015). As versions were revised, classifications became more specific. For example, a hand fracture is coded and identified by multiple factors, such as right or left, the specific bone, the affected area of the bone, whether it is a closed or open fracture, and so forth. ICD-10 also allowed for more details to be included about injuries, external causes, and poisonings, such as severity/complexity and where and how injuries occurred (CDC, 2015). The WHO has now completed work on the next version, ICD-11, which is effective January 1, 2022, but does not yet have a mandatory implementation date (Chaplain, 2020; WHO, 2021). It is projected the United States will begin using ICD-11 no earlier than 2023, transitioning initially to implementation of mortality data (Chaplain, 2020). ICD-11 is fully digital, more compatible with EHR systems, and designed to be user-friendly with online resources (Chaplain, 2020). This new version is also more comprehensive than ICD-10. It incorporates new codes and classifications, additional chapters and allows for more flexibility and detailed reporting of clinical modifications or specialty adaptations (Chaplain, 2020; WHO, 2021).

Healthcare Common Procedure Coding System

The CMS established the mandatory **Healthcare Common Procedure Coding System (HCPCS)** to enable physicians and other health care providers to use common language and standardized codes (CMS, 2009b, 2022a). These codes are used to identify and bill health services, medical products, and to collect data. The system consists of two parts: Level I and Level II codes. Level I codes, each consisting of five numbers, are called **Current Procedural Terminology (CPT)** codes and maintained by the American Medical Association (CMS, 2022a). These Level I codes are used to bill for individual procedures that a patient receives such as doctor visits and skilled therapy. Level II codes are maintained by CMS. These codes are alphanumeric (one letter followed by four digits) and used for health products such as DME, prosthetics, orthotics, and supplies (DMEPOS), drugs, biologicals, along with certain services (e.g., ambulance) not included in the Level I codes (CMS, 2022a).

Modifiers are supplemental letter codes included with standard CPT codes to provide additional information about the claim, such as to identify which therapy discipline implemented the specific therapy service (in accordance with the respective discipline's plan of care). For example, for outpatient rehabilitation claims, the modifier *GO* is used to identify occupational therapy services, *GP* for physical therapy services, and *GN* for speech-language pathology services (CMS, 2019e). As of January 1, 2020, CMS is also requiring use of *CO* modifiers for services provided, in whole or part, by OTAs and *CQ* modifiers for services of PTAs (CMS, 2019e). These CO and CQ codes are used alongside the corresponding GO or GP therapy modifier to identify those OTA or PTA services implemented under an OT or PT plan of care (CMS, 2019e). Beginning in 2013, CMS mandated that therapists report non-payable, functional limitation G-codes and severity modifiers for therapy services at specified times during the therapy process, but this requirement was discontinued at the end of 2018 (CMS, 2021f).

Prospective Payment System

Inpatients with Medicare Part A benefits in settings such as hospitals, skilled nursing facilities, inpatient rehabilitation centers, and home health agencies come under the federal **Prospective Payment System (PPS)**, which pays a predetermined and fixed payment for total care of a client's condition according to diagnoses and overall level of care needed (CMS, 2013a, 2020b, 2021b, 2021d). CMS uses different classification systems and reporting measures for each kind of institutional health setting when categorizing conditions and care levels for reimbursement (Fearon & Levine, 2016). As of January 1, 2020, the original PPS system for home health was modified to include the **Patient-Driven Groupings Model (PDGM)** which provides a greater focus on clinical and other patient characteristics to better align Medicare payments with clients' care needs (CMS, 2019f, 2021g). Under the prospective payment system, therapy sessions and other services are typically consolidated or bundled into the daily per-diem rate or are part of an episode-based payment for total care rather than reimbursed separately. However, any services or products covered under Medicare Part B benefits rather than Part A for that setting are not included in the PPS payment and billed separately. These Medicare Part B services are reimbursed for each individual item or type of service according to the **Medicare Physician Fee Schedule (MPFS)**, described in the following section, if all the criteria are met (CMS, 2003b, 2009b). Other payers establish their own criteria for what services and medical equipment/supplies are covered and the specific reimbursement rates. The documentation needed to meet payer and legal requirements for different practice settings is explained further in Chapter 17.

Fee Schedules

Insurers establish a **fee schedule** that delineates benefits provided (e.g., health services and equipment/supplies) and specifies the maximum rates that will be paid for each of these covered items, according to the specific plan. Health providers and vendors who accept assignment are reimbursed at no more than that insurer's preset rates for medical products and services rendered. Even if the provider submits a higher priced claim based on their typical charges for a covered service or product, the actual payment required of the insurer and patient combined cannot exceed contractual price limits. Medicare Part B covered products and services (including occupational therapy) are reimbursed according to current **established rates** in the MPFS as part of HCPCS (CMS, 2003b, 2009b). The MPFS applies to a variety of settings such as occupational therapy private practices, comprehensive outpatient rehabilitation facilities, in addition to clients in hospitals and skilled nursing facilities who are not covered with a Medicare Part A stay (CMS, 2009b). Part B services provided to the same patient on the same day (including select timed and untimed therapy services from one or multiple disciplines) might have to be bundled together and reimbursed by CMS at a reduced rate, called the **multiple procedure payment reduction (MPPR;** CMS, 2016a).

Many insurers require that the patient pay a predetermined amount of initial out-of-pocket expenses each year, called a **deductible**, for health services or supplies received before the insurer will begin paying for covered services. However, there may be mandated exceptions to the deductible requirement for certain preventative services (CMS,

2010). Depending on the specific plan, a deductible can range from around $100 to thousands of dollars per person. Some funding sources also mandate that clients pay an out-of-pocket preset dollar amount, called a **copayment**, directly to the provider at each health care visit or for each covered medical supply. For example, a copayment (ranging from about $5 to $50 depending on the plan) for an occupational therapy outpatient visit would supplement what the funding source also pays the occupational therapy provider for that visit. A copayment for a medication at an approved pharmacy might, for example, be $10 for generic or $20 for a brand-name drug each time that medication is refilled. Again, actual costs are plan specific.

For various insurers (including Medicare), patients may be responsible for paying a **coinsurance** amount after meeting their deductible, which is a *percentage* of the *allowable* reimbursement rate (CMS, 2003b, 2009b). To help clarify insurance concepts, Box 3-1 presents various payment scenarios for a pretend client receiving therapy services. The numbers used in these examples are for illustrative purposes only:

Box 3-1

EXAMPLES OF BILLING AND REIMBURSEMENT

Coinsurance

- Occupational therapy service—$50 charged by occupational therapy clinic
- Medicare B allowable amount (MPFS)—$40
- Medicare B pays 80% of the $40, which equals $32
- Patient is responsible for paying remaining 20% coinsurance of the $40, which equals $8.
- Total reimbursement to occupational therapy clinic for this service is $40 ($32 + $8)

Deductible

- Occupational therapy service—$120 charged by outpatient clinic
- Insurance company allowable amount—$90

plus

- Physical therapy service—$80 charged by outpatient clinic
- Insurance company allowable amount—$68
- However, patient has a remaining $200 deductible so is responsible for paying $90 + $68 ($158) to outpatient clinic
- Insurance company pays $0
- Total reimbursement to outpatient clinic for both services is $158

(continued)

Coinsurance amounts are determined by the insurer according to the specific plan benefits. Often, the beneficiary pays a lower percentage out-of-pocket if using an **in-network provider** that is part of a group contracted with and preferred by the insurance company. For example, although actual percentages will depend on the specific plan, an individual might be responsible for a coinsurance of 10% if using an in-network provider for a particular service but might, instead, be required to pay a coinsurance of 20% or 30% for the very same service if using an **out-of-network provider**. Complete Worksheet 3-4 to test your knowledge of reimbursement principles.

Box 3-1 (continued)
Examples of Billing and Reimbursement

Coordination of Benefits

- Occupational therapy service—$85 charged by occupational therapy clinic
- Medicare B allowable amount (MPFS)—$50
- Medicare B pays 80% of the $50, which equals $40
- Patient also has Medigap insurance that pays the remaining 20% of $50 which equals $10
- Patient owes clinic $0
- Total reimbursement to occupational therapy clinic for this service is $50 ($40 + $10)

Co-Pay

- Occupational therapy service—$75 charged by occupational therapy clinic
- Insurance company allowable amount paid at 100%—$32

plus

- Physical therapy service—$75 charged by outpatient clinic
- Insurance company allowable amount paid at 100%—$32
- Patient has a co-pay of $20 per therapy session
- Insurance company pays $62 to outpatient clinic ($32 + $32)
- Patient is responsible for paying $40 to outpatient clinic ($20 + $20)
- Total reimbursement to outpatient clinic for both services is $102 ($62 + $40)

Timed and Untimed Services

Many CPT codes for therapy are based on time using 15-minute intervals. Other CPT therapy codes are considered untimed procedures and billed at a fixed amount (for that specific procedure) regardless of how much time is used (CMS, 2009a, 2016b). An occupational therapy evaluation (an untimed procedure) is only billed 1 unit regardless of how much time was needed or how many different assessment tools were used to complete the evaluation that day (CMS, 2009a, 2016b). Some codes are mutually exclusive and cannot be billed together (CMS, 2009a, 2016b). For example, codes requiring constant attendance or direct one-on-one patient contact (such as self-care training, ultrasound, or neuromuscular reeducation) cannot be billed together for one or two clients during the same 15-minute time-period (CMS, 2009a, 2016b). Some passive types of interventions, such as hot and cold packs, may have CPT codes but are not individually reimbursable as they are bundled into other therapy procedures (Scott, 2013). Additionally, there are strict billing rules regarding treating more than one client at a time, which might require a cheaper concurrent rate or group rate (CMS, 2006, 2009a).

Units are always based on services provided per *single calendar day* (CMS, 2016b). It is important to understand that although all timed services (e.g., therapeutic exercise, ADL instruction, wheelchair management training) are billed as 15-minute units, they are actually regarded by Medicare to be anywhere from 8 minutes to 22 minutes as per the following CMS chart in Box 3-2 (CMS, 2016b):

Box 3-2
TIMED UNITS OF THERAPY

Units	Number of Minutes
1 unit	≥ 8 minutes through 22 minutes
2 units	≥ 23 minutes through 37 minutes
3 units	≥ 38 minutes through 52 minutes
4 units	≥ 53 minutes through 67 minutes
5 units	≥ 68 minutes through 82 minutes
6 units	≥ 83 minutes through 97 minutes
7 units	≥ 98 minutes through 112 minutes
8 units	≥ 113 minutes through 127 minutes
	The pattern remains the same for treatment times in excess of 2 hours.

Reproduced from Centers for Medicare & Medicaid Services. (2016b). *Medicare claims processing manual* (Pub. 100-04: Ch. 5, Section 20.2). Author. Retrieved October 15, 2021 from https://www.cms.gov/Regulations-and-Guidance/Guidance/Manuals/Downloads/clm104c05.pdf

Thus, if a client received skilled instruction and practice in transfers for 10 minutes in addition to working on therapeutic exercise for 11 minutes, the total billable time would be 21 minutes, which equals only 1 billable unit. The service that consisted of the most time is billed, which is therapeutic exercise in this case. However, if the time spent on transfers was 10 minutes and therapeutic exercise was 25 minutes, total time equals 35 minutes, which is 2 units billed as 1 unit of each of the two services. Services cannot be billed if the therapy session was less than 8 minutes (CMS, 2016b).

Although CMS does not require that the time for each individual intervention be recorded, CMS does require that the **total *timed* code treatment minutes and total treatment time in minutes** be recorded (CMS, 2016b). Total treatment time consists of the number of treatment minutes for both timed and untimed skilled services combined but does *not* include any non-billable time (such as chart review and rest periods; CMS, 2019c). When two disciplines perform a joint skilled service to one client, CMS does not allow duplicate billing of units for a single time frame. For example, if an OTA and physical therapist assistant (PTA) team up to implement a timed intervention together for 30 minutes with a client, such as transfer training, those disciplines should either divide the time spent in half with each billing for 15 minutes (1 unit) or one discipline can bill 2 units while the other does not bill any (CMS, 2006, 2009a). However, the practitioners should still document separately in a contact or progress note, describing what transpired during the entire time spent with the client.

The occupational therapy practitioner should only bill for actual treatment time, not ancillary tasks such as preparing the treatment area, transporting the client, reviewing charts, documenting, allowing for client toilet breaks or rest periods, etc. (CMS, 2003a). However, if your time transporting the client is also used for a pertinent intervention outlined in the OT's intervention plan (i.e., skilled instruction in wheelchair mobility or cognitive retraining such as functional problem solving or topographical orientation), then that time could potentially be billable. If the client's intervention plan includes areas such as dressing and transfers, you might take the opportunity of the client's necessary toilet break to work on skilled toilet transfers, managing clothing, and safety education.

Therapy Students

As only qualified practitioners can bill Medicare for skilled services, strict criteria must be followed regarding treatment rendered by therapy students (CMS, 2006). The rules differ for Medicare Part A and B. Students require *appropriate supervision* by the qualified practitioner for the intervention to qualify as a Part B reimbursable skilled service. This means a supervisor's mere presence in the room, such as line-of-sight supervision, is not sufficient (CMS, 2006). Student participation in Part B skilled service delivery is allowable in situations such as if the qualified practitioner is present in the room, directly involved in the client's care, responsible for the services, and not performing other tasks or treating other clients at the same time (CMS, 2006). Part A requirements are discussed further in the skilled nursing facility section in Chapter 17.

Financial Limitation Legislation

Therapy cap refers to the mandated monetary limits for Medicare Part B outpatient therapy services (excluding hospital outpatient settings prior to 2012) originally set in 1999 at $1500 for physical therapy (PT) and speech-language pathology (SLP) services combined plus an additional $1500 for occupational therapy (CMS, 2019d). Subsequently, Congress enacted several moratoria and periodic exceptions to these caps based on medical necessity and eventually signed into law the Bipartisan Budget Act of 2018 (PL 115-123) with Section 50202 repealing these monetary caps (CMS, 2019d, 2021e). However, this legislation required that claims for incurred expenses above the former cap amounts include a modifier to confirm that the therapy services are medically necessary as justified by health record documentation; this is referred to as the **KX modifier threshold** (CMS, 2015, 2019d). In 2021, these KX modifier threshold amounts were $2110 for occupational therapy and $2110 for physical and speech therapy combined (CMS, 2021e). In addition, the law designates a targeted medical review process at a $3000 threshold amount for PT and SLP combined and $3000 for occupational therapy (CMS, 2019e) for select claims. Section 53107 of the Bipartisan Budget Act of 2018 mandates CMS pay a reduced amount (85% of the MPFS rate) for therapy services provided, in whole or part, by an OTA or PTA, effective January 1, 2022 (CMS, 2021e). This reduced reimbursement rate applies if an OTA or PTA implements more than 10% of a furnished therapy service (CMS, 2021e).

Advanced Beneficiary Notice of Noncoverage (ABN), otherwise known as CMS-R-131 form, must be issued to notify Part B beneficiaries in advance of services that are likely to be denied by Medicare. Clients must be informed that Medicare is not expected to pay for services that are not reasonable or medically necessary, not a covered service, or exceed the KX modifier threshold for which Medicare may deny payment for continued services (CMS, 2013b, 2018). Clients are informed with the ABN that if they choose to continue therapy, they will have a financial obligation to pay for services Medicare denies, for example, in that outpatient setting or skilled nursing facility (CMS, 2013b, 2018). The ABN Form CMS-R-131 can be found on the CMS website (www.cms.gov).

Medical Supplies and Durable Medical Equipment

The health record validates the client's need for reimbursable and non-reimbursable medical equipment and supplies based on the client's pertinent medical condition and circumstances. Routine supplies (e.g., Band-Aids, tongue depressors, exam gloves) are not reimbursable as they are factored into the rate paid for a particular procedure (such as an evaluation or basic wound care). Certain equipment, such as a commode used in a hospital, is also deemed routine for the care already being paid for in that setting and, as such, is not reimbursed separately. However, that same type of item could potentially be reimbursed for home use upon discharge if medically necessary criteria are met.

DME is equipment that is reasonable and medically necessary for the individual to use at home. "Durable" means that the equipment can be used repeatedly (such as an item typically available for rental; CMS, 2014d, 2021a). Third-party payers will usually provide coverage for the purchase (or rental as appropriate) of items the payer designates as DME or reimbursable supplies so long as specific criteria are met and usually requiring that a physician prescribe the item (CMS, 2021a). CMS delineates the following four criteria that must be met for items to be considered DME (CMS, 2014d, 2021a):

1. Can withstand repeated use
2. Is primarily and customarily used to serve a medical purpose
3. Generally is not useful to a person in the absence of an illness or injury
4. Is appropriate for use in the home

Some items such as orthotics and prosthetics are categorized differently and not considered as DME. **Medical supplies** such as ostomy supplies, wound care dressings, blood glucose test strips, gloves, incontinence pads, and so forth are expendable and, as such, normally do not meet the DME criteria (CMS, 2021a). However, some of these items may be covered as *non-routine* medical supplies if the plan offers that benefit and the items are substantiated in the record as reasonable and medically necessary for the client's condition (i.e., diabetic testing supplies for use by an individual at home). In determining the "reasonableness" of an item for Medicare to pay for it, CMS specifies the following considerations (CMS, 2021a):

1. Would the expense of the item to the program be clearly disproportionate to the therapeutic benefits that could ordinarily be derived from use of the equipment?
2. Is the item substantially more costly than a medically appropriate and realistically feasible alternative pattern of care?
3. Does the item serve essentially the same purpose as equipment already available to the beneficiary?

Box 3-3 provides examples of items that can and cannot qualify as DME.

Box 3-3 DURABLE MEDICAL EQUIPMENT	
Examples of Health-Related Equipment and Supplies for Home Use	*Can Item Meet the CMS Criteria to Qualify as DME?*
Grab bars	No (considered self-help device, non-medical in nature)
Raised toilet seat	No (considered a convenience item)
Long handle sponge	No
Tub seat	No (considered a comfort or convenience item)
Therapy putty	No
Resting hand orthosis	No (orthotic devices are a different category)
Air conditioner	No
Commode	Yes (if patient confined to bed or room)
Reacher	No
Glucose monitoring strips	No (medical supplies are a different category)
Prosthetic limb	No (prosthetic devices are a different category)
Walker	Yes (must meet mobility assistive equipment clinical criteria)
Wheelchair	Yes (must meet mobility assistive equipment clinical criteria)
Exercise bike	No
Plate guard	No
Telephone alert system	No

Adapted from Centers for Medicare & Medicaid Services. (2014d). *Medicare national coverage determinations manual* (Pub. 100-03: Ch. 1, Part 4, Section 280.1). Retrieved October 15, 2021 from https://www.cms.gov/Regulations-and-Guidance/Guidance/Manuals/Downloads/ncd103c1_Part4.pdf

Fraud and Abuse

OTs and OTAs must adhere to established legal and ethical standards in place when billing for occupational therapy services and supplies. CMS defines fraud as "*making false statements or representations of material facts in order to obtain some benefit or payment for which no entitlement would otherwise exist … and performed knowingly, willfully, and intentionally*" (CMS, 2002b). Abuse is defined by CMS as "*practices that, either directly or indirectly, result in unnecessary costs to the Medicare program*" (CMS, 2002c). Standards that CMS uses to judge if abusive billing acts were committed or not include the following (CMS, 2002c):

- *Were the billed services/items reasonable and necessary?*
- *Did the billed services/items conform to professionally recognized standards?*
- *Were the billed services/items provided at a fair price?*

Examples of fraud and abuse as delineated by CMS are presented in Box 3-4. Health care providers and suppliers who commit fraud and abuse by not conforming to third-party-payer requirements (e.g., CMS regulations) may be subject to prosecution and could have penalties imposed such as fines, payment of restitution, or even imprisonment (CMS, 2002a). Fraud and abuse might also result in various administrative sanctions, such as being excluded from program participation or having to pay civil monetary penalties (CMS, 2002a).

Box 3-4	
CMS Examples of Fraud	**CMS Examples of Abuse**
Billing for services and/or supplies that were not furnished or provided	Billing excessive charges for supplies or services
Billing for missed client appointments	Providing and billing for services that are not medically necessary
Paying or receiving bribes or kickbacks for client referrals or goods/services used	Providing services that do not meet recognized standards of professional care
Misrepresenting and describing a furnished service as a covered service when it is not	Billing Medicare using a higher fee schedule than the one used for non-Medicare clients
Duplicate billing, such as additionally billing the client or another payer, to obtain more than the allowable amount	Billing Medicare for services that are the responsibility of other insurers according to the Medicare secondary payer regulation
Using someone else's Medicare card to obtain services	Participants violating the provider/supplier agreement
Adapted from Centers for Medicare & Medicaid Services. (2002b). *Medicare general information, eligibility and entitlement manual* (Pub. 100-01: Ch. 1, Section 20.3.1). Retrieved September 27, 2021 from https://www.cms.gov/Regulations-and-Guidance/Guidance/Manuals/Downloads/ge101c01.pdf; Centers for Medicare & Medicaid Services. (2002c). *Medicare general information, eligibility and entitlement manual* (Pub. 100-01: Ch. 1, Section 20.3.2). Retrieved September 27, 2021 from https://www.cms.gov/Regulations-and-Guidance/Guidance/Manuals/Downloads/ge101c01.pdf	

Helpful Resources for Billing and Reimbursement

This chapter has presented an overview of the complex and ever-changing billing and reimbursement process. It is imperative that occupational therapy practitioners be knowledgeable regarding current payer regulations and ethical occupational therapy practice (AOTA, 2020a). A good information source is the AOTA website (www.aota.org), which contains a section on reimbursement and regulatory policy and is a useful resource to help practitioners keep current with new health care legislation and payer requirements. The Medicare Learning Network, part of the CMS website (www.cms.gov), contains web-based educational videos, fact sheets, and booklets regarding health benefits, documentation, billing, and reimbursement. In addition, CMS regulatory forms and manuals can be accessed easily on the CMS website. Some sections of CMS manuals particularly applicable to occupational therapy include the following:

- *Publication 100-02: Medicare Benefit Policy Manual*
  - Chapter 1—Inpatient Hospital Services Covered Under Part A (Section 110: Inpatient Rehabilitation Facility [IRF] Services)
  - Chapter 7—Home Health Services (Section 40.2: Skilled Therapy Services)
  - Chapter 8—Coverage of Extended Care Services (SNF) Under Hospital Insurance
  - Chapter 15—Covered Medical and Other Services (Section 220: Coverage of Outpatient Rehabilitation Therapy Services [Physical Therapy, Occupational Therapy, and Speech-Language Pathology Services] Under Medical Insurance)

- ***Publication 100-04: Medicare Claims Processing Manual***
  - ○ Chapter 5—Part B Outpatient Rehabilitation and CORF/OPT Services (Sections 10, 20, 30)

Information regarding early intervention and special education eligibility and services can be found at the U.S. Department of Education website at www.ed.gov. An organization called The American Health Information Management Association (AHIMA; www.ahima.org) offers information and professional articles on a large list of topics pertaining to aspects of the health record such as legislation, code sets, EHR requirements and standards, etc. In addition, the American Academy of Professional Coders (AAPC) website (www.aapc.com) contains a medical terminology glossary of billing and coding language, other informational resources, and offers training materials for billing and coding.

Complete Worksheets 3-2 and 3-3 to test your knowledge of billing and coding terms and basic concepts. In subsequent chapters of this manual, you will learn more about the professional language, standards, and the specific formats used by occupational therapy practitioners to communicate and substantiate client care and meet third-party-payer requirements.

Worksheet 3-2
Billing and Reimbursement Terms

Match the following terms to the appropriate descriptions. Use each term only once.

a. Third-party payer   k. Medicare Advantage Plan
b. GO modifier   l. Workers' Compensation
c. Copayment   m. ABN
d. Deductible   n. CMS-1500
e. IDEA Part C   o. IDEA Part B
f. Medicaid   p. Medicare Part D
g. Medigap insurance   q. CPT codes
h. Coinsurance   r. ICD codes
i. KX modifier   s. CO modifier
j. Fee schedule   t. Beneficiary

1. _____ The 20% out-of-pocket expense that a Medicare Part B beneficiary pays for a covered service
2. _____ A combined federal-state health program with income eligibility guidelines
3. _____ Mandates an appropriate and free public education in the least restrictive environment for children with disabilities
4. _____ A claim form
5. _____ The person covered by an insurance plan
6. _____ The initial out-of-pocket expenses an individual must pay to providers before the insurance company begins paying for those covered services
7. _____ Medicare Part C
8. _____ Used by insurers to indicate set prices for covered services
9. _____ Used on claim forms to identify specific therapy services provided based on units of time
10. _____ Used to indicate services provided by an OTA under an OT plan of care
11. _____ A prescription drug program
12. _____ An entity that pays for health services that is not the individual or provider
13. _____ Used to indicate a client's specific diagnosis or condition
14. _____ A mandatory insurance that businesses pay to cover employees injured on the job
15. _____ Establishes early intervention services up to age 3 years
16. _____ A set amount individuals pay to a health provider at each visit, in addition to what the insurer pays
17. _____ Used to indicate therapy services that exceed financial threshold limits
18. _____ A plan that helps pay for out-of-pocket Medicare expenses
19. _____ This must be provided prior to therapy exceeding Medicare Part B financial limits
20. _____ Used to indicate that occupational therapy services were provided

Worksheet 3-3
Billing and Coding

For each of the statements below, indicate if it is true (T) or false (F).

1. _____ Tub seats and elevated toilet seats meet the CMS criteria for DME.

2. _____ A sock aid and long shoehorn for a client with total hip precautions are billed as DME.

3. _____ Billing CMS for missed client appointments is fraud.

4. _____ For a client in occupational therapy, ADL practice supervised by an aide for 18 minutes should be billed as 1 unit.

5. _____ The modifier on claim forms that indicates an occupational therapy service is "GO."

6. _____ For Medicare Part B, a covered timed 25-minute occupational therapy skilled procedure is billed as 2 units.

7. _____ An OT who performs an occupational therapy evaluation (for a client with Medicare Part B) for 60 minutes should bill 4 units.

8. _____ The yearly financial limitation in 2021 for Medicare Part B therapy services is $2110 combined for physical, occupational, and speech therapy before any exceptions are applied.

9. _____ CPT codes are maintained by the American Medical Association.

10. _____ HCPCS Level I codes are used to bill for items such as prosthetics and DME.

11. _____ An OT and PT work together simultaneously with a client (skilled transfer training) for 15 minutes, which allows them to each bill Medicare Part B 1 unit of therapy.

12. _____ ICD Codes are established by CMS.

13. _____ Total timed treatment time in minutes includes the time spent providing skilled interventions and documenting in the client's health record.

14. _____ Twenty-one minutes of transfer training plus 8 minutes for client rest periods is billed as 1 unit.

15. _____ The bundling of services reimbursed at a reduced rate is called the multiple procedure payment reduction.

Morreale, M. J. (2023). *The OTA's guide to documentation: Writing SOAP notes* (5th ed.). SLACK Incorporated.

Worksheet 3-4
Billing and Reimbursement Scenarios

For each scenario, fill in the blanks with the correct dollar amounts that the third-party payers and client would each have to pay for services furnished. Realize the numbers used are for illustrative purposes only.

1. *Client has Medicare Part A and B and has already met deductibles.*
   - Occupational therapy outpatient service—$90 charged by occupational therapy clinic
   - Medicare B allowable amount (MPFS)—$68
   - Medicare B pays _____
   - Medicare A pays _____
   - Patient is responsible for paying _____
   - Total reimbursement to occupational therapy clinic for this service is _____

2. *Client has private insurance that pays 90% of allowable amount. Client also has a remaining $150 deductible.*
   - Occupational therapy service—$60 charged by outpatient clinic
   - Insurance company allowable amount—$55
   - Physical therapy service—$60 charged by outpatient clinic
   - Insurance company allowable amount—$55
   - Insurance company pays _____
   - Patient pays _____
   - Total reimbursement to outpatient clinic for both services is _____

3. *Client has Medicare Part B, Medigap insurance, and no deductible.*
   - Occupational therapy outpatient service —$110 charged by occupational therapy outpatient clinic
   - Medicare B allowable amount (MPFS)—$82
   - Medicare B pays _____
   - Medigap insurance pays _____
   - Patient pays clinic _____
   - Total reimbursement to occupational therapy clinic for this service is _____

4. *Client has private insurance which pays 80% of covered services in-network and 75% out-of-network at allowable rates.*
   - Occupational therapy service—$120 charged by outpatient therapy clinic in-network provider
   - Insurance company allowable rate—$96
   - Insurance company pays _____
   - Client pays _____
   - Total reimbursement to occupational therapy clinic for this service is _____

5. *Client has private insurance which requires a co-pay of $15 per outpatient therapy session.*
   - Occupational therapy service—$90 charged by occupational therapy outpatient clinic
   - Insurance company allowable amount—$72
   - Physical therapy service—$90 charged by outpatient clinic
   - Insurance company allowable amount—$72
   - Insurance company pays _____
   - Patient pays _____
   - Total reimbursement to outpatient clinic for both services is _____

Morreale, M. J. (2023). *The OTA's guide to documentation: Writing SOAP notes* (5th ed.). SLACK Incorporated.

References

American Occupational Therapy Association. (2018). Physical agents and mechanical modalities. *American Journal of Occupational Therapy, 72*(Suppl.2), 7212410055. https://doi.org/10.5014/ajot.2018.72S220

American Occupational Therapy Association. (2020a). AOTA 2020 occupational therapy code of ethics. *American Journal of Occupational Therapy, 74*(Suppl. 3), 7413410005. https://doi.org: 10.5014/ajot.2020.74S3006

American Occupational Therapy Association. (2020b). Guidelines for supervision, roles, and responsibilities during the delivery of occupational therapy services. *American Journal of Occupational Therapy, 74*(Suppl. 3), 7413410020. https://doi.org/10.5014/ajot.2020.74S3004

American Occupational Therapy Association. (2020c). Occupational therapy in the promotion of health and well-being. *American Journal of Occupational Therapy, 74*, 7403420010 https://doi.org: 10.5014/ajot.2020.743003

American Occupational Therapy Association. (2020d). Occupational therapy practice framework: Domain and process (4th ed.). *American Journal of Occupational Therapy, 74*(Suppl. 2), 7412410010. https://doi.org: 10.5014/ajot.2020.74S2001

American Occupational Therapy Association. (2021a). Medicaid. Retrieved September 28, 2021 from https://www.aota.org/Advocacy-Policy/Federal-Reg-Affairs/Pay/medicaid.aspx#SchoolBasedMedicaid

American Occupational Therapy Association. (2021b). Occupational therapy scope of practice. *American Journal of Occupational Therapy, 75*(Suppl. 3), 7513410020. https://doi.org/10.5014/ajot.2021.75S3005

American Occupational Therapy Association. (2021c). Standards of practice for occupational therapy. *American Journal of Occupational Therapy, 75*(Suppl. 3), 7513410030. https://doi.org/10.5014/ajot.2021.75S3004

Center for Parent Information and Resources. (2017). Key terms to know in early intervention. Retrieved September 18, 2021 from https://www.parentcenterhub.org/keyterms-ei/

Centers for Disease Control and Prevention. (2015). International classification of diseases (ICD-10-CM/PCS) Transition-Background. Retrieved September 29, 2021 from https://www.cdc.gov/nchs/icd/icd10cm_pcs_background.htm

Centers for Medicare & Medicaid Services. (n.d.a). How Medicare works with other insurance. Retrieved May 26, 2022 from https://www.medicare.gov/supplements-other-insurance/how-medicare-works-with-other-insurance

Centers for Medicare & Medicaid Services. (n.d.b) What's Medicare Supplement Insurance (Medigap)? Retrieved May 26, 2022 from https://www.medicare.gov/supplements-other-insurance/whats-medicare-supplement-insurance-medigap

Centers for Medicare & Medicaid Services. (2002a). *Medicare general information, eligibility and entitlement manual* (Pub. 100-01: Ch. 1, Section 20.3). Retrieved September 27, 2021 from https://www.cms.gov/Regulations-and-Guidance/Guidance/Manuals/Downloads/ge101c01.pdf

Centers for Medicare & Medicaid Services. (2002b). *Medicare general information, eligibility and entitlement manual* (Pub. 100-01: Ch. 1, Section 20.3.1). Retrieved September 27, 2021 https://www.cms.gov/Regulations-and-Guidance/Guidance/Manuals/Downloads/ge101c01.pdf

Centers for Medicare & Medicaid Services. (2002c). *Medicare general information, eligibility and entitlement manual* (Pub. 100-01: Ch. 1, Section 20.3.2). Retrieved September 27, 2021 from https://www.cms.gov/Regulations-and-Guidance/Guidance/Manuals/Downloads/ge101c01.pdf

Centers for Medicare & Medicaid Services. (2003a). *Medicare claims processing manual* (Pub. 100-04: Ch. 5, Section 20.3). Retrieved October 15, 2021 from https://www.cms.gov/Regulations-and-Guidance/Guidance/Manuals/downloads//clm104c05.pdf

Centers for Medicare & Medicaid Services. (2003b). *Medicare claims processing manual* (Pub. 100-04: Ch. 5, Section 100.2). Retrieved September 29, 2021 from https://www.cms.gov/Regulations-and-Guidance/Guidance/Manuals/downloads//clm104c05.pdf

Centers for Medicare & Medicaid Services. (2006). *Medicare benefit policy manual* (Pub. 100-02: Ch. 15, Section 230). Retrieved September 29, 2021 from https://www.cms.gov/Regulations-and-Guidance/Guidance/Manuals/Downloads/bp102c15.pdf

Centers for Medicare & Medicaid Services. (2009a). 11 Part B billing scenarios for PTs and OTs. Retrieved October 29, 2021 from https://www.cms.gov/Medicare/Billing/TherapyServices/Downloads/11_Part_B_Billing_Scenarios_for_PTs_and_OTs.pdf

Centers for Medicare & Medicaid Services. (2009b). *Medicare claims processing manual* (Pub. 100-04: Ch. 5, Section 20). Retrieved September 29, 2021 from https://www.cms.gov/Regulations-and-Guidance/Guidance/Manuals/Downloads/clm104c05.pdf

Centers for Medicare & Medicaid Services. (2010). Background: The Affordable Care Act's new rules on preventative care. Retrieved September 28, 2021 from https://www.cms.gov/CCIIO/Resources/Fact-Sheets-and-FAQs/preventive-care-background

Centers for Medicare & Medicaid Services. (2013a). *Medicare claims processing manual* (Pub. 100-04: Ch. 3, Section 140) retrieved September 29, 2021 from https://www.cms.gov/regulations-and-guidance/guidance/manuals/downloads/clm104c03.pdf

Centers for Medicare & Medicaid Services. (2013b). *Medicare claims processing manual* (Pub. 100-04: Ch. 5, Section 10.5). Retrieved September 30, 2021 from https://www.cms.gov/Regulations-and-Guidance/Guidance/Manuals/Downloads/clm104c05.pdf

Centers for Medicare & Medicaid Services. (2014a). *Medicare benefit policy manual* (Pub. 100-02: Ch. 15, Section 230.2). Retrieved September 27, 2021 from https://www.cms.gov/Regulations-and-Guidance/Guidance/Manuals/Downloads/bp102c15.pdf

Centers for Medicare & Medicaid Services. (2014b). *Medicare claims processing manual* (Pub. 100-04: Ch. 25, Section 70.1). Retrieved September 28, 2021 from https://www.cms.gov/Regulations-and-Guidance/Guidance/Manuals/Downloads/clm104c25.pdf

Centers for Medicare & Medicaid Services. (2014c). *Medicare claims processing manual* (Pub. 100-04: Ch. 26, Section 10). Retrieved September 28, 2021 from https://www.cms.gov/Regulations-and-Guidance/Guidance/Manuals/Downloads/clm104c26.pdf

Centers for Medicare & Medicaid Services. (2014d). *Medicare national coverage determinations manual* (Pub. 100-03: Ch. 1, Part 4, Section 280.1). Retrieved October 15, 2021 from https://www.cms.gov/Regulations-and-Guidance/Guidance/Manuals/Downloads/ncd103c1_Part4.pdf

Centers for Medicare & Medicaid Services. (2015). *Medicare claims processing manual* (Pub. 100-04: Ch. 5, Section 10.3.1). Retrieved September 30, 2021 from https://www.cms.gov/Regulations-and-Guidance/Guidance/Manuals/Downloads/clm104c05.pdf

Centers for Medicare & Medicaid Services. (2016a). *Medicare claims processing manual* (Pub. 100-04: Ch. 5, Section 10.7). Retrieved September 30, 2021 from https://www.cms.gov/Regulations-and-Guidance/Guidance/Manuals/Downloads/clm104c05.pdf

Centers for Medicare & Medicaid Services. (2016b). *Medicare claims processing manual* (Pub. 100-04: Ch. 5, Section 20.2). Retrieved September 27, 2021 from https://www.cms.gov/Regulations-and-Guidance/Guidance/Manuals/Downloads/clm104c05.pdf

Centers for Medicare & Medicaid Services. (2018). *Medicare claims processing manual* (Pub. 100-04: Ch. 30, Section 70.2). Retrieved May 24, 2022 from https://www.cms.gov/Regulations-and-Guidance/Guidance/Manuals/Downloads/clm104c30.pdf

Centers for Medicare & Medicaid Services. (2019a). *Medicare benefit policy manual* (Pub. 100-02: Ch. 15, Section 220). Retrieved September 27, 2021 from https://www.cms.gov/Regulations-and-Guidance/Guidance/Manuals/Downloads/bp102c15.pdf

Centers for Medicare & Medicaid Services. (2019b). *Medicare benefit policy manual* (Pub. 100-02: Ch. 15, Section 220.2). Retrieved September 27, 2021 from https://www.cms.gov/Regulations-and-Guidance/Guidance/Manuals/Downloads/bp102c15.pdf

Centers for Medicare & Medicaid Services. (2019c). *Medicare benefit policy manual* (Pub. 100-02: Ch. 15, Section 220.3). Retrieved September 27, 2021 from https://www.cms.gov/Regulations-and-Guidance/Guidance/Manuals/Downloads/bp102c15.pdf

Centers for Medicare & Medicaid Services. (2019d). *Medicare claims processing manual* (Pub. 100-04: Ch. 5, Section 10.2). Retrieved September 30, 2021 from https://www.cms.gov/Regulations-and-Guidance/Guidance/Manuals/Downloads/clm104c05.pdf

Centers for Medicare & Medicaid Services. (2019e). *Medicare claims processing manual* (Pub. 100-04: Ch. 5, Section 10.3.3). Retrieved September 30, 2021 from https://www.cms.gov/Regulations-and-Guidance/Guidance/Manuals/downloads//clm104c05.pdf

Centers for Medicare & Medicaid Services. (2019f). Medicare Learning Network: Overview of the Patient Driven Groupings Model. Retrieved September 29, 2021 from   https://www.cms.gov/files/document/se19027.pdf

Centers for Medicare & Medicaid Services. (2020a). *Medicare benefit policy manual* (Pub. 100-02: Ch. 7, Section 40.2.1). Retrieved September 27, 2021 from https://www.cms.gov/Regulations-and-Guidance/Guidance/Manuals/Downloads/bp102c07.pdf

Centers for Medicare & Medicaid Services. (2020b). *Medicare claims processing manual* (Pub. 100-04: Ch. 3, Section 20). Retrieved September 28, 2021 from https://www.cms.gov/Regulations-and-Guidance/Guidance/Manuals/downloads//clm104c03.pdf

Centers for Medicare & Medicaid Services. (2021a). *Medicare benefit policy manual* (Pub. 100-02: Ch. 15, Section 110.1). Retrieved May 26, 2022 from https://www.cms.gov/Regulations-and-Guidance/Guidance/Manuals/Downloads/bp102c15.pdf

Centers for Medicare & Medicaid Services. (2021b). *Medicare claims processing manual* (Pub. 100-04: Ch. 10, Section 20). Retrieved September 29, 2021 from https://www.cms.gov/regulations-and-guidance/guidance/manuals/downloads/clm104c10.pdf

Centers for Medicare & Medicaid Services. (2021c). National Health Expenditures 2020 Highlights. Retrieved May 24, 2022 from https://www.cms.gov/files/document/highlights.pdf

Centers for Medicare & Medicaid Service. (2021d). Skilled nursing facility PPS. Retrieved September 29, 2021 from https://www.cms.gov/Medicare/Medicare-Fee-for-Service-Payment/SNFPPS

Centers for Medicare & Medicaid Services. (2021e). Therapy services. Retrieved September 30, 2021 from https://www.cms.gov/Medicare/Billing/TherapyServices

Centers for Medicare & Medicaid Services. (2021f). Therapy services: Functional reporting. Retrieved October 2, 2021 from https://www.cms.gov/Medicare/Billing/TherapyServices/Functional-Reporting

Centers for Medicare & Medicaid Services. (2021g). The role of therapy under the home health patient-driven groupings model (PDGM). Retrieved May 27, 2022 from https://www.cms.gov/files/document/se20005.pdf

Centers for Medicare & Medicaid Services. (2022a). Healthcare Common Procedure Coding System (HCPCS) Level II Coding Procedures. Retrieved May 24, 2022 from https://www.cms.gov/Medicare/Coding/MedHCPCSGenInfo/Downloads/2018-11-30-HCPCS-Level2-Coding-Procedure.pdf

Centers for Medicare & Medicaid Services. (2022b). What is a MAC. Retrieved May 24, 2022 from https://www.cms.gov/Medicare/Medicare-Contracting/Medicare-Administrative-Contractors/What-is-a-MAC

Chaplain, S. (2020). Rules are changing: The impending transition to ICD-11. American Academy of Professional Coders: Salt Lake City, UT. Retrieved September 29, 2021 from https://www.aapc.com/blog/51622-rules-are-changing-the-impending-transition-to-icd-11/

DeJong, G. (2016). Coming to terms with the IMPACT Act of 2014. *American Journal of Occupational Therapy, 70*(3), 7003090010p1-7003090010p6. doi: 10.5014/ajot.2016.703003

Fearon, H. M., & Levine, S. M. (2016). Payment policy and coding. In L. Quinn & J. Gordon (Eds.), *Documentation for rehabilitation: A guide to clinical decision making in physical therapy* (3rd ed., pp. 35-55). Elsevier.

Frolek Clark, G., & Holahan, L. (2015). Medicaid FAQ for school occupational therapy practitioners. *OT Practice, 20*(20), 18-20.

Gateley, C. A., & Borcherding, S. (2017). *Documentation manual for occupational therapy: Writing SOAP notes* (4th ed.). SLACK Incorporated.

HealthCare.gov. (n.d.). No health insurance? See if you'll owe a fee. Retrieved May 26, 2022 from https://www.healthcare.gov/glossary/fee/

Scott, R. W. (2013). *Legal, ethical, and practical aspects of patient care documentation: A guide for rehabilitation professionals* (4th ed.). Jones & Bartlett Learning.

U.S. Department of Education. (n.d.a). IDEA: Statute and regulations. Retrieved May 26, 2022 from https://sites.ed.gov/idea/statuteregulations/

U.S. Department of Health & Human Services. (2021). About the Affordable Care Act. Retrieved September 27, 2021 from https://www.hhs.gov/healthcare/about-the-aca/index.html

World Health Organization. (2021). International statistical classification of diseases and related health problems (ICD). Retrieved September 29, 2021 from https://www.who.int/classifications/classification-of-diseases

Chapter 4

Using Professional Terminology

Abbreviations and Symbols

Health care professionals are often pressed for time but are still obligated to complete documentation within established time frames. While the use of symbols and abbreviations can be timesavers, practitioners must use them very carefully and judiciously. Remember that your notes may be read by someone who knows little about occupational therapy and who will determine whether to pay for your services. In addition, other disciplines such as teachers and aides may not be familiar with specific medical jargon and may have difficulty interpreting what you have recorded. Remember that you are permitted to write out any word rather than shortening it or using a symbol. In this manual and in clinical practice, you will find that some settings or disciplines use more abbreviations and symbols than others. Many examples of common abbreviations and symbols used in health care are presented in Table 4-1 but this should not be considered an all-inclusive list. Also realize that some of these items could differ in composition or use from the abbreviations and symbols approved and used in a particular setting. However, for learning purposes, only the specific abbreviations and symbols contained in Table 4-1 will be utilized in the worksheets and documentation examples throughout this manual.

Use Only Approved Abbreviations and Ensure Accuracy

Your facility will be able to furnish a list of the abbreviations it allows so that the abbreviations and symbols you use will be validated if there is a question. **Do not make up your own abbreviations, and do not use any abbreviation that is not on your facility's approved list**. The Joint Commission, which accredits hospitals and other health care facilities, does not maintain an approved list of acceptable abbreviations and symbols for use in documentation, but it does specify and update an _Official "Do Not Use" List_ of those items that are prohibited (Joint Commission, 2022). This list can be referred to at the Joint Commission website (https://www.jointcommission.org). For example, the abbreviations QD (daily) and QOD (every other day) are prohibited because each can be easily mistaken as the other or confused with QID (four times a day; Institute for Safe Medication Practices [ISMP], 2021; Joint Commission, 2022).

Health professionals can also refer to the nonprofit ISMP website (https://www.ismp.org) for additional safety recommendations and a much larger list of abbreviations and symbols that are prone to error and miscommunication, pertaining primarily to medications and their use. ISMP advises that these listed items should not be used for medical communication such as written or verbal prescriptions, drug labels, or notations for medication management (ISMP, 2021). In addition, ISMP has compiled a lengthy list of "look-alike and sound-alike" drug names to increase awareness of those that may be confused easily with another medication, for example, close-sounding Darvon/Diovan/Dioval or Diazepam/Diltiazem (ISMP, 2019). It is also recommended that health professionals avoid using

Morreale, M. J. _The OTA's Guide to Documentation:_
Writing SOAP Notes, Fifth Edition (pp. 71-86).
© 2023 Taylor & Francis Group.

abbreviations for medication names and spell out the entire word instead (ISMP, 2021, Davis, 2020). For example, the use of "OXY" for Oxytocin could easily be mistaken as Oxycontin or Oxycodone (ISMP, 2019, 2021). Of course, health providers should always try to ensure accuracy when interviewing clients and documenting reported medication use and other data. Confirm or clarify information verbally rather than just guessing at items written down by clients on intake forms. Always use extreme care when typing or pointing and clicking on items in EMR check-off lists and drop-down menus to help prevent errors.

An Abbreviation Could Have Multiple Meanings

In order to maintain uniformity and clarity in the health record, each health care facility or agency establishes a list of approved abbreviations and symbols that may be used in documentation. An abbreviation may have more than one meaning so you must know which meaning is approved by your facility for the use of that abbreviation. Davis (2020) identifies some anatomical abbreviations that are especially problematic due to multiple meanings; these include the letter B (bladder, brain, or breast), letter H (hip or hand) and letter C (carotid, cerebral, or coronary) along with several others. Davis (2020) also presents a list of other abbreviations requiring caution due to ambiguity, for example, LL (can refer to lower lid, lip, or leg; left lung or leg) and ED (can indicate emotional disorder, eating disorder, erectile dysfunction, or elbow disarticulation). It is important to consider the context in which an abbreviation is used, such as for the following example:

Client needed HOH assist to hold the spoon and bring food to her mouth.

As *HOH* is an abbreviation for *hard of hearing* and *hand-over-hand*, the only phrase that would make sense for that specific statement is:

*Client needed **hand-over-hand** assist to hold the spoon and bring food to her mouth.*

As another example, consider this statement:

The student created fundraising flyers for the PTA.

The abbreviation PTA can represent several different meanings, such as *Parent Teacher Association, physical therapist assistant*, or *prior to admission*. Thus, the correct intention of the sentence could be ambiguous to the reader. Although "prior to admission" can obviously be disregarded in this instance, consider several possible scenarios that could be relevant to the other meanings of the abbreviation *PTA*: 1) Perhaps the school-related organization (PTA) is having a fundraiser (which is likely the intended meaning); or 2) the health practitioner (PTA) working at that school is in charge of a fundraising event and needs help creating flyers; or 3) a fundraising event might be planned to provide financial assistance to the physical therapist assistant (PTA) such as if that person's house burned down recently. Be cognizant of instances where a particular abbreviation may not be clearly understood by intended audiences and write out the word or phrase instead.

Abbreviations Are Case Sensitive

It is also important to note that abbreviations are case sensitive, so you must always write or enter them carefully to ensure accuracy of upper and lower-case letters. For example, *ADD* stands for "attention deficit disorder" yet *add* means "adduction." *PT* is "physical therapy" or "physical therapist" whereas *pt.* refers to "patient." Be especially careful with software programs that autocorrect. For example, the abbreviation *EHR* might incorrectly be converted to *HER*. For purposes of using this manual, the following list of abbreviations in Table 4-1 will be permitted. Realize that this list is not all inclusive and that there are entire books devoted to medical abbreviations. It is also possible that some of the abbreviations presented may not be on the approved list of a specific facility or agency. As an OTA, you will certainly encounter many other commonly used and acceptable abbreviations for anatomical structures that are not specifically delineated in this manual, such as for specific nerves, spinal segments, ligaments, and muscles (i.e., flexor carpi ulnaris [FCU] or ulnar collateral ligament [UCL]). Also, this manual cannot possibly include all the diagnoses and specialized medical or rehabilitation tests and terms that might be specific to a particular practice area or geographic region.

Use Relevant Terminology

As health care evolves, medical terms and abbreviations can become obsolete and be replaced by new terminology, as shown in the Chapter 2 examples of respectful language. Sames (2015) suggests that using buzzwords helps to demonstrate that one is up to date. In clinical practice it is likely you will notice trendy terms such as *evidence-informed-practice; interprofessional collaboration; diversity, equity, and inclusion; quality measures; sustainable outcomes; episode based-management*; and *value-based care*. Global health care trends include more collaboration between disciplines, a focus on functional outcomes, healthy communities, inclusiveness, and providing services that are proven to work with lasting effects (Sames, 2015).

The American Occupation Therapy Association reviews Official Documents at regular intervals to revise content and update professional language to make information more compatible with current legislation, payer requirements, global health care trends, values, and best practices. OTAs can keep current by joining professional associations, attaining continuing education, using a mentor, and reading up-to-date professional books and journals. Again, always check with your facility regarding acceptable terms and abbreviations appropriate for your work setting.

Table 4-1		
Abbreviations and Symbols		
Abbreviations		
Ⓐ assistance	ATNR asymmetrical tonic neck reflex	CMS Centers for Medicare & Medicaid Services
$\bar{a}$ before	Ⓑ bilateral	CNS central nervous system, clinical nurse specialist
AA Alcoholics Anonymous	BADLs basic activities of daily living	CO_2 carbon dioxide
AAROM active assisted range of motion	BE below elbow	C/O complains of
abd abduction	BK below knee	cont. continued; continue
add adduction	BKA below knee amputation	COPD chronic obstructive pulmonary disease
ADD attention deficit disorder	BM bowel movement	COPM Canadian Occupational Performance Measure
ADHD attention deficit hyperactivity disorder	BMI Body Mass Index	COTA Certified Occupational Therapy Assistant
ADLs activities of daily living	BP blood pressure	CP cerebral palsy
ad lib. as desired	BRP bathroom privileges	CPAP continuous positive airway pressure
AE above elbow	°C Celsius	CPM continuous passive motion
AFO ankle-foot orthosis	$\bar{c}$ with	CPR cardiopulmonary resuscitation
AIDS acquired immunodeficiency syndrome	C&S culture and sensitivity	CPT Current Procedural Terminology
AK above knee	CA carcinoma; cancer	CRPS complex regional pain syndrome
AKA above knee amputation	CABG coronary artery bypass graft	CSF cerebrospinal fluid
ALS amyotrophic lateral sclerosis	CAD coronary artery disease	CST craniosacral therapist
am, AM morning	CAT computerized axial tomography	CT computed tomography
AMA against medical advice; American Medical Association	CBC complete blood count	CTD cumulative trauma disorder
AMB ambulation	CCU coronary (cardiac) care unit	CTR carpal tunnel release
amt. amount	CGA contact guard assist	CTRS Certified Therapeutic Recreation Specialist
ant anterior	CHF congestive heart failure	CTS carpal tunnel syndrome
AP anterior-posterior	CHI closed head injury	
appt. appointment	CHT Certified Hand Therapist	
AROM active range of motion	CIMT Constraint Induced Movement Therapy	
ASAP as soon as possible	cm centimeter	
ASHD arteriosclerotic heart disease	CMC carpometacarpal	

(continued)

Table 4-1 (continued)
Abbreviations and Symbols

Abbreviations

CVA	cerebrovascular accident	F	Fair (muscle strength grade of 3)	HS	bedtime
CXR	chest x-ray			Ht	height
d	day	f	female	HTN	hypertension
Ⓓ	dependent	FBS	fasting blood sugar	HVPC	high volt pulsed current
D&C	dilation and curettage	FCE	functional capacity evaluation	Hx	history
DD	developmental disability			Ⓘ	independent
DIP	distal interphalangeal joint	FERPA	Family Educational Rights and Privacy Act	I&O	intake and output
DJD	degenerative joint disease	FIM™	Functional Independence Measure	IADLs	instrumental activities of daily living
DME	durable medical equipment	flex.	flexion	ICU	intensive care unit
		fl oz	fluid ounce	i.e.	that is
DMEPOS	durable medical equipment, prosthetics, orthotics, and supplies	FM	fine motor	IEP	Individualized Education Program
		ft.	foot; feet (the measurement, not the body part)	IFSP	Individualized Family Service Plan
DNR	do not resuscitate	F/U	follow-up	IM	intramuscular
D.O.	Doctor of Osteopathic Medicine	FUO	fever of unknown origin	in.	inches
		FWB	full weightbearing	int.	internal
DOA	date of admission; dead on arrival	Fx	fracture	IP	inpatient; interphalangeal
DOB	date of birth	G	Good (muscle strength grade of 4)	IR	internal rotation
DOE	dyspnea on exertion			IRF	inpatient rehabilitation facility
DPT	Doctor of Physical Therapy	GAD	generalized anxiety disorder		
Dr.	doctor	GI	gastrointestinal	IV	intravenous
DRG	diagnostic related group	gm	gram	KAFO	knee-ankle-foot orthosis
DRUJ	distal radioulnar joint	GSW	gunshot wound	kg	kilogram
DTR	deep tendon reflex	GYN	gynecology	Ⓛ	left
DVT	deep vein thrombosis	HA, H/A	headache	lb.	pound
Dx	diagnosis	H&P	history and physical	LBP	low back pain
ECG	electrocardiogram	HBV	hepatitis B virus	LD	learning disability; learning disorder
ECHO	echocardiogram	HEENT	head, eyes, ears, nose, throat	LE	lower extremity
ECT	electroconvulsive therapy			LGBT	lesbian, gay, bisexual, transgender
EEG	electroencephalogram	HEP	home exercise program		
EHR	electronic health record	HHA	home health agency	LLQ	left lower quadrant
EKG	electrocardiogram	HIPAA	Health Insurance Portability and Accountability Act	LOC	loss of consciousness; level of consciousness
EMG	electromyogram				
ENT	ear, nose, throat			LPN	Licensed Practical Nurse
EOB	edge of bed; explanation of benefits	HIB	harassment, intimidation, and bullying	LRTI	ligament reconstruction tendinous interposition
		HIV	human immunodeficiency virus	LTC	long-term care
ER	external rotation; emergency room			LTG	long-term goal
		HOB	head of bed	LUQ	left upper quadrant
e-stim	electrical stimulation	HOH	hand-over-hand; hard of hearing	LVAD	left ventricular assist device
etc.	etcetera				
ETOH	ethyl alcohol	HP	hot pack		
eval.	evaluation	hr.	hour	m	murmur; meter; male
exam	examination	HR	heart rate	max	maximum
ext.	extension	HRT	hormone replacement therapy	MCP, MP	metacarpophalangeal
°F	Fahrenheit				

(continued)

Table 4-1 (continued)
Abbreviations and Symbols

Abbreviations

MD	muscular dystrophy; medical doctor	NS	no show; not seen	PHI	protected health information
MDS	Minimum Data Set	NSAID	non-steroidal anti-inflammatory drug	PHR	personal health record
meds.	medications	NSR	normal sinus rhythm	PIP	proximal interphalangeal
MET	basal metabolic equivalent	OCD	obsessive-compulsive disorder	PLOF	prior level of function
mg	milligram	OOB	out of bed	pm, PM	afternoon
MHz	megahertz	OP	outpatient	PMH	past medical history
MI	myocardial infarction	OR	operating room	PNF	proprioceptive neuro-muscular facilitation
min	minutes; minimum	ORIF	open reduction, internal fixation	PNI	peripheral nerve injury
ml	milliliter	OT	occupational therapist; occupational therapy	PNS	peripheral nervous system
mm	millimeter				
MMT	manual muscle test	OTA	occupational therapy assistant	POC	plan of care
mo.	month	OTAS	occupational therapy assistant student	POMR	problem-oriented medical record
mod	moderate				
MRI	magnetic resonance imaging	OTC	over the counter	pos.	positive
		OTD	Doctor of Occupational Therapy	post op	postoperative
MS	multiple sclerosis			PPS	Prospective Payment System
MSW	Master of Social Work	OTR	Registered Occupational Therapist		
MVA	motor vehicle accident			PRE	progressive resistive exercise
N	Normal (muscle strength grade of 5)	OX4	oriented to time, place, person, situation	pre op	preoperative
NA	not applicable; not available	oz	ounce	PRN	as needed
		$\bar{p}$	after	pro	pronation
N/A	not applicable	P	plan; posterior; pulse; Poor (muscle strength grade of 2)	PROM	passive range of motion
NAD	no acute distress			pt.	patient
NBQC	narrow base quad cane			PT	physical therapist; physical therapy
NDT	neurodevelopmental treatment	PA	posterior-anterior; physician's assistant	P/T	part time
neg.	negative			PTA	physical therapist assis-tant; prior to admission
NG	nasogastric	PAM	physical agent modality		
NICU	neonatal intensive care unit	PDD	pervasive developmental disorder	PTSD	post-traumatic stress disorder
NKA	no known allergy	PDPM	patient-driven payment model	PWB	partial weightbearing
NKDA	no known drug allergy			qt.	quart
NMES	neuromuscular electrical stimulation	PE	physical examination	Ⓡ	right
		PEG	percutaneous endoscopic gastrostomy	R	respiration
NOS	not otherwise specified			RA	rheumatoid arthritis
NP	nurse practitioner	per	by	RBC	red blood cell count
NPO	nothing by mouth	peri.	perineal	re:	regarding
NPP	nonphysician practitioner; notice of privacy practices	PET	positron emission tomography	rehab	rehabilitation

(continued)

Table 4-1 (continued)
Abbreviations and Symbols

Abbreviations

reps	repetitions	SOAP	subjective, objective, assessment, plan	TTWB	toe-touch weightbearing
resp	respiratory; respiration	SOB	shortness of breath	tx	treatment; traction
RICE	rest, ice, compression, elevation	S/P	status post	UA	urinalysis
RLQ	right lower quadrant	SSN	Social Security number	UE	upper extremity
RN	Registered Nurse	STAT	immediately	UMN	upper motor neuron
R/O	rule out	STD	sexually transmitted disease	URI	upper respiratory infection
ROM	range of motion			US	ultrasound
ROS	review of symptoms	STG	short-term goal	UTI	urinary tract infection
RTC	return to clinic	STM	short-term memory	VAD	ventricular assist device
RTO	return to office	sup	supination	VC	vital capacity
RUGS	Resource Utilization Groups	suppos	suppository	VD	venereal disease
RUQ	right upper quadrant	T	temperature; Trace (muscle strength grade of 1)	v.o.	verbal orders
RSD	reflex sympathetic dystrophy			vol.	volume
		TAM	total active motion	VS	vital signs
Rx	prescription	TB	tuberculosis	W	watt
Ⓢ	supervision	TBI	traumatic brain injury	W/cm²	watt per centimeter squared
s̄	without	TEDS	thromboembolic disease stockings	WBAT	weightbearing as tolerated
S	subjective				
SBA	stand-by assistance	TENS	transcutaneous electrical nerve stimulation	WBC	white blood cell; white blood count
SCI	spinal cord injury				
SH	social history	TFCC	triangular fibrocartilage complex	WBQC	wide base quad cane
SI	sensory integration			w/c	wheelchair
SIDS	sudden infant death syndrome	ther ex	therapeutic exercise	WDWN	well developed, well nourished
		THR	total hip replacement		
Sig:	instruction to patient	TIA	transient ischemic attack	wk	week
SLE	systemic lupus erythematosus	TKR	total knee replacement	WFL	within functional limits
		TM(J)	temporomandibular (joint)	WNL	within normal limits
SLP	speech-language pathologist; speech-language pathology			wt	weight
		t.o.	telephone order	x, X	times
		TOS	thoracic outlet syndrome	y.o.	year old
SNF	skilled nursing facility	TPM	total passive motion	yr	year
SOC	start of care	TPR	temperature, pulse, and respiration		

Symbols

1°	primary	↓	down; downward; decrease	–	minus; negative (also abbreviated neg.)
2°	secondary; secondary to	↑	up; upward; increase		
Δ	change	↔	to and from	#	number (#1); pounds
x1, x2	of 1 person; of 2 people *Example*: "transferred to toilet c̄ min Ⓐ x2"	→	to; progressing forward; approaching	%	percent
				&	and
		~	approximately	°	degree
♀	female	@	at	"	inches
♂	male	=	equals	'	feet
>	greater than	+	plus; positive (also abbreviated pos.)	/	per
<	less than				

Client Instructions and Home Programs

OTs and OTAs provide specialized instruction and home programs to teach clients, their support persons (e.g., parents, family/significant others, caregivers), and/or other disciplines (e.g., teachers, nurses) methods to promote the client's health, function, occupational participation, safety, and enhance/maintain gains made in therapy. Education and training can include instruction in home exercise programs (e.g., strength, ROM, coordination); safe protocols for transfers, functional mobility, or feeding; suggestions for proper positioning in wheelchair or bed; energy conservation or joint protection techniques; recommendations for the classroom; instructions for adaptive equipment, assistive technology, or orthotic device use/care; strategies to improve behavior, sensory processing, or coping mechanisms; and so forth.

OTs and OTAs should individualize home programs and instructions for each client and ensure the directions are easily understandable, keeping in mind the learner's primary language, level of education, and health literacy. Instructions and home programs can include pictures, diagrams, or other visual representations to make the information easier to remember and understand. Use professional judgment to avoid the use of terms and abbreviations that may be intimidating or not understandable to the learner. Box 4-1 lists several examples of professional jargon converted to lay terminology.

Box 4-1 EXAMPLES OF LAY TERMINOLOGY FOR HOME PROGRAMS	
Rather Than Writing …	*You Might Write …*
Flex shoulder 10X. Extend elbow to max 10X.	Lift your arm overhead and bring it back down by your side 10 times. Bend your elbow (touching palm to shoulder) then straighten elbow as much as you can in front of you with forearm facing up 10 times.
Pronate and supinate forearm 10X with elbow add/flexed 90°.	While keeping elbow at your side and bent at a right angle, turn your palm all the way facing up and then turn palm facing back down. Do 10 repetitions.
Provide verbal cues to minimize Mason's kyphotic posture when seated at his desk.	Give Mason verbal reminders not to slouch/slide forward while he is seated at his desk.
Bed ↔ w/c provide Sam with SBA and verbal cues for center of gravity before rising.	When transferring Sam from the bed to wheelchair and back, stand next to him for safety and remind him to lean forward ("nose over toes") before standing up.
Encourage Marisa to use a dynamic tripod grasp for graphomotor activities rather than gross movements of her UE.	When Marisa is writing, remind her to hold the pencil with the tips of her thumb, index, and long fingers. Encourage her to use small movements of those fingers to write instead of moving her entire arm.
During supervised play, position Kaylee Ⓛ sidelying and facilitate bimanual activities. Provide HOH assist PRN.	During supervised play, place Kaylee on her left side and encourage her to use both hands together to hold and manipulate toys. Gently use your hands to help position Kaylee's hands as needed.

Instructions and home programs should also specify relevant precautions/contraindications along with the health provider's name and contact information. Provide a hard copy or digital version of the written instructions or program to the persons being taught and keep a copy in the client's medical chart (Fairchild et al., 2018). Complete Learning Activity 4-1 to practice converting instructions into more easily understood language. Refer to Chapter 8 to learn more about the necessity of documenting client or family/significant others' understanding of instructions/home program, identifying barriers to their learning and any follow-up that may be needed.

LEARNING ACTIVITY 4-1: LAY TERMINOLOGY

Convert the following home program instructions into terminology that clients/caregivers can more easily understand.

1. Left shoulder 2X daily: protraction/retraction (slide towel on tabletop) 10X, abduct shoulder 10X while standing then IR/ER 5X with shoulder add. Do Ⓑ flex. 10X with cane.

2. During supervised play, position Ben prone on elbows and weight shift to left by having him ext Ⓡ UE for toys. Facilitate three-jaw chuck (i.e., pegs, shape sorter) with tactile cues.

3. When Dorothy is in w/c, provide verbal cues and min Ⓐ to minimize posterior pelvic tilt and kyphotic posture. If asymmetrical, provide lateral support with pillow PRN for midline orientation. Elevate RUE on arm trough to ↓ edema.

4. Logan's mealtimes: Supported sitting, no trunk rotation, feet flat. Have Logan use built-up utensils and provide HOH assist for wrist ext and cylindrical grasp to pick up food and maintain on utensil. Encourage active elbow flex. food → mouth.

Worksheet 4-1
Using Abbreviations

Translate each sentence written with abbreviations into full English phrases or sentences.

1. Pt. Ⓘ ADLs.

2. Client reports ↓ pain Ⓡ shoulder p̄ HP.

3. Resident w/c ↔ EOB with SBA.

4. Client c/o pain in Ⓡ index MCP joint p̄ ~ 2 min PROM.

5. Client w/c → mat c̄ sliding board max Ⓐ x2.

6. Pt. O x 4.

7. Client has SOB p̄ 30 reps of UE PRE.

8. Pt. has ↓ STM and OCD which limit IADLs.

9. Pt. min Ⓐ AMB bed → toilet 2° ↓ balance.

10. Child's FM WFL to don AFO Ⓘ.

Morreale, M. J. (2023). *The OTA's guide to documentation: Writing SOAP notes* (5th ed.). SLACK Incorporated.

Worksheet 4-2
Using Abbreviations—Additional Practice

Shorten these statements using only the standard abbreviations in this chapter.

1. Client requires minimal assistance to stand and pull up clothing with partial weight-bearing status of right lower extremity.

2. Patient is able to feed herself independently with the use of built-up utensils.

3. Client has intact sensation in both upper extremities but reports minimal pain.

4. Client has fifty-five degrees of passive range of motion in the left index distal interphalangeal joint, which is within functional limits.

5. While sitting on edge of bed, client is able to put on her socks with standby assistance, but requires moderate assistance with putting on and taking off left shoe.

6. Student is independent in wheelchair mobility and activities of daily living.

7. Patient requires moderate assistance of two people to transfer from wheelchair to toilet and from toilet to wheelchair.

8. Patient's toe-touch weight-bearing status limits her performance of instrumental activities of daily living.

9. Constraint induced movement therapy protocol was initiated to improve function of weak left upper extremity for activities of daily living.

10. Client was lying on her back with head of bed raised. Client was able to correctly state her own name, the name of facility, and today's date. Neuromuscular electrical nerve stimulation was applied for 10 minutes to right glenohumeral joint to help minimize subluxation.

Worksheet 4-3
Deciphering Doctors' Orders and Abbreviations

Translate the following abbreviations into full English phrases or sentences.

1. Dx s/p Ⓡ TKR 2° OA, WBAT
    OT 2x/wk for BADLs, IADLs

2. X-ray + Ⓛ index finger MCP Fx 2° GSW

3. 5 y.o. child has pain 2° bone CA Ⓛ LE

4. Dx Ⓡ DRUJ Fx c̄ ORIF
    OT 3x/wk for PAMs PRN, P/AROM, ADLs, CPM

5. 1° Dx PTSD, 2° Dx HTN

6. 1° Dx DJD Ⓡ hip, 2° Dx COPD & CHF

7. Dx CAD, TIA, PEG

8. Dx Ⓡ BKA, CABG, HBV

9. s/p Ⓛ TKR, PWB, OOB c̄ walker

10. Dx: C6 SCI, HTN, UTI
    OT: eval for w/c and DME

Morreale, M. J. (2023). *The OTA's guide to documentation: Writing SOAP notes* (5th ed.). SLACK Incorporated.

Worksheet 4-4
Deciphering Abbreviations—More Practice

Translate the following abbreviations into full English phrases or sentences.

1. The infant remained in the NICU for 2 wks 2° to low birth wt of 2100 gm.

2. The resident reported LBP. He needed mod Ⓐ to don Ⓡ KAFO and CGA to transfer safely EOB → w/c using WBQC and FWB Ⓡ LE.

3. To ↓ pain and edema Ⓛ elbow, client was instructed in RICE.

4. Client needs DME recommendations and ADL instruction following LVAD.

5. This yr the OT and PT were part of the school district committee that developed new policies and procedures regarding HIB and IEPs.

6. Dx: PDD-NOS, ADHD
   OT: ADLs, SI, FM
   2 x/wk X 12 wks

7. EMG pos. Ⓡ CTS and neg. TOS

8. Dx: s/p Ⓛ THR, pt. NWB Ⓛ LE
   OT eval. and tx; ADLs, Ⓑ UE PREs
   3x/wk X 4 wks

9. MRI + TBI, VS stable, BRP c̄ assist

10. CXR neg. TB but pos. URI. Pt. has DOE and FUO.

Morreale, M. J. (2023). *The OTA's guide to documentation: Writing SOAP notes* (5th ed.). SLACK Incorporated.

Worksheet 4-5
Additional Practice

Shorten these notes using only the standard abbreviations in this chapter.

1. The patient participated in occupational therapy session bedside for instruction in activities of daily living. She was lying on her back and was able to go from a supine position to a sitting position on the edge of the bed with minimum assistance. She needed maximum assistance to put on her lower body garments over her feet. She went from a sitting position to a standing position with moderate assistance to pull up lower body clothing. Moderate assistance was needed for the client to be able to put on upper body garments.

2. The resident came to the occupational therapy clinic via wheelchair escort. The resident was observed to lean to his left while sitting in his wheelchair. The resident needed verbal cues and minimum assistance in positioning his body in the wheelchair to maintain midline orientation and symmetrical posture. The resident transferred from his wheelchair to the toilet with moderate assistance of one person to help him keep his balance using a standing pivot transfer. He needed verbal cues and visual feedback from a mirror to maintain upright posture.

3. The patient was seen in the occupational therapy clinic for treatment of his left distal radioulnar joint fracture. Patient is now 10 weeks status-post wrist fracture. Patient also has an upper respiratory infection. He was seen for assessment of selected, relevant client factors for a total of 40 minutes. His left upper extremity shoulder flexion was a grade of 4 out of 5, shoulder extension was a grade of 4 out of 5, elbow flexion was a grade of 4 out of 5, elbow extension was a grade of 4 out of 5, wrist extension was a grade of 3 minus out of 5, wrist flexion was a grade of 3 minus out of 5, and grip strength was 8 pounds. The patient's left upper extremity light touch is intact. The patient's right upper extremity muscle strength and sensation are noted to be within functional limits.

4. The occupational therapy evaluation for the 65-year-old female client with multiple sclerosis and low vision included assessments such as the Canadian Occupational Performance Measure, visual acuity, visual perception, range of motion, and manual muscle test. When asked about past medical history, the client reported she was diagnosed with sleep apnea approximately 18 months ago and uses a continuous positive airway pressure machine nightly. She also reported a 5-year history of hypertension.

5. The 10-year-old student is a boy who is in the fourth grade. He is diagnosed with attention deficit hyperactivity disorder because he has poor attention and exhibits hyperactivity at times. A long-term goal written in the student's Individualized Education Program is for him to be able to maintain sitting at his desk for 30 minutes without getting out of his seat during class and without the teacher having to remind him to stay in his seat. Another long-term goal in this student's Individualized Education Program is for him to be able to finish his project in art class during the time allotted without the art teacher having to redirect him to the task.

Morreale, M. J. (2023). *The OTA's guide to documentation: Writing SOAP notes* (5th ed.). SLACK Incorporated.

Worksheet 4-6
Generating Abbreviations

Using the list of abbreviations in this chapter, list appropriate abbreviations for the following categories:

Lower extremity weight-bearing status

1.

2.

3.

4.

5.

Different types of range of motion

1.

2.

3.

4.

5.

Physical agent modalities

1.

2.

3.

4.

5.

Morreale, M. J. (2023). *The OTA's guide to documentation: Writing SOAP notes* (5th ed.). SLACK Incorporated.

References

Davis, N. M. (2020). Medical abbreviations that have contradictory or ambiguous meanings. Institute for Safe Medication Practices. Retrieved June 13, 2022 from https://www.ismp.org/resources/medical-abbreviations-have-contradictory-or-ambiguous-meanings

Fairchild, S. L., O'Shea, R. K., & Washington, R. D. (2018). *Pierson and Fairchild's principles & techniques of patient care* (6th ed.). Elsevier.

Institute for Safe Medication Practices. (2019). List of confused drug names. Author. Retrieved October 11, 2021 from https://www.ismp.org/recommendations/confused-drug-names-list

Institute for Safe Medication Practices. (2021). List of error-prone abbreviations. Author. Retrieved October 11, 2021 from https://www.ismp.org/recommendations/error-prone-abbreviations-list

Joint Commission. (2022). Official "do not use" list. Author. Retrieved May 26, 2022 from https://www.jointcommission.org/resources/news-and-multimedia/fact-sheets/facts-about-do-not-use-list/

Sames, K. M. (2015). *Documenting occupational therapy practice.* (3rd ed.). Pearson Education, Inc.

Chapter 5

Avoiding Common Documentation Mistakes

Throughout your career as an OTA, you will encounter many opportunities to use your professional documentation skills. Of course, one essential responsibility of the OTA is to enter information in the health or education record. In addition, OTAs provide clients with individualized written instructions for home exercise programs, occupational adaptations, safety techniques, adaptive equipment use, or other recommendations in collaboration with the OT. Other documentation tasks might include writing notes and memos to colleagues and staff. You may even be involved with composing letters, reports, or marketing materials to send to insurance companies, school administrators, or other health care professionals.

Your written and verbal communication is a reflection of you, the occupational therapy practitioner. It also reflects on your department and the profession of occupational therapy as a whole. Think about what someone will infer about you from documentation that has numerous cross-outs/corrections, incomplete information, or errors in spelling and grammar (Sames, 2015). Perhaps your colleagues or clients will question your credibility, competence, or even your intelligence. They may regard your work as sloppy and unprofessional, which could result in less respect for you. In a litigation situation, an attorney might even accuse you of being careless or providing inferior care (Sames, 2015). However, well-written documentation that is grammatically correct, well organized, accurate, and neat demonstrates professionalism and pride in your work.

A careless error in just one letter or word can change the meaning of a sentence or make it sound silly, such as, *"Client requires increased time to transfer into the commode"* or *"The client reported hypersensitivity when his scar was palpitated."* Of course, the correct version of these two sentences should be, *"Client requires increased time to transfer **onto** the commode"* or *"The client reported hypersensitivity when his scar was **palpated.**"* Make use of readily available resources such as a dictionary, thesaurus, software program, or smartphone app to assist you with spelling and grammar as needed. Also, take the necessary time to write carefully and proofread your work. Rushing to complete documentation too quickly may result in substandard work and inaccuracies in copying or recording information. This could possibly lead to serious consequences for you or the client. Errors can be made very easily by clicking on the wrong item in a drop-down menu, hitting the wrong key on a keyboard, or inadvertently tapping the wrong place on a touch screen. Also, be vigilant when using electronic devices that correct spelling automatically as you are composing notes, emails, or text messages. The auto-correction feature could very easily substitute unintended and erroneous words or information. Thus, it is always prudent to double-check your work.

Morreale, M. J. *The OTA's Guide to Documentation: Writing SOAP Notes, Fifth Edition* (pp. 87-98).
© 2023 Taylor & Francis Group.

Quoting and Paraphrasing

There are several ways to document what your client or another person has said. It is important to objectively and accurately convey that person's intent as it relates to the client's situation. Do not embellish the information or guess at what the person might be thinking or feeling. You can quote or state what the person said exactly word for word, or you can paraphrase or summarize it. Direct quotes are preferable in many instances because they depict the client's actual reporting of pain level, emotional components or concerns, carryover of home programs, understanding of instructions/precautions, perception of how the individual is progressing in therapy, etc. When quoting someone exactly, the person's specific words are used between a set of quotation marks. Remember that the punctuation to end the sentence stays within the quotation marks. If you are referring to the client's statement in the first person (I), the use of the word "I" should be within the quotation marks. For example, to use a first person quote, you might write:

The client stated, "I will never be able to go back to work."

Use clinical reasoning to determine the extent of a quotation for a particular client. Consider what is clear and meaningful to enter into the health record and pertinent to the client's situation.

The client stated, "I will never be able to go back to work. My job is very stressful."

If you, the OTA, are referring to the client in the third person (he, she), that pronoun will be outside of the quotation marks and you will just quote the exact words said. For example:

The client stated that he "will never be able to go back to work."

You can also use a combination of quotes and paraphrasing to effectively summarize and document the client's communication. For example:

The client stated that he "will never be able to go back to work" because he considers his job too stressful.

Sometimes, you might just want to quote or emphasize a significant word or phrase. For example:

The client stated that he "will never" be able to return to his job.

The client expressed that he will not be able to resume his "very stressful" job.

If you are just paraphrasing or summarizing what another person said, you do not have to use quotation marks. Here are some examples of paraphrasing:

- *The client expressed doubts about returning to work.*
- *The client stated he was uncertain about his ability to return to work.*
- *The client stated that his job was too stressful for him to return to work.*

Also, remember that an indirect question does not require a question mark. Here are some examples:

- *The client asked if he would ever be able to return to work.*
- *The client inquired about returning to work.*
- *The client asked about coping strategies to enable return to work.*

LEARNING ACTIVITY 5-1: QUOTING AND PARAPHRASING

Ask a partner a question about leisure interests. Document your partner's response by using a quote. Then rewrite your sentence by paraphrasing what your partner said. Which of the two statements would you choose for a "real" intervention note?

Ask a partner a question about how that person's day is going. Document your partner's response by using a quote. Then rewrite your sentence by paraphrasing what your partner said. Which of the two statements would you choose for a "real" intervention note?

Ask a partner a question about a desired personal or professional goal to attain within a year from now. Document your partner's response by using a quote. Then rewrite your sentence by paraphrasing what your partner said. Which of the two statements would you choose for a "real" intervention note?

The following examples of quoting and paraphrasing demonstrate common documentation errors and how information can be recorded in different ways. Pay close attention to punctuation.

- Correct:
  - *Patient stated, "I didn't sleep well last night."*
  - *Patient stated that he "didn't sleep well last night."*
  - *Patient stated that last night he did not sleep well.*
  - *Patient stated that he slept poorly last night.*
- Incorrect:
  - *Patient stated, "he didn't sleep well last night."*
  - *Patient stated, he "didn't sleep well last night".*
  - *Patient stated, I "didn't sleep well" last night.*
  - *Patient stated "he slept poorly last night."*
- Correct:
  - *Mary stated she has "an ache" in her right hip.*
  - *Mary stated, "I have an ache in my right hip."*
  - *Mary stated she has discomfort in her right hip, which she describes as an ache.*
  - *Mary stated that her right hip aches.*
- Incorrect:
  - *Mary stated, "I have an ache in her right hip."*
  - *Mary stated, I have "an ache" in my right hip.*
  - *Mary stated "her right hip aches."*
  - *Mary stated "she has an ache in her right hip."*
- Correct:
  - *The client asked, "Will I be able to walk soon?"*
  - *The client inquired if she would soon be able to ambulate.*
  - *The client asked if she would "be able to walk soon."*
  - *The client asked when she would be able to walk again.*
- Incorrect:
  - *The client asked "if she would be able to walk soon."*
  - *The client asked if she would "be able to walk soon?"*
  - *The client asked, Will I be able to walk soon?*
  - *The client asked when will I walk again?*

Worksheet 5-1
Quoting and Paraphrasing

Identify which of the following statements are correct (C) or incorrect (I). Pay close attention to punctuation.

1.   ___ The child stated that she was extremely hungry.
2.   ___ The child stated that "she was starving."
3.   ___ The child "stated I am starving."
4.   ___ The child verbalized that she was "starving."
5.   ___ The child stated "I am starving".
6.   ___ The patient asked how to put her orthosis on?
7.   ___ The patient asked "How do I put my orthosis on"?
8.   ___ The patient asked about the proper way to put on her orthosis.
9.   ___ The patient asked, "How do I put my orthosis on?"
10. ___ The patient asked "how to put her orthosis on."
11. ___ The client requested a new buttonhook.
12. ___ The client asked if "she could have a new buttonhook."
13. ___ The client asked, "Can I have a new buttonhook"?
14. ___ The client asked for a new buttonhook.
15. ___ The client asked, "Can I have a new buttonhook?"
16. ___ The client stated "he felt dizzy" as he stood at the kitchen counter.
17. ___ The client reported feeling "dizzy" while standing at the kitchen counter.
18. ___ While standing at the kitchen counter, the client stated "he felt dizzy."
19. ___ The client, while standing at the kitchen counter, stated I feel "dizzy."
20. ___ The client reported dizziness while standing at the kitchen counter.

© 2023 Taylor & Francis Group.
Morreale, M. J. (2023). *The OTA's guide to documentation: Writing SOAP notes* (5th ed.). SLACK Incorporated.

Worksheet 5-2
Spelling

Some common words used in occupational therapy documentation are often misspelled. For each of the word pairs below, place a check mark next to the word or phrase that is spelled correctly.

1. ____ defered   ____ deferred
2. ____ definately   ____ definitely
3. ____ dining   ____ dinning
4. ____ excercise   ____ exercise
5. ____ parraffin   ____ paraffin
6. ____ transfering   ____ transferring
7. ____ recieve   ____ receive
8. ____ pnumonia   ____ pneumonia
9. ____ rotator cup   ____ rotator cuff
10. ____ tolorate   ____ tolerate
11. ____ therapy puddy   ____ therapy putty
12. ____ independent   ____ independant
13. ____ tremors   ____ tremers
14. ____ phlegm   ____ phlem
15. ____ diaphram   ____ diaphragm
16. ____ urinary track   ____ urinary tract
17. ____ anasthesia   ____ anesthesia
18. ____ brachial plexus   ____ brachial plexis
19. ____ incontinence   ____ incontinents
20. ____ illiac crest   ____ iliac crest
21. ____ oculomotor   ____ occulomotor
22. ____ vitiligo   ____ vitilago
23. ____ diaphorretic   ____ diaphoretic
24. ____ boutonniere deformity   ____ boutinniere deformity
25. ____ homonymous hemianopsia   ____ homonomous hemianopsia

Morreale, M. J. (2023). *The OTA's guide to documentation: Writing SOAP notes* (5th ed.). SLACK Incorporated.

Worksheet 5-3
Spelling—More Practice

For each of the word pairs below, place a check mark next to the word that is spelled correctly.

1. _____ counseling   _____ counselling
2. _____ diarrhea   _____ diarrea
3. _____ hemhorrage   _____ hemorrhage
4. _____ benefit   _____ benifit
5. _____ interfered   _____ interferred
6. _____ eyesite   _____ eyesight
7. _____ pullies   _____ pulleys
8. _____ extention   _____ extension
9. _____ hygeine   _____ hygiene
10. _____ preparation   _____ preperation
11. _____ therapeutic   _____ theraputic
12. _____ flexability   _____ flexibility
13. _____ strength   _____ strenth
14. _____ assymetrical   _____ asymmetrical
15. _____ toilet   _____ toliet
16. _____ leisure   _____ liesure
17. _____ nauseous   _____ nauseus
18. _____ eccymosis   _____ ecchymosis
19. _____ paresthesia   _____ parasthesia
20. _____ pulse oximeter   _____ pulse oxymeter
21. _____ glycometer   _____ glucometer
22. _____ bollis   _____ bolus
23. _____ jejunostomy   _____ jujenostomy
24. _____ sphygmomanometer   _____ sphygnomanometer
25. _____ electromyelogram   _____ electromyogram

Worksheet 5-4
Using Words Correctly

Students often misuse certain words that sound similar. Complete the following sentences by choosing the correct word from the two choices provided in parentheses.

1. The home health _____ gave the patient a shower. (aid or aide)

2. The client refused to _____ the doctor's diagnosis. (accept or except)

3. The traumatic brain injury will have a tremendous _____ on activities of daily living. (affect or effect)

4. If the client falls, she probably will _____ her hip due to osteoporosis. (brake or break)

5. The patient became short of _____ after ambulating to the bathroom. (breath or breathe)

6. The client stated she wanted to _____ 10 pounds. (lose or loose)

7. The patient injured her _____ right hand, which prevented her from writing. (dominant or dominate)

8. The occupational therapy room is _____ down the hallway than the physical therapy room. (farther or further)

9. The _____ caseload consists of 10 clients, as compared to 15 clients last week. (currant or current)

10. The OT asked the patient to _____ the scissors down on the table. (lay or lie)

11. The weight of the pan was more _____ the patient could manage. (than or then)

12. The clients in the craft group put _____ projects away in the closet. (their or there)

13. The child was able to remain quiet and _____ while standing in line. (stationary or stationery)

14. The _____ of the school attended the IEP meeting. (principal or principle)

15. The resident regained _____ of bowel and bladder. (continents or continence)

Morreale, M. J. (2023). *The OTA's guide to documentation: Writing SOAP notes* (5th ed.). SLACK Incorporated.

Worksheet 5-5
Using Words Correctly—More Practice

Choose the correct word from the two choices provided in parentheses.

1. The client has difficulty _____ the steering wheel. (griping or gripping)
2. The client was able to navigate his wheelchair throughout the store's _____ without knocking anything over. (isles or aisles)
3. The patient refused to take _____ responsibility for his actions. (personal or personnel)
4. The patient reported pain when his biceps muscle was _____ by the OTA. (palpitated or palpated)
5. The client was able to _____ all bathing tasks without assistance. (perform or preform)
6. The child asked for a _____ of candy. (peace or piece)
7. The client had difficulty swallowing liquids due to _____. (dysphagia or dysphasia)
8. The student was denied _____ to the client's medical record. (excess or access)
9. The client followed the OTA's _____ and purchased a shower chair. (advice or advise)
10. A buttonhook can be a useful assistive _____ for clients with impaired dexterity. (device or devise)
11. The student was _____ at playing the violin. (adapt or adept)
12. The client developed a lung infection due to _____ of food. (aspiration or inspiration)
13. The resident was very _____ during transfers as she would not wait for the wheelchair to be properly positioned and locked before trying to stand up. (compulsive or impulsive)
14. The occupational therapy assistant handed the client a(n) _____ basin because the client was nauseous. (nemesis or emesis)
15. The child's _____ was unsafe due to the presence of lead. (residents or residence)

Morreale, M. J. (2023). *The OTA's guide to documentation: Writing SOAP notes* (5th ed.). SLACK Incorporated.

Capitals

When in doubt regarding the use of capitals, always refer to a style guide, medical/college dictionary, or spell-checking app. Some of the more commonly confused situations regarding capitals are listed in the following chart and, according to American Psychological Association (APA) Style (2020, 2022) and *Merriam-Webster's Guide to Punctuation and Style* (Merriam-Webster, 2001), the following rules pertain:

Capitalized	Example	Not Capitalized	Example
Proper names in medical terminology	Parkinson disease, Babinski sign, Heimlich maneuver	Common nouns in medical terminology	measles, virus, flu, hysterectomy, biceps
Trade names of products and medications	Pampers diapers, Jobst glove, Advil, Velcro, Theraband	Generic drugs and products	disposable diapers, compression glove, ibuprofen, hook and loop fastener, resistance band
Specific organizations	American Occupational Therapy Association, Rotary Club	Generic organizations	study group, a book club, craft group
Academic degrees and professional designations after the person's name	Hans Handfixer, OTR/L, Lilly Lifesaver, RN	General degrees or generic professional designations	an associate's degree, an occupational therapist, an emergency room nurse
Exact test titles	Canadian Occupational Performance Measure	Generic tests	range of motion assessment, a cognitive evaluation, a short-term memory test
Specific department proper names	Healthy Hospital Occupational Therapy Department	Generic department names	an occupational therapy department, rehab department, rehab facility
Official titles as part of a name	Dr. Jones, Reverend Smith, Professor Jenkins	Generic or descriptive titles	the doctor's office, an orthopedic surgeon, the priest, a college professor

Verb Tenses

Choose and use one verb tense within a paragraph. Consider the following paragraph which is *not* well written:
*The OTA **has helped** Joe's fine motor skills; the PT **helped** Joe's balance. The special educator **had worked** with Joe so he could learn the school routine. The classroom aide **works** very closely with him every day.*

The above paragraph uses four different verb tenses: present perfect, past, past perfect, and present. Instead, it is better to choose and use only one verb tense.

The OTA has helped Joe's fine motor skills; the PT has helped Joe's balance. The special educator has worked with Joe so he could learn the school routine. The classroom aide has worked very closely with him every day.

Pronouns

Use the pronoun for the gender that the individual identifies as or use gender neutral language instead. Be careful to make the pronoun reference clear in a sentence. If you say, *"Jane and Mary agree that her skills are improving,"* it is not clear if the "her" refers to Jane or Mary. It is better to say, *"Jane and Mary agree that Mary's skills are improving."* Another incorrect example is *"The OT's student put his goniometer in his lab coat pocket,"* as it is not clear whose goniometer or whose pocket is being referred to. It would be better to say, *"The OT student put the OT's goniometer in the OT's lab coat pocket."*

Worksheet 5-6
Capitals

Underline the words that do not correctly follow the rules for capitals.

1. The OTA put the chart on the Occupational Therapist's desk.

2. The Patient was going to see his Doctor this afternoon.

3. The OT Aide used velcro and Scotch Tape to fix Mrs. Smith's lapboard during the occupational therapy session.

4. The Doctor spoke to the child who has Chicken Pox.

5. The OTA Student performed a Sensory Test on the client.

6. The client took Tylenol and Antacids before his Business Meeting.

7. The Nurse told the new mother that the infant has down syndrome.

8. The Physical Therapist informed the OTA that their client was admitted to the Hospital due to Pneumonia.

9. The Occupational therapy assistant worked in the outpatient department.

10. The OT used the Miller assessment for preschoolers to assess the child with Autism.

11. The Skilled Nursing Facility Resident diagnosed with guillain-barre syndrome also has Dementia.

12. The OT club at the local Community College volunteered at a Food pantry last weekend and donated canned goods, kleenex, band-aids, and paper towels.

13. The OTA Student attended an Inservice to learn more about kinesiology.

14. The OTA students had opportunities to observe OTs working in Hand Therapy Clinics, Long-Term Care facilities, and Elementary schools.

15. The local newspaper wrote an article about We-Care Rehabilitation Hospital occupational therapy department.

Match the pronoun appropriately to the subject. Also, you must determine if the subject and pronoun are singular or plural for consistency, for example, "*Emily dressed herself independently,*" or "*Emily and Samantha dressed themselves independently.*"

Plurals and Possessives

In regard to plurals or possessives, we will now look at several situations that are commonly prone to errors. According to the Publication Manual of the APA (2020), to indicate the plural of an abbreviation, usually just the letter "s" is added without an apostrophe. For example:

- *The OTs each supervised two OTAs.*
- *The MDs wanted to use the conference room.*
- *The three OTAs all graduated from the same college.*
- *The OTA presented an in-service on body mechanics to the four RNs.*

When you are indicating that something belongs to one person or object (singular possessive), most of the time an apostrophe is used before the letter "s." Here are some examples:

Worksheet 5-7
Pronouns, Plurals, Possessives

Look at the following sentences and determine the incorrect components in each sentence.

1. The three client's appointments were all rescheduled because their OTA was ill.

2. The OTAs lab coat was new.

3. The OTA students résumé was reviewed by the OT.

4. The childs parent's attended most therapy session's.

5. The children almost hurt himselves when they collided with each other in the hallway.

6. The nurses patient gave them all flowers.

7. The PT's and OT's had the day off.

8. The occupational therapists' paperwork was on the administrative assistants desk.

9. One of the client's left an orthotic's device on the food tray.

10. The OT took the OTAs lab coat home by mistake.

11. Sarah told her math and social studies teachers she did the homework by themselves.

12. The broken wheelchairs were repaired by the two PTA's.

13. The student had difficulty opening the combination's lock on the locker.

14. The client diagnosed with depression completed a three-step's craft projects independently.

15. The parents was given a variety of equipments to help improve the triplets motor skills.

Morreale, M. J. (2023). *The OTA's guide to documentation: Writing SOAP notes* (5th ed.). SLACK Incorporated.

- *The client's right hand was minimally edematous.*
- *That chair's armrests are broken.*
- *The OTA's goniometer is in her desk.*
- *The patient's commode was placed next to his bed.*

When you have more than one person or object and want to indicate that something belongs to all of them (plural possessive), the apostrophe goes after the letter "s." For example:

- *The clients' charts were in the file cabinet.*
- *The OTA students' lunches were free in the hospital cafeteria.*
- *The occupational therapy assistants' treatment notes were cosigned by their supervisors.*
- *The OTAs' patients were all in the waiting room.*
- *Three of the patients' lunch trays were missing utensils.*

Conclusion

Now you are ready to begin the process of writing SOAP notes. Always remember that your documentation is a reflection of you as both an individual and occupational therapy professional. Make a concerted effort to use correct spelling, punctuation, and grammar in all of your professional writing. When in doubt, refer to a dictionary, spell-checking program, or style manual to ensure accuracy. The rest of this manual will take you step-by-step through the process of writing SOAP notes and help you to practice using clinical reasoning skills. You will soon be thinking and writing like an OTA.

References

American Psychological Association. (2022). *APA Style: Capitalization.* Retrieved May 25, 2022 from https://apastyle.apa.org/style-grammar-guidelines/capitalization

American Psychological Association. (2020). *Publication manual of the American Psychological Association (7th ed.).* Author.

Merriam-Webster. (2001). *Merriam-Webster's guide to punctuation and style (2nd ed.).* Author.

Sames, K. M. (2015) *Documenting occupational therapy practice (3rd ed.).* Pearson Education, Inc.

Chapter 6

Writing the "S"—Subjective

The first section of the SOAP note contains **SUBJECTIVE** information obtained from the client. This "S" section expresses the client's perspective regarding their condition or treatment. Subjective data is information that cannot necessarily be verified or measured during the intervention session. In this section, the occupational therapy practitioner records the client's report of limitations, concerns, and problems, as well as what the client communicated that was relevant to treatment. This can include statements regarding significant complaints of pain, fatigue, or expressions of feelings, attitudes, concerns, goals, and plans. Appropriate, direct quotes are often used in the subjective section of the SOAP note. In this case, it is understood that the statement comes from the individual receiving the therapy, unless otherwise stated. This subjective information will have more significance and relevance to the rest of your note if it specifically pinpoints an issue rather than just noting a vague or general comment from the client. For instance, if the client tells you, "My hand hurts," you may probe further, asking, "Where does it hurt?" or "When does it hurt?" or "Describe what it feels like." This will allow your note to communicate more detailed information on the individual's condition by recording the client's own description or perception: *Client states he has sharp pain in his Ⓡ thumb CMC joint when he uses a hammer or wrench.* You may quote, paraphrase, or summarize what the client said. Review Chapter 5 for detailed information regarding the use of proper grammar and punctuation for direct and indirect quotes.

Examples of "S" Statements

- *"I don't need therapy."*
- *Student stated she has difficulty changing in and out of her gym clothes within the allotted time in class.*
- *Client reports "pins and needles" in Ⓡ hand when driving > 15 minutes.*
- *Client reports feeling "frustrated" because her short arm cast interferes with ability to perform home management tasks.*
- *Patient expressed doubts about ever getting better and then began to cry.*
- *Client reports, "I keep losing my patience at home and yelling at my family, and I don't know what to do about it."*
- *"I can't tie my shoes or zip my coat because my thumb is too stiff."*
- *Veteran reports that he has frequent flashbacks of combat duty that wake him up at night.*
- *Child reports that she is too embarrassed to wear her leg brace and orthotic devices because the other students make fun of her.*

Morreale, M. J. *The OTA's Guide to Documentation: Writing SOAP Notes, Fifth Edition* (pp. 99-103). © 2023 Taylor & Francis Group.

- *Patient expresses a desire to return to her factory job as soon as possible. She also states concern about the financial implications of her inability to work 2° her injury.*
- *Client reports being fearful of leaving her family and moving to a group home.*
- *Client reports that his doctor has ordered "some home care for a few days to work on transfers."*
- *Client reported that she has been performing her shoulder exercises twice daily without any discomfort. She also stated that she can now reach items in her upper kitchen cabinets with her ® UE.*
- *Client called the emergency line last night to report a burning sensation in her "gut," which made her afraid she was going to die. Today she reports that she has been worrying about dying and has not showered since the day before yesterday.*
- *Resident expressed that she has had several episodes of urinary incontinence recently and, therefore, does not like leaving her room.*
- *Client stated, "I feel so stressed out about losing my job that I can't concentrate or sleep. I don't feel like myself anymore." She also reported that gardening and volunteer work are her primary coping strategies, and that she would like to learn more about relaxation techniques.*
- *Student stated that her hand gets very tired when she writes.*
- *Client reports that stress and anxiety about losing his job are the reasons he drinks alcohol excessively.*

Sometimes the client is not able to speak or does not make any relevant comments. In such cases, include that information in the "S" section. For example:

- *Client unable to communicate due to aphasia.*
- *Client did not speak without cueing.*
- *Patient communicated using his message board that he wants to be able to walk again.*
- *Resident does not clearly verbalize during treatment, but smiles and nods appropriately when asked questions.*

In certain instances, the "S" part of the SOAP note might reflect an important statement, problem, or concern that the client's caregiver, family members, or significant others communicate to the OTA regarding the client. Also, when working with infants and very young children, you may report what the parent or guardian says. For example:

- *Mother reports child will only tolerate mashed or pureed foods due to child's oral sensitivity.*
- *Caregiver reports client refuses to wear her orthosis.*
- *Although client denies taking alcohol and drugs, her husband states, "I am really concerned that she is eventually going to kill herself. She will not stop drinking and taking cocaine."*
- *Parent reported child has an ear infection and is "very cranky today." She also expressed concern that the child's recurrent ear infections may necessitate surgery.*
- *Daughter reports client lives with her and sometimes forgets to turn off the stove. Daughter states she works full-time and is concerned that her mother is home alone during the day and could hurt herself or start a fire.*

The "S" section is usually reserved for the client's point of view except for situations with infants/young children, people who are unable to communicate, and special circumstances. If a client is deaf or only speaks a different language, it is important to know your facility's protocol for this type of situation. Someone should be present who can interpret or translate all communication between the client and occupational therapy practitioner. This should also be recorded in the note.

Common Errors

Not Using Communication Time With the Client Effectively

A common error that new OTAs make in gathering subjective information is in failing to make good use of communication with the client during intervention sessions. Of course, it is important to make the client feel comfortable and at ease. However, rather than using most of the therapy time to talk socially, a good OTA will use the time to listen effectively and to ask questions that will elicit pertinent information about the client's attitudes and concerns. This information can then be used to ensure effective intervention as well as appropriate documentation. Instead of discussing the weather or a professional sporting event, why not ask clients how they think they are doing in therapy or what their feelings are related to their upcoming discharge placement? As OTAs gain experience, they begin to use the intervention session to obtain relevant data regarding important areas such as occupational history, functional abilities, prior level of functioning, priorities, motivation, and family support. Effective communication during intervention sessions can seem just like a conversation on the surface. However, skilled OTAs carefully direct the conversation to topics that are meaningful to client care rather than allowing it to remain superficial. Use this opportunity to expand the client's occupational profile and gather information that is vital to providing the very best occupational therapy possible. When conversing with your client, guide the discussion to your client's history, problems, needs, concerns, strengths, support systems, living situation, and desired therapy goals. Without knowing these things from your client's point of view, you will have difficulty planning effective interventions. When an OTA does not listen effectively during treatment, the "S" may read:

- *Client talked about grandchildren visiting.*
- *Resident reported she was wearing a new dress today.*
- *Pt. stated that his lunch tasted very good.*

While these statements are within the scope of the "S," they are not particularly helpful pieces of information to spend time and space reporting.

Not Writing Concise, Coherent Statements

Another common error new OTAs make when writing the subjective section of the note is that of simply listing any remarks clients make about their condition.

For example, during one intervention session, the client said all of the following:

- *"I'm wobbly as can be today."*
- *"I can't feel anything with my hands."*
- *Client expressed dizziness after bending down to touch the floor while in a seated position.*
- *Client acknowledged improvement in his sitting balance in comparison to the previous week.*

These statements generally involve stability, balance, and safety issues. While the quotations are a very objective way of reporting information and all of the remarks are relevant to the intervention session, it is more effective to summarize the client's statements more concisely and coherently. Rather than listing each of these statements separately in the "S" section of the note, organize and record them in a more professional manner. For example:

- *Client reported lack of sensation in both hands and dizziness in sitting position with dynamic movement (a "wobbly" sensation). He also acknowledged improvement in sitting balance since last week.*

  —or—

- *Client acknowledged improved sitting balance as compared to previous week. However, he expressed dizziness after bending down while sitting, and reported feeling "wobbly." Client also reported inability to feel anything with his hands.*

In the next two exercises, you will have the opportunity to select coherent and concise "S" statements.

Worksheet 6-1
Choosing a Subjective Statement

A female client is recovering after a Ⓛ CVA. This contact note was written after one of her occupational therapy intervention sessions.

O: *Client participated in 45-minute OT session in hospital room to ↑ AROM in Ⓡ shoulder and improve activity tolerance, UE strength, and dynamic standing balance, in order to ↑ independence in ADL tasks.*

ADL: Client was instructed on safety techniques and adaptive equipment use for toileting. Client required use of bilateral grab bars in bathroom to sit ↔ stand safely. Client first attempted to stand while pulling on walker and one grab bar. Client was instructed on proper procedures for safe transfers and the use of bilateral grab bars, which she reported understanding.

Performance Skills: Client sit → stand CGA for balance. Client worked on activity tolerance, dynamic standing balance, and ↑ AROM in Ⓡ shoulder by moving personal hygiene items from bathroom counter to medicine cabinet for 5 minutes before needing to sit and rest 2 minutes. She then participated in activities to ↑ dynamic standing balance by pouring liquid from a pitcher while standing CGA for balance. After a 1-minute rest, client continued activities to ↑ dynamic standing balance and safety in ADL activities by pushing wheeled walker while picking up objects from floor with a reacher.

Client Factors: AROM right shoulder abduction < 90°. PROM Ⓡ shoulder abduction WNL.

The intervention session included all of the following. Which would be best to use as the subjective section of the SOAP note?

1. *Client remarked that her grandson will be coming to visit later in the week, and that she will be very glad to see him.*
2. *Client was cooperative and engaged in social conversation throughout the intervention session.*
3. *Client reports that she feels "pretty good" today.*
4. *Client says she has difficulty moving Ⓡ UE, although she does not know why it will not move. She reports, "It really doesn't hurt. It's just tight."*
5. *Nursing staff report client is unsafe to toilet self independently.*

Worksheet 6-2
Writing Concise, Coherent Statements

Your client is recovering from a Ⓛ total hip replacement. During an occupational therapy intervention session, the client makes the following statements.

- *"I used that dressing stick and sock aid like you showed me to get dressed without bending down this morning."*

- *"It's getting easier for me to get dressed now."*

- *"My hip doesn't hurt when I stand up or sit down, especially with that new toilet seat you got for me."*

- *"My daughter said they delivered all that bathroom equipment to her house yesterday."*

Using these statements, write your own concise and organized version for the "S" portion of the SOAP note.

S:

Morreale, M. J. (2023). *The OTA's guide to documentation: Writing SOAP notes* (5th ed.). SLACK Incorporated.

Chapter 7

Writing the "O"—Objective

The second part of the note is the **OBJECTIVE** section. This is where you will record all measurable, quantifiable, and observable data obtained during your client's occupational therapy session. In this section, your note presents a mental picture or synopsis of the entire encounter. Once you begin viewing things with your professional eyes, these observations can look and seem quite different. Instead of simply seeing a child playing with a toy, you now begin to make skilled observations, such as noting the child's asymmetrical posture, hand preference, balance, ability to cross midline, and specific pinch and grasp patterns. A student or new OTA may have difficulty deciding what kind of material to include and what to omit in the "O" section. At first your "O" may tend to be longer than that of an experienced OTA, but with time you will learn to write notes that are both complete and concise.

If you are entering information into an electronic documentation system, you will need to follow the integrated prompts, sequence of templates, and organizational format for that specific software program. Some practitioners choose to also include a SOAP note in the comments section to ensure that all the necessary client data is entered and to substantiate care in case the claim is reviewed by the payer later on. Even if you are not writing SOAP notes per se, the information presented in this chapter will help you to learn what is important to look for, how to organize client data, and what is essential to include in your documentation.

Guidelines for Writing Good Observations

Begin With a Statement About the Setting and Purpose of the Activity

Start with the term for *client* that is most appropriate for your facility, such as resident, infant, child, student, patient, veteran, consumer, etc. Follow that with terminology noting the client's active participation in therapy (Sames, 2015). For example, instead of writing that the client was "seen" during the session, it is preferable to use the words "participated in" (Sames, 2015, p. 15). As third-party payers may balk at paying for continued therapy if it appears the client just attended as a passive observer; this is an important distinction (Gateley & Borcherding, 2017; Sames, 2015). You may use similar words in the opening sentence such as *"client engaged in"* or *"client worked on."* Next, indicate where the therapy took place and the purpose of the therapy session.

If your interventions are **occupations or activities**, use the following format for your opening sentence:

Client participated in _____ -minute session in _____ for _____.
                   #   *(in what setting)*   *(purpose of the intervention session)*

Morreale, M. J. *The OTA's Guide to Documentation: Writing SOAP Notes, Fifth Edition* (pp. 105-127). © 2023 Taylor & Francis Group.

For example:

- *Resident participated in 45-minute session bedside for instruction in compensatory dressing techniques.*
- *Child engaged in 30-minute OT session in classroom to improve ability to use computer keyboard in class.*
- *Client participated in 30-minute cooking group in OT kitchen for skilled instruction in compensatory techniques for meal preparation.*

Facilities and payers may require that OT practitioners document the number of minutes for the entire occupational therapy session and/or each specific occupational therapy service the client receives. These recorded minutes are typically used for billing purposes, such as determining the correct Current Procedural Terminology (CPT) codes and verifying that required therapy time was implemented for designated levels of care (such as for CMS Patient-Driven Payment Model groupings in skilled nursing facilities). Also, if questions arise regarding the amount or specific type of occupational therapy intervention the client received, the recorded minutes will help verify the amount of services provided. For example, for an OT session that lasted 40 minutes, the OT or OTA who implemented the session might document that the client received 18 minutes of ADL training, 12 minutes of therapeutic exercise, and 10 minutes of cryotherapy. Time notations may also be used to track the productivity of individual staff members or the entire department. Facilities that do not charge for occupational therapy by the number of minutes may not require that you document the length of time a client was seen. However, you do still need to document the skilled services that were provided.

If the session is centered on improving **client factors and skills** such as active range of motion, strength, activity tolerance, dexterity, or dynamic balance, then add a reference to the **relevant occupation** in the opening line:

Client participated in ____ -minute session in _____ to work on _____ for _____.
    #   (in what setting)   (purpose)   (for what expected
                                                              functional gain)

For example:

- *Student engaged in 30-minute therapy session in OT room to promote development of dynamic tripod grasp for **handwriting**.*
- *Child engaged in 45-minute OT session at his home to work on increasing selective attention and fine motor manipulation as a prerequisite to **enhanced play and ADL tasks**.*
- *Client participated in 20-minute session in hospital room for skilled instruction in energy conservation for **IADLs**.*
- *Consumer participated in role-play activity for 30 minutes in assertion group in order to explore alternative ways to get his **social needs** met.*
- *Client participated in 30-minute current events group to decrease social anxiety when **interacting with peers**.*
- *Pt. participated in 60-minute OT session in clinic for application of moist heat, P/AROM, and strengthening exercises to ®️ UE in order to restore skills needed for **return to work**.*
- *Resident participated in ½ hour UE exercise group to ↑ strength for **w/c mobility**.*

Occupational therapy practitioners do not always write the "O" this exact way. In some instances, you might choose to switch your sentence around slightly:

- *In sensory integration playroom, child participated in 30 minutes of OT activities to address sensory defensiveness in classroom activities.*
- *In OT kitchen, client worked 15 minutes on standing activities in order to increase activity tolerance for cooking.*
- *In order to improve interpersonal skills and promote leisure skills development, pt. participated in 30-minute OT craft group.*

Show Your Skill

It is important to show the need for your skill as an OTA in the very first sentence of your "O." As previously mentioned, instead of saying, *"Client seen for 45 minutes bedside for dressing,"* it is better to indicate active client engagement (Gateley & Borcherding, 2017; Sames, 2015) and then clearly identify the specific skilled occupational therapy services implemented. You might say:

- *Client participated in 45-minute ADL session bedside for **instruction in compensatory dressing techniques**.*
- *Client engaged in therapy 35 minutes bedside to **facilitate attention to** Ⓛ **side during self-care activities**.*
- *Resident participated in therapy 45 minutes bedside for **instruction in adaptive equipment use to increase safety in ADL tasks**.*

Here are some more examples showing the skill of an occupational therapy practitioner:

- *Client engaged in 30 minutes of therapy in OT kitchen to work on **improving time management for IADLs**.*
- *For 30 minutes in technology clinic, child and parents participated in **assistive technology training for classroom activities**.*
- *Pt. participated in 1-hour session in OT clinic for **fabrication of Ⓛ thumb spica orthosis to ↓ pain during ADLs**.*
- *In classroom, child participated in OT session 30 minutes for **adaptation of backpack to enable Ⓘ use**.*
- *Resident participated 40 minutes in OT life skills group for **instruction in stress management techniques**.*

Follow the Opening Sentence With a Summary of What You Observed

After the setting and purpose have been established, you will discuss the intervention you have just completed, either in chronological order or organized into categories. Some notes work best when reported chronologically and others work better with categories.

Organization of the "O"

Electronic documentation programs typically have a structured series of drop-down menus or templates. These programs might also allow for brief comments or possibly lengthier narratives or supplemental SOAP notes to be entered by the health practitioner. There are different ways to organize the information gleaned from your observations. One way is to present the information chronologically and discuss each intervention or event in the order it occurred during that particular session.

Resident participated in 45-minute OT session bedside for skilled instruction in ADLs and to ↑ activity tolerance. Once set up, resident was able to wash face and upper body with min Ⓐ and use of a wash mitt while sitting on EOB and using bedside table. 3 verbal cues were required to avoid excessive right shoulder elevation during washing task. Client also was instructed in use of long handle hairbrush and electric toothbrush. She demonstrated ability to use these items to perform grooming tasks with min Ⓐ needed to open toothpaste and two 60-second rest periods. Next, while sitting up in bed with head of bed raised, resident applied make-up with min Ⓐ to open containers.

Alternately, you may choose to organize your information into categories.

When categorizing your information, choose the categories that make the most sense for your note. For example, suppose that today you saw a female home care client for a cooking session in her kitchen. She is recovering from a total hip replacement (THR) and needs to be able to prepare a light meal independently once her home health aide is discontinued. You do not know her level of safety awareness or her ability to perform all steps of the activities while using a wheeled walker. You wonder if her activity tolerance and upper extremity function are adequate for functional mobility and cooking, and you also want to assess her judgment, problem solving, and ability to adhere to THR precautions. You choose the following categories:

- Functional mobility
- Upper extremity AROM and strength
- Activity tolerance
- Cognition

Your note might look like this:

> **O**: *Client participated in 60-minute OT session at home for skilled instruction in compensatory cooking techniques and safety assessment.*
>
> ***Functional Mobility**: Client used wheeled walker to maneuver throughout kitchen and she needed min verbal cues to position walker appropriately for reaching objects in cabinets and refrigerator. Client was instructed in use of walker basket and wheeled cart to transport items.*
>
> ***UE AROM and Strength**: WFL for reaching items in drawers and upper cabinets and putting dishes in the sink Ⓘ. UE strength adequate for opening refrigerator door, using manual can opener, and pouring soup in and out of small pot. Client required min Ⓐ to use reacher to obtain item from bottom shelf in refrigerator.*
>
> ***Activity Tolerance**: Client demonstrated ability to stand Ⓘ for 10 minutes to heat soup at stove and make sandwich at counter. Client required a 5-minute break then stood at sink for 5 minutes to wash dishes.*
>
> ***Cognitive**: Client able to respond to verbal instructions and questions with correct response 3/3 times. Client stated she did not think it would be safe for her to use the oven at this time and would use the toaster oven instead. Client able to problem solve and safely adhere to all THR precautions.*

There is no list of "correct" categories. You must use your clinical judgment to determine what is appropriate to include, summarize, or categorize. If the client has no deficits in a particular area, it is not necessary to address that category in the note. In choosing categories, you could use the following *Occupational Therapy Practice Framework: Domain and Process, 4th Edition (OTPF-4)* categories (AOTA, 2020) as these are useful in any practice setting:

- Occupations
- Performance skills
- Performance patterns
- Client factors
- Activity demands
- Contexts

In some instances, these *OTPF-4* categories may be too broad for your purposes. You might choose subcategories or other areas that relate more specifically to your client and your practice setting. You may want to consider some of the following:

- **ADL and IADL task performance**: Note how each of the performance skills and client factors observed impact completion of specific ADL/IADL tasks. Include assist levels and required set-up, adaptive equipment/durable medical equipment, positioning, compensatory techniques, and methods used. Also include extent and type of cuing and response, rest periods needed, family/caregiver education, and client's response to the intervention provided.

- **Education and work**: Note activity demands and any adaptive equipment, assistive technology, or modifications needed for school, work, or volunteer activities. Address time management, organizational skills, and ability to perform educational or job-related tasks. Consider career and transitional planning as well as the development of vocational skills.

- **Leisure and play**: Consider physical, cognitive, psychosocial, and developmental factors regarding participation in leisure activities. Note barriers to play and leisure, skill development, and appropriateness of leisure time and choices.

- **Rest and sleep**: Note any physical, emotional, contextual/environmental concerns or barriers regarding proper rest and sleep.

- **Posture and balance**: Note whether balance was static or dynamic for sitting and standing. Consider whether the client leans in one direction, has rotated posture, or has even or uneven weight distribution. Notice position of the head, upper extremities, trunk, and overall symmetry. Note what feedback, cues, or devices were needed to maintain or restore midline orientation or balance.

- **Coordination and dexterity**: Note if dominant hand is affected, the type of prehension patterns used, ability to grasp and maintain grasp of objects without dropping, functional reach and purposeful release, proximal control, precision handling, in-hand manipulation, and gross versus fine motor ability. Determine ability to manage bimanual tasks.

- **Swelling or edema**: Describe location and type of edema and give girth or volumetric measurements if possible.

- **Pain**: Describe or quantify the pain and note the frequency and anatomic location. Consider how pain impacts occupations, performance patterns, and try to determine what makes the pain better or worse.

- **Muscle, bone, joint, and sensory functions**: Describe specific type and location of sensory losses and consider whether PROM, AROM, strength, and structural alignment are adequate for performing occupational tasks. Note if client uses hearing aids, assistive listening devices, orthosis, sling or compression device, eyeglasses/contact lenses or optical devices.

- **Movement patterns in affected extremities**: Note motor planning, ataxia, tremors, tone (i.e., rigidity, flaccidity, hypotonicity, hypertonicity, and synergy pattern). Also describe facilitation or stabilization required, unwanted body movements, primitive reflexes, substitution, or compensatory motions.

- **Ability to follow instructions**: Note attention, behavior, type and amount of instruction required (such as physical, verbal or visual cuing), and ability to follow one-, two-, or three-step directions.

- **Cognition and perception**: Report on task initiation; appropriateness of verbal, written, or motor responses; approach to the task; ability to stay on task; sequencing; problem solving; orientation (identifying time, place, person, and situation); requirements for cuing; number of steps successfully completed in task; judgment (recognition of impairments, impulsivity, safety); and ability to correct errors. Note if client has unilateral neglect, impaired spatial relations, or difficulty crossing midline.

- **Health management:** Note relevant physical, cognitive, and emotional components supporting or hindering the individual's ability to monitor and self-manage symptoms of their condition or situation for occupational participation. Consider ability to procure, handle and care for personal care devices, comply with health provider recommendations, and self-determination to improve/maintain one's health and wellness (AOTA, 2020).

- **Functional mobility**: Note the kind of assistance, cues, adapted technique, special devices, or equipment required for the client to reposition self in bed, walk, transfer, propel a wheelchair, and use public transportation or drive.

- **Activity tolerance**: Note level of energy and endurance during tasks (indicate if sitting, standing, lying in bed, etc.) and impact on occupational performance.

- **Psychosocial factors**: Note client's overall appearance, hygiene, affect, mood, body image, and appropriateness of behavior. Also note family or community support, coping strategies, intra- and interpersonal skills, and ability to adapt and make realistic discharge decisions for self.

Look at the following client situation and two different examples of how the "O" part of the note might be written for this client.

Julie is a 27-year-old mother of two children ages 2 and 4. She is employed in a manufacturing job that involves lifting 30-pound boxes. She is currently unable to work due to back pain from a herniated disc in her lumbar area. She complains of pain when doing her housework and says that she wants to be able to perform IADLs and work tasks without pain. To assist in intervention planning, the OT delegates several tasks to the OTA that need to be observed and modified. You, the OTA, are asked to have this client demonstrate some performance skills for IADLs and work. You watch her take items from the refrigerator, wash the dishes, sweep and vacuum the floor, and lift a box from the floor to a chair. You observe that her body mechanics are poor and determine that she would benefit from client education. If you reported on your session using chronological order, you might say:

O: *Client participated in 30-minute session in OT clinic for assessment of low back pain and instruction in proper body mechanics. Client sits asymmetrically with weight shifted to her Ⓛ hip. Client demonstrated incorrect body mechanics in the way she usually removes items from the refrigerator, washes dishes, cleans the floors, and lifts. She was then instructed in proper body mechanics for completing those tasks (using a golfer's lift, squats, stepping toward the item she wishes to retrieve, facing the load and keeping it close to her body). Client demonstrated techniques correctly and was given education materials to remind her of correct positioning.*

If you wanted to put the same information into categories, you might say:

O: *Client participated in 30-minute session in OT clinic for assessment of low back pain and instruction in proper body mechanics for IADL and work.*

***Bending and Lifting**: Client demonstrated her usual way of moving items from low surfaces to higher ones, demonstrating incorrect body mechanics in back extension and bending at the waist. After instruction in using golfer's lift or squat, client demonstrated ability to use these techniques correctly in lifting and work activities after two attempts.*

***Transporting**: Client exhibited torque in the spine in transporting items such as dishes. After instruction in sidestepping, facing the load and keeping it close to the body, client demonstrated proper use of these techniques with less reported pain.*

***Reaching**: IADL tasks such as sweeping and vacuuming also habitually performed with rotation and over-extension of the back. After instruction and demonstration of moving the body rather than overextending the arms, and keeping the load close to the body, client demonstrated correct body mechanics in performing reaching tasks with decreased pain.*

***Client Education**: Client given educational material to remind her of correct positioning for task and client reported that she understood what to do.*

In this case, the chronological note works better because there is some repetition in the categorized version, and the categorized version is also longer. However, some notes are better if they are divided into sections. Categories help an inexperienced OTA to focus on the performance skills the client is demonstrating rather than the treatment media that is being used to facilitate these skills. It also helps other professionals to find pertinent information more quickly when they read your note. Complete Worksheet 7-1 to review a chronological note that would work better in categories.

Worksheet 7-1
Organizing the "O" With Categories

Consider the following chronological observation:

Child engaged in 60-minute OT session in daycare setting to work on reach/grasp/release and feeding skills. With min Ⓐ for facilitation of movement at elbow, child demonstrated ability to use Ⓛ UE to reach, grasp, and release 5 objects with 1-2 verbal cues per object and used Ⓡ UE to stabilize self for unsupported sitting at table. Child was able to feed self Ⓘ with ~50% spillage, but demonstrated significant limitations in chewing action with ~3 rotary chews & swallowing ~90% of food without chewing. Child required verbal cues throughout session to maintain attention to task. Child wore Ⓛ soft thumb spica orthosis for entire session.

How would you divide this information into categories to make it more organized and easier to read? Choose three to four categories and redistribute the information above into the categories you have chosen to write the "O" part of the note.

Morreale, M. J. (2023). *The OTA's guide to documentation: Writing SOAP notes* (5th ed.). SLACK Incorporated.

Additional Guidelines for Writing Good Observations

Do Not Duplicate Services

Make sure that your intervention is **specific to occupational therapy** as third-party payers will not pay for duplication of services. While there will naturally be some overlap among rehabilitation disciplines, it is important to record what occupational therapy is doing differently. For example, the physical therapist might be working with a client on ambulation with the goal of teaching the use of an ambulation device or working on improving ambulation distance. Occupational therapy might work with this same client using the ambulation device for a **specific activity or occupation**, such as loading the dishwasher safely or getting clothes out of a closet without becoming short of breath. If both occupational therapy and physical therapy are working on transfers, perhaps physical therapy is working on transfers to the mat or wheelchair and occupational therapy is working on transfers to the toilet or tub using adaptive equipment. If the speech therapist has the client reading a newspaper to facilitate articulation and language, the occupational therapy practitioner might be using the newspaper to facilitate cognitive skills and functional problem solving for specific occupations/activities, such as locating classified ads or the weekend entertainment.

Organize Assessment Data

The "O" section does not always need to be written in complete sentences, but it does need to be organized and make sense. Give complete information in the most concise form possible. It is imperative that certain details be included. For example, ROM must be specified as passive, active, or assistive and must indicate the action and joint at which the movement occurred. UE or LE must indicate which UE or LE. Level of physical or verbal assistance must be specified if assistance was given.

When you are documenting test results, it is helpful to put them into a chart like the following examples, rather than burying them in a narrative.

Sensation in Ⓛ hand:	
Hot/cold:	*Intact*
Sharp/dull:	*Impaired over volar surface, intact over dorsal surface*
Stereognosis:	*Absent*
Light touch:	*Absent*

Hand Strength	Left	Right
Grip	30 lb	62 lb
3 point pinch	11 lb	18 lb
Lateral pinch	16 lb	19 lb
Tip pinch	9 lb	14 lb

Use Professional Language

As demonstrated in the following examples, appropriate changes in wording can make your notes sound more professional and succinct.

Rather than saying: *Resident flopped down onto bed short of breath, closed her eyes, and moaned. Resident reclined in bed with min Ⓐ to position herself.*

You might say: *Client observed to be fatigued following therapy session and required min Ⓐ for positioning in bed.*

Rather than saying: *Veteran grabbed onto the trapeze and used it in order to sit up.*

You might say: *Supine → sit using trapeze.*

Rather than saying: *OTA put her hand over the client's bad hand to help client hold onto the toothbrush.*

You might say: *Client needed hand-over-hand assist to maintain grasp on toothbrush using affected hand.*

Rather than saying: *Client put the board in place to make a sliding board transfer.*

You might say: *Client positioned sliding board for transfer.*

Tables 7-1 and 7-2 provide suggestions for professional terms and language commonly used in occupational therapy. You might also review the information in Chapter 2 to help ensure your documentation vocabulary is respectful. Additional lists of professional terminology are presented in Chapter 12. **It is important to understand that your documentation should describe the actual behaviors or symptoms you observe but not assign diagnostic terms**. For example, if you notice a client on your caseload having trouble with memory, do not presume and document that this client has "Alzheimer's disease" unless the client has been diagnosed specifically with this condition. Rather, you would document how this client's apparent memory loss is interfering with ability to perform a specific activity/occupation or creates a safety concern at this time. As another example, avoid documenting "client is depressed" as that is also a diagnostic term. However, you should document any pertinent behaviors and concerns, for example, if the client is expressing severe sadness or remaining in bed all day for extended periods without showering or dressing. Of course, you should discuss your findings with the OT to determine if further evaluation, medical referral, or other recommendations are warranted in these kinds of situations. **Always use professional reasoning to choose the most appropriate word choice and course of action for the client's particular condition or situation**. Complete Worksheets 7-2 and 7-3 to help you practice the use of professional language. Worksheet 7-4 will assess your knowledge of appropriate, alternate terms for common brand-name health items.

Table 7-1 Using Professional Language		
Rather than saying …	*You might say …*	
Good arm (or leg)	Strong arm (or leg) Strong upper (or lower) limb Unaffected extremity Uninvolved extremity	
Bad arm (or leg)	Weak arm (or leg) Weak upper (or lower) limb Affected arm (or leg)	Involved extremity Non-functional extremity
Suffers from (i.e., disease or condition) Victim (i.e., stroke/cancer victim, victim of MS)	Diagnosed with Has a diagnosis of Has side effects from Experiencing symptoms of	
Client did	Client performed Client demonstrated Client participated	Client engaged in Client worked on
Client said Client told	Client stated Client reported Client expressed Client described	Client articulated Client indicated Client verbalized
Client walked	Client ambulated Client performed functional mobility Functional ambulation to …	
Client went up the stairs Client went up the ramp Client went up the curb	Ascended stairs/ramp/curb	
Client went down the stairs Client went down the ramp Client went down the curb	Descended stairs/ramp/curb	
Client ambulated in wheelchair Wheelchair ambulation	Performed wheelchair mobility Self-propelled wheelchair Propelled wheelchair (i.e., independently, with min assist, etc.) Ambulated while pushing wheelchair	
Gave client (item such as buttonhook, therapy putty, orthotic device)	Client was issued Client was provided	
Gave client (i.e., test, procedure, medication) —or— Did (specific method to client as intervention to support occupation)	Administered Applied (i.e., hot pack, paraffin, bandage, orthotic device) Implemented	Performed (i.e., PROM, stump wrapping, wound care, retrograde massage) Client received
Client took off (i.e., shirt, orthosis)	Client doffed	
Client put on (i.e., pants, orthosis)	Client donned	
Showed client Helped client	Client was instructed Skilled instruction provided Client was taught	Client was educated regarding Training provided for … Recommended (i.e., a device or technique)
Made (i.e., orthosis)	Fabricated Customized	
Made (i.e., exercise program)	Designed Developed Created	

(continued)

Table 7-1 (continued)
Using Professional Language

Rather than saying …	You might say …	
Changed	Modified Adapted Customized	Updated Revised
Looked at (i.e., for safety, ability, or sizing)	Observed Assessed Reassessed Evaluated	Examined Measured for … Fitted for … Determined
Feel (i.e., muscle, joint)	Palpate Assess Examine	
Put	Positioned Set-up	
Upper extremity dressing/bathing Lower extremity dressing/bathing	Upper body dressing/bathing Lower body dressing/bathing	
Treatment	Intervention Skilled services	
Splint	Orthosis Orthotic device	
Splinting	Fabrication of orthotic device Fitting of orthotic device Orthosis modified to allow for …	
Can't walk	Unable to ambulate Non-ambulatory Wheelchair user Confined to bed	
Senile	Has dementia Diagnosed with Alzheimer's disease Impaired cognition Altered mental status Memory deficits	
Mentally retarded	Intellectual disability Has Down syndrome Has an IQ of …	
Brain-damaged	Diagnosed with traumatic brain injury/acquired brain injury Sustained closed head injury/head trauma Cognitive impairment/cognitive disability	
Addict Alcoholic Crackhead Junkie Drug abuser	Person with substance use disorder Individual with alcohol use disorder Has a problem with unhealthy use of … Struggling with addiction/maintaining sobriety Client is using …	
Normal child (development)	Child with typical development Neurotypical	
Abnormal child (development)	Child with atypical development Challenges in age-appropriate developmental skills Toddler diagnosed with developmental delay Infant with congenital limb differences Neurodivergent	
Weaknesses (child)	Challenges Delayed skills acquisition Has not yet attained ability to …	

Table 7-2
Using Professional Language: Anatomy and Bodily Function Terms

Rather than saying ...	You might say ...	
Arm	Upper extremity Upper limb	
Leg	Lower extremity Lower limb	
Underarm Armpit	Axilla	
Under the tongue (i.e., medication)	Sublingual	
Pinky	Small finger Fifth digit	
Knuckle	Metacarpal head MP joint	
Pointer finger	Index finger Second digit	
Stomach	Abdomen	
Rear end Bottom Bum Sit bones	Buttocks Rectum Ischial tuberosity Sacrum	
Belly button	Navel	
Fat Obese Heavy	Client has a body mass index of ... Client is _____ tall and weighs _____ pounds. Child is in _____ percentile for weight.	
Sweat Sweating	Perspire Strong body odor Perspiring profusely	Diaphoretic Has hyperhidrosis
Client had to go to the bathroom	Needed to use restroom Felt need to have a bowel movement Needed to urinate Felt urge to urinate Urinary urgency	
Poop	Bowel movement Defecate Stool	Loose stools Diarrhea Feces
Pee	Urine Urinate Void	
Burp Belch	Eructation	
Fart Gassy Pass gas	Flatulence Flatus	
Throw up Puke	Vomit Emesis Regurgitate Gagging (i.e., on own saliva, due to aversion of specific food, etc.)	Projectile vomit Retching Nausea
Pass out Woozy	Episode of syncope Fainted Lightheaded Vertigo Dizziness	

(continued)

Table 7-2 (continued)

Using Professional Language: Anatomy and Bodily Function Terms

Rather than saying ...	You might say ...	
Had an accident (urine or feces) Wets self Pooped/peed in Leaks urine pants Soiled pants/diaper	Episode of incontinence Incontinent of urine Stress incontinence Urinary incontinence	Accidental bladder leakage Incontinent of feces Fecal incontinence Accidental bowel leakage
Period Time of the month	Menses Menstrual cycle Menstruation	
Swelling Swollen	Edema noted (location) Edematous (quantify/describe) Lymphedema	
Black and blue	Ecchymosis Bruise	
Blood clot	Thrombus Embolus	
Blind spot in eye	Scotoma	
Double vision	Diplopia	
Bedsore	Decubitus ulcer Pressure injury	
Runny nose Snot	Rhinorrhea Rhinitis Clear nasal discharge Nasal mucus (color)	
Earwax	Cerumen	
Bones rubbing together Crackling joints	Crepitation Crepitus	
Pins and needles sensation	Paresthesia	
Low muscle tone Limp/floppy muscles	Flaccidity Hypotonicity Has hypotonia	
High muscle tone	Hypertonicity Spasticity Rigidity Unwanted movements	

Slumps
Can't sit/stand up straight
Sits crooked
Bent/humped over when standing/sitting
	Kyphosis
	Posterior pelvic tilt
	Unable to maintain upright
	  trunk posture/midline
	  orientation (i.e., in wheelchair,
	  when standing, sitting on edge
	  of bed)
	Leans to left or right when ...
	  (i.e., lying supine with head of
	  bed raised, sitting on toilet)
		Poor postural alignment/
		  asymmetrical
		Unable to sit/stand
		  unsupported
		Forward head posture
		Slides forward in seat

Front of body	Anterior trunk (or torso)	
Back of body	Posterior trunk (or torso)	
Side of (part of body such as arm, leg)	Lateral aspect of ... Medial aspect of ...	
Side of hand	Ulnar aspect of hand Radial aspect of hand	
Front of hand Back of hand	Volar hand Dorsal hand	
Close to (part of body) Farther away from (part of body)	Proximal to (i.e., wound is 1 cm proximal to ulnar head) Distal to (i.e., numbness distal to elbow)	

Worksheet 7-2
Using Professional Terminology

Rewrite these sentences to make them sound more professional in a contact note.

1. The client said she had pain just past the pinky knuckle in her bad hand.

2. Five minutes after the treatment session started, the patient said he had to go to the bathroom.

3. The client afflicted with Alzheimer's occasionally has an accident in his diaper.

4. The OTA gave the client therapy putty for home use.

5. The teenager complained of cramps because it was that time of the month for her.

6. The client's left glenohumeral joint crackled when passive range of motion was done to it.

7. The client suffers from multiple sclerosis and says she has difficulty putting on her lower extremity garments.

8. The OTA gave the senile client a mental status exam.

9. It was determined that the very obese client needed an oversized electric wheelchair and he was instructed in wheelchair ambulation.

10. The dyspraxic child said she tripped on her shoelaces and fell on her bottom, sustaining a large black and blue.

Morreale, M. J. (2023). *The OTA's guide to documentation: Writing SOAP notes* (5th ed.). SLACK Incorporated.

Worksheet 7-3
Using Professional Terminology—More Practice

Rewrite these sentences to make them sound more professional in a contact note.

1.   On the way to school, the child threw up on the school bus and became sweaty and clammy.

2.   The paraplegic client developed a bedsore on his sit bones.

3.   The preschool accepted normal and abnormal children.

4.   The client was unable to wash her right armpit because she could not actively lift her bad right shoulder.

5.   The OTA showed the client a different way to put on upper extremity clothes so that the client could do this by herself.

6.   The child asked for a tissue because he had snot running down his face.

7.   The client's hearing improved after the doctor removed excessive earwax.

8.   After going to the bathroom the autistic child rubbed some poop on the bathroom wall.

9.   The brain-damaged client said he has double vision.

10. The client takes nitroglycerin under his tongue and takes an insulin shot in his stomach.

Morreale, M. J. (2023). *The OTA's guide to documentation: Writing SOAP notes* (5th ed.). SLACK Incorporated.

Worksheet 7-4
Trademarked Versus Generic Therapy Terms

For each of the following brand names, indicate the generic equivalent term you might use in documentation. Use an internet search engine if you need help in determining the appropriate term.

1. _____ Purell
2. _____ Velcro
3. _____ Dycem
4. _____ Polyform, Aquaplast, Ezeform
5. _____ Ace bandage
6. _____ Kinesio Tape
7. _____ Pampers
8. _____ Theraputty
9. _____ Theraband
10. _____ Neosporin
11. _____ Advil
12. _____ Tylenol
13. _____ Q-tip
14. _____ Chux
15. _____ Nerf ball
16. _____ Thick-It
17. _____ TED stockings
18. _____ Hoyer lift
19. _____ Jobst glove
20. _____ Coban, CoFlex

Morreale, M. J. (2023). *The OTA's guide to documentation: Writing SOAP notes* (5th ed.). SLACK Incorporated.

Make Your Note Specific and Concise

When first learning to write client observations, it is often hard to decide what to include and what to leave out. Initially, it is better to include too much information, rather than take a chance on omitting something important. As your observational skills become more refined, it will become second nature to include all of the important data and instinctively eliminate the "fluff." Then, the "O" section of your notes will begin to be more professional and concise. Here is a client observation written by an inexperienced OTA. In an effort to include all of the necessary data, this note is too wordy and needs some improvement.

O: *Client was seen in rehab gym for hot pack and ⓡ UE strengthening. Session lasted 50 minutes. Client first had a hot pack applied to ⓡ shoulder for 20 minutes. After the hot pack came off, client was asked to clasp hands together and raise arms above head 30X. Pt was then instructed to cross her midline and touch her opposite shoulder with ⓡ UE. Client required six rest periods for completion. Client completed tasks ⓘ. Client was then introduced to weight and pulley system. Client was asked to specify how much weight she thought she could do. She responded with 5 lb. Client did 30 reps of the pulley system with 5 lb in shoulder flexion to strengthen her rotator cuff in order to decrease the probability of dislocating her shoulder again.*

An OTA with more experience might have written a more concise note:

O: *Client participated in 50-minute OT session in rehab gym to prevent further ⓡ shoulder dislocation. Hot pack applied to ⓡ shoulder for 20 min followed by the following ⓡ UE strengthening exercises for rotator cuff:*

- *ⓑ clasped hand shoulder flexion and extension x 30 repetitions*
- *Horizontal adduction ⓡ hand to ⓛ shoulder x 30 repetitions*
- *6 rest periods were needed to complete above exercises.*
- *ⓡ shoulder flexion using pulleys with 5 lb wt. x 30 repetitions*

You will notice, however, that there is still another problem with this note. It sounds like a physical therapy note rather than an occupational therapy note. This note needs to have functional components added, although they do not have to be in the "O." A statement from the client in the "S" about what she is unable to do with an injured rotator cuff and a statement in the "A" and/or "P" indicating functional problems/goals would suffice to make it a good occupational therapy note. Notice that being more concise means knowing what information can be omitted without compromising the quality of the observation.

It is possible to be **too** succinct, thereby omitting necessary information. For example, consider the following "O" from an inpatient occupational therapy session:

O: *Client seen bedside for instruction in dressing techniques.*

This "O" does not provide much information. When additional information is added, we learn quite a bit more about the session with this client:

O: *Client participated in 45-minute OT session bedside for skilled instruction in dressing techniques. Client exhibited some difficulty with sequencing and attempted to don slacks before underwear. Client also required min verbal cues to attend to ⓛ side to place ⓛ arm in shirt sleeve. Fine motor skills were WFL to manage buttons, but moderate ⓐ was needed to line up and fasten buttons properly 2° inattention to detail.*

It is a matter of carefully balancing the need to be complete when writing the "O" with the need to be concise. In Worksheet 7-5, you will have an opportunity to make an observation more concise, without losing any of its informational content. Worksheets 7-6 and 7-7 provide additional opportunities to practice using professional language.

Conclusion

This chapter has explained the basic components for writing the *objective* part of your SOAP note. The "O" section requires proper organization and a succinct summary describing what skilled occupational therapy services were provided in what setting. It is important that occupational therapy practitioners use professional language and not duplicate services of another discipline. To make your documentation even better, the next chapter will provide you with additional tips for writing the "O" and making your notes more accurate, professional, and complete. Remember, as you practice composing notes and gain clinical experience, your documentation will improve and become much easier.

Worksheet 7-5
Being More Concise

Revise the following treatment observations to make the note complete but more concise and professional.

O: *Pt seen 30 minutes in his hospital room for ADLs. Client ambulated ~36 inches to shower stall with SBA for safety. Client instructed to complete shower while sitting. Client has an IV in place. Client performed shower with SBA to manage IV line. Client able to wash upper and lower body Ⓘ and dry entire body after completing shower. Client required ~20 minutes to complete shower. Client then ambulated ~36 inches to chair and sat. Client needed verbal cues to remain seated while donning underwear and pants. Client able to dress UE Ⓘ and lower body after verbal cues for sitting. Client demonstrated good sitting balance, but needed SBA for standing balance. Following shower, client stated he would like to take a nap. Client walked to his bed with SBA and was assisted back into bed.*

Morreale, M. J. (2023). *The OTA's guide to documentation: Writing SOAP notes* (5th ed.). SLACK Incorporated.

Worksheet 7-6
Using Professional Language

Rewrite the following paragraphs to make them sound more concise and professional.

1. The resident suffers from Parkinson disease and is confused sometimes about the date. Resident uses a rolling walker and walks by shuffling her feet across the floor. I am concerned that when she goes home she may fall because she tends to grab onto the walker to stand up. She cannot always hold her urine well and rushes to the bathroom because she is afraid she will have an accident.

2. Client was asked by OTA to put on a bathrobe and slippers to determine the client's ability to perform dressing. The client needed three verbal cues to tie the bathrobe belt and she needed two verbal cues to figure out which was the right slipper and which was the left. Client walked from her bed to a chair using a rolling walker and OTA had to give her CGA because client was wobbly. OTA propped up client with pillows so that client's bad arm would be supported and elevated and she would no longer lean to the right while sitting in the chair.

3. Client said he has pain and numbness in his ®️ hand due to his diagnosis of carpal tunnel syndrome. An orthotic device called a volar wrist extension orthosis was made by the OTA today to support the client's right wrist and help make his hand feel better. During today's session the OTA provided instruction and had the client practice putting on and taking off his orthosis. OTA observed that client was able to put the orthosis on and remove it independently.

Morreale, M. J. (2023). *The OTA's guide to documentation: Writing SOAP notes* (5th ed.). SLACK Incorporated.

4. Logan was born with cerebral palsy and is in the second grade. He was seen by the OTA today for 30 minutes in the classroom to work on ways to help him use a computer tablet better. Logan has excess tone and decreased voluntary control in his upper extremities. His wild and jerky arm movements cause many mistakes when Logan tries to use the tablet and touch screen keyboard for classroom tasks. Logan does have good head control. He is also able to maintain a fairly good upright position in his wheelchair for most of the time. Methods attempted during today's session included him using a mouthstick while the tablet was positioned upright with a support on the desk. Logan did a good job following instructions for how to use the mouthstick. He was able to write his name five times using the tablet touchscreen keyboard without making any mistakes. He received a sticker as a reward for doing so well.

Morreale, M. J. (2023). *The OTA's guide to documentation: Writing SOAP notes* (5th ed.). SLACK Incorporated.

Worksheet 7-7
Understanding Health Care Terms

Answer the following multiple-choice questions to test your knowledge of various health care terms. Use an internet search engine or medical dictionary if you need help in determining the correct answer

1. An OTA reviewing a client's chart sees the term "malaise" in the list of the client's signs and symptoms. The OTA should interpret this as which of the following?
    a. The client is malnourished and underweight
    b. The client has a general feeling of unwellness
    c. The client has maladaptive coping skills
    d. The client has trouble sleeping

2. An OTA reviewing a client's chart sees that the physician documented a "syncopal episode" today. The OTA should interpret this as which of the following?
    a. The client had fainted
    b. The client had dangerously high blood pressure
    c. The client had vomited excessively
    d. The client had blood in urine

3. An OT practitioner might use the term "turgor" when referring to which of the following in documentation?
    a. Cognition
    b. Muscle strength
    c. Skin elasticity
    d. Ambulation

4. Which of the following examples is a possible fit with using the term "perseveration" in documentation?
    a. A child with autism fixated on doing a non-productive task repeatedly
    b. A client perspiring excessively while performing therapy tasks
    c. A client living in poverty
    d. A child removed from unfit parents and placed in foster care

5. Echolalia refers to which of the following?
    a. A type of cardiac test
    b. Licking non-food objects or surfaces
    c. Repetition of speech
    d. Slow movements

6. A client on the behavioral health unit has an intense fear of getting sick and is unable to stop thinking about germs getting on his hands. Which of the following terms is suitable to use in documentation regarding this client?
    a. Self-injurious behavior
    b. Anhedonia
    c. Obsession
    d. Compulsion

Morreale, M. J. (2023). *The OTA's guide to documentation: Writing SOAP notes* (5th ed.). SLACK Incorporated.

7. In documentation, an OTA might use the term "midline orientation" when referring to which of the following?
   a. Ability to state person, place, and time accurately
   b. Psycho-social skills for waiting in line
   c. Vocational ability to work at a middle-manager level
   d. Ability to sit upright in wheelchair

8. The term "scotoma" relates to which of the following?
   a. Cancer
   b. Vision
   c. Hearing
   d. Skin lesion

9. Which of the following is a fit with determining if a client has crepitation?
   a. Measuring girth
   b. Passive range of motion
   c. Sensory assessment
   d. Pulse oximeter

10. A client with excessive cerumen might have challenges with which of the following?
    a. Coordination
    b. Acne
    c. Hearing
    d. Blood glucose levels

11. When a client reports a "pins and needles" sensation in the hand, an OTA might use which of the following terms in documentation?
    a. Paresthesia
    b. Ecchymosis
    c. Eructation
    d. Flatus

12. An emesis basin is more suitable to use for which of the following?
    a. Handwashing a piece of clothing
    b. Sponge bathing
    c. Feeding self with use of only one hand
    d. Vomiting

13. An OTA is reviewing a child's chart and reads that the child has a PEG tube. The OTA can expect that this is due to challenges with which of the following?
    a. Urinating
    b. Ear infections
    c. Respiration
    d. Eating

14. Which of the following is an example of what an OTA might expect to see in a client with documented anhedonia?
    a. Difficulty with speech
    b. Gagging or spitting out food
    c. Loss of pleasure
    d. Problems with memory

Morreale, M. J. (2023). *The OTA's guide to documentation: Writing SOAP notes* (5th ed.). SLACK Incorporated.

15. The term "hippotherapy" in an intervention plan refers to which of the following?
    a. Maintaining patient privacy
    b. Horseback riding program
    c. Instruction in total hip precautions
    d. Using hip-hop music for expression of feelings

16. An OTA sees that a child's intervention plan includes goals to improve finger to palm translation. Which of the following is a possible intervention for the OTA to choose to address this?
    a. Picking up marbles and moving them into same hand
    b. Stacking 1-inch cubes with one hand
    c. Holding an open book with both hands
    d. Using tweezers to pick up small objects embedded in sand

17. The OT intervention plan indicates that the client needs to be measured for a bariatric wheelchair. Which of the following would be a more suitable choice for this client?
    a. Ultralight wheelchair
    b. Sports wheelchair
    c. Geri-chair
    d. Oversized wheelchair

18. An OTA reviewing a client's chart reads that the client has a halo. The OTA should understand this to mean which of the following?
    a. The client needs stabilization of cervical spine
    b. The client has an implanted cardiac device
    c. The client uses a heel-ankle-leg orthosis
    d. The client uses a power mobility scooter

19. A client with dysphasia has challenges with which of the following?
    a. Eating
    b. Speaking
    c. Hearing
    d. Coordination

20. For a client diagnosed with presbycusis, which of the following is a fit as a possible choice to be included in the intervention plan?
    a. Magnifying glass
    b. Exercise bands
    c. Telephone relay service
    d. Memory aids

References

American Occupational Therapy Association. (2020). Occupational therapy practice framework: Domain and process (4th ed.). *American Journal of Occupational Therapy, 74*(Suppl. 2), 7412410010. https://doi.org: 10.5014/ajot.2020.74S2001

Gateley, C. A., & Borcherding, S. (2017). *Documentation manual for occupational therapy: Writing SOAP notes* (4th ed.). SLACK Incorporated.

Sames, K. M. (2015). *Documenting occupational therapy practice* (3rd ed.). Pearson Education, Inc.

Chapter 8

Tips for Writing a Better "O"

This chapter contains additional tips to improve your clinical reasoning and documentation skills. By incorporating these principles, your notes will appear more professional and complete, and you will be more likely to comply with third-party payer guidelines.

Focus on Function

Make certain that occupation is integral to the note. In an intervention session devoted to activities/occupations such as self-care or home management tasks, function is obvious. In other circumstances, **function must be addressed separately** in order to justify skilled occupational therapy. Interventions to support occupations, such as physical agent modalities (PAMs) or methods addressing client factors/skills (such as strength, range of motion, dexterity, balance, and endurance) all need function emphasized in the therapy note. For example, although the following note is an observation of a session that was devoted to client factors, it contains a statement about the functional intent of the exercises.

O: *Client worked on Ⓛ UE AROM and strengthening exercises 20 minutes at bedside **in order to regain ability to dress self**. Following skilled instruction, client performed self-ranging exercises sitting on EOB with standby Ⓐ for balance and verbal instructions to correct errors. Client was verbally cued 5 times to reach higher with Ⓛ UE during shoulder flexion AROM to attain range needed for **donning a pullover shirt**.*

Write From the Client's Point of View and Avoid Mentioning Yourself

The focus of good professional writing should be on the client and not the OTA. Turn your sentences around so that the client is the subject of your sentence.

Rather than saying: *The OTA put the client's shoes on for him.*
You might say: *Client Ⓓ in donning shoes.*
Rather than saying: *OTA instructed the client and family in energy conservation techniques for self-care.*
You might say: *Client and family were instructed in energy conservation techniques for self-care and demonstrated understanding by performing correctly.*

129

Morreale, M. J. *The OTA's Guide to Documentation:*
Writing SOAP Notes, Fifth Edition (pp. 129-150).
© 2023 Taylor & Francis Group.

Rather than saying:	*To compensate for low vision during bill-paying tasks, client was educated by OTA in use of a lighted tabletop 3X magnification lamp.*
You might say:	*To compensate for low vision during bill-paying tasks, client was educated in use of a lighted tabletop 3X magnification lamp.*
Rather than saying:	*The OTA told the client that, due to his unilateral neglect and spatial relations deficits, it would be unsafe for him to drive at this time.*
You might say:	*Client was educated that driving would be unsafe for him to do at this time because of his unilateral neglect and spatial relations deficits.*

Focus on the Client's Response to the Intervention Provided Rather Than on What the OTA Did

Rather than saying:	*Client was reminded about hip precautions.*
You might say:	*Attempting to don shoes, client required 3 verbal cues to keep hip in correct alignment.*
Rather than saying:	*Client was asked orientation questions pertaining to the time of day.*
You might say:	*When verbally cued to look at watch, client was unable to correctly identify time.*
Rather than saying:	*Client reminded to relax when interacting with sales clerk.*
You might say:	*When interacting with sales clerk, client exhibited signs of anxiety. She started to tremble, breathe rapidly, and required 2 verbal cues to relax.*
Rather than saying:	*Child was asked a series of yes/no questions.*
You might say:	*Child responded correctly to 2 out of 10 yes/no questions.*

De-Emphasize the Treatment Media

To improve a client's abilities for occupational performance and participation, OTAs often use various media, such as exercise equipment, worksheets, playthings, or other methods/tasks to help the client reach desired functional goals. When recording the use of such interventions to support occupations, an OTA uses skilled observations and professional reasoning to determine the relevant client factors, performance patterns, and skills to describe in documentation. As notes must reflect the skilled therapy that is happening, the OTA should de-emphasize the media used and focus instead on the areas being addressed that are working toward the client's established goals. For example, an inexperienced OTA might write the following:

Client worked on placing pegs into a pegboard.

This sentence may accurately describe what a casual observer would see. However, as a trained professional, the OTA needs to look beyond the media used and see what the client was really accomplishing. The treatment media used here are pegs and a pegboard, but what is the performance skill? Placing pegs into a pegboard is not a practical skill an adult needs in order to be able to care for oneself. However, the performance skill practiced during this activity may well be crucial to achieving independence. Suppose the OTA had written:

Client worked on tripod pinch using pegs and a pegboard.

Notice that in this example the OTA did not simply add the performance skill to the statement *"Client worked on placing pegs into a pegboard to increase tripod pinch"* but actually turned the sentence around so that the tripod pinch received the emphasis and the treatment media was mentioned only for clarification. Suppose that the OTA had written:

Client worked on tripod pinch in order to be able to grasp objects needed for ADL tasks.

In this case, mention of the media becomes optional. The OTA might also have written:

Client worked on tripod pinch using pegs and a pegboard in order to be able to grasp objects needed for ADL tasks.

Which of the three preceding examples do you think best describes the skilled occupational therapy instruction that is occurring in this intervention session? This may seem like a minor distinction, but it is very important in demonstrating the need for skilled occupational therapy and the emphasis on functional outcomes in therapy.

One of the most common errors that inexperienced OTAs make is focusing on the media used rather than on the performance skill that is being improved by use of the media. Consider this OTA's written observation, which could use some improvement:

Client seen 30 minutes in rehab gym for standing balance activities. Client stood to walker with min Ⓐ for balloon toss. Client used Ⓡ UE to hit balloon and was able to reach to Ⓡ and Ⓛ sides approximately 7 out of 10 tries. Activity was continued for 3 minutes. Client requested rest-break and sat for 30 seconds. Client then stood with mod Ⓐ to walker and hit balloon with Ⓛ UE for 3 minutes. Client was able to hit balloon approximately 6 out of 10 times and spontaneously switched to Ⓡ hand x2 when balloon was to her far right. Client sat for another break and to switch activities. Client stood CGA to toss beanbags with Ⓡ hand for 4 minutes. Client scored 240 points with Ⓡ hand by throwing beanbags at target. Once all beanbags were thrown, client sat for a 30-second break. Client stood with CGA for balance to toss beanbags with Ⓛ hand for 3½ minutes. Client scored 150 points with Ⓛ hand by throwing beanbags at scoring target. Once all beanbags were thrown, client sat and session was ended.

When this note is rewritten to focus on the performance skills instead, notice the significant difference in professionalism in the way the note reads:

Client engaged in 30-minute OT session in rehab gym to work on dynamic and static standing balance activities needed for ADL and IADL tasks. Pt. stood to walker with mod Ⓐ for dynamic standing balance necessary for Ⓘ showering using a balloon toss activity. Client held walker with Ⓛ hand and used Ⓡ UE to reach both Ⓡ and Ⓛ sides approximately 7/10 attempts. Client sustained activity for 3 minutes continuously, took a 30-second rest break, then stood to walker again with mod Ⓐ for 3 minutes of continuous activity involving weight shifting and balance required in balloon tossing. Client demonstrated ability to reach to Ⓡ and Ⓛ sides to reach for moving object approximately 6/10 times and was able to spontaneously shift weight 2 times to reach object. After taking 30-second rest break, client stood to walker for 4 more minutes of dynamic balance activity with CGA to perform beanbag toss activity with target. She sat for a 30-second rest, then stood again with CGA for 3½ minutes of continuous dynamic balance activity.

This note has now also indicated the relevant occupations that are being addressed as part of the client's intervention plan (ADL/showering and IADL tasks).

Make It Very Clear That You Were Not Just a Passive Observer in the Session

This will be a critical factor in reimbursement. OTAs do not get paid to just **watch** a client do something. To demonstrate that the skill of an occupational therapy practitioner is needed, you must be **actively involved** in intervention, such as providing client/family education; assessing safety, client factors, and skills; or modifying the activity. Otherwise, the intervention will be considered unskilled.

Rather than saying: *Client compensated for shoulder flexion by leaning forward with whole body during prehension activities.*

You might say: *Client required skilled instruction to avoid compensation at the shoulder during prehension activities.*

Rather than saying: *Client completed a worksheet on identifying road signs and got 4/10 correct.*

You might say: *To assess skills needed as a prerequisite for driving, client was asked to complete a worksheet on identifying road signs. Client only correctly identified 4/10 items, which is a safety concern for operating a motor vehicle.*

Rather than saying: *Client performed home exercise program.*

You might say: *Home exercise program was observed for accurate movement patterns and updated to accommodate for progress.*

Worksheet 8-1
De-Emphasizing the Treatment Media

Rewrite the following statements to concisely emphasize the skilled occupational therapy that is actually occurring in the intervention session.

1. Client played a game of catch using bilateral UEs to facilitate grasp and release patterns.

2. Resident put dirt into pot to halfway point, added seedling, and filled remainder of pot with dirt, which was transferred by cup. Resident completed three more pots while standing 8 minutes before requiring a 5-minute rest. Resident then resumed standing position for approximately 5 minutes to water completed pots.

3. Client painted some picture frames in crafts group to be able to see that she could do something successfully.

4. Child traced around a can to make a circle and then cut out the circle to work on his visual-motor skills. He also drew a face in the circle and glued it onto a paper bag to make a puppet.

Morreale, M. J. (2023). *The OTA's guide to documentation: Writing SOAP notes* (5th ed.). SLACK Incorporated.

Although You Will Assess the Information You Observed and Make a Professional Judgment About It, Avoid Judging the Client

Rather than saying: *Client was compliant.*
                         —or—
                         Client was cooperative.

You might say: *Client demonstrated ability to follow 3-step directions and sequence WFL.*

Rather than saying: *Child was difficult to treat today because she did not want to use a built-up spoon for self-feeding.*

You might say: *Child required four verbal prompts to pick up and use built-up spoon to begin self-feeding.*

Rather than saying: *Resident has a very negative attitude about therapy and poor attendance.*

You might say: *Resident refused therapy 3 out of 5 days this week.*

Rather than saying: *Child is fat.*

You might say: *Luca weighs 110 lb. and is in 95th percentile for BMI.*

When working with a client who exhibits peculiar or difficult personality traits, behavior, or whose opinions or values you do not agree with, it is easy to judge the client and to reflect your judgments in the "O." However, you must be careful to maintain your professional attitude and avoid personal or emotional bias. The following is an example of a note written by an OTA who was experiencing a difficult client situation. The client "went off on" the OTA. The client refused to get out of bed, lied about having already performed grooming tasks, threw her toothpaste on the floor, refused to brush her teeth or comb her hair, and cursed at the OTA. In spite of all of this, the OTA wrote this part of the "O" that was nonjudgmental of the client:

Client initially declined therapy several times, but after 5 minutes of encouragement, agreed to participate. Client demonstrated Ⓘ supine → sit on EOB with good dynamic sitting balance to perform grooming. Client exhibited frustration regarding her condition by saying several profane words and throwing an item on floor. Following skilled instruction, client demonstrated ability to use reacher Ⓘ to retrieve toothpaste tube from floor. Client was issued non-slip matting to stabilize grooming items on bedside table and client verbalized, "I don't want to do this" 3 times, while keeping her eyes closed.

Indicate Client/Family Understanding

If you are instructing the client or family/significant others in a home program of exercises, transfers, positioning, methods of self-care, or other procedures, it is important to document this in the record. Note the kinds of education and practice provided and the specific recommendations or methods you are asking the client or others to follow-through with at home. Your documentation in the health record should also indicate that the client/family *demonstrated understanding* such as via *return demonstration* (Scott, 2013). As appropriate, document that the task was observed and that the client or caregiver demonstrated *ability to perform task safely, accurately,* or *adhered to all medical precautions, followed all procedures or steps correctly,* etc. However, if specific challenges are evident with the client/family learning and performing the particular task properly, this should be noted in the chart and followed-up with additional education and practice. A copy of the written home program or instructions given to the client/family (such as specific exercises, transfer procedures, use/care of orthotic device, list of recommended equipment, etc.) should be placed in the chart. The instructions should also include any precautions (such as if pain or swelling might occur) and a method of follow-up (Fairchild et al., 2018; Scott, 2013). The following are some examples that demonstrate client/family understanding:

- *Caregiver demonstrated ability to transfer client safely from wheelchair ↔ toilet using proper body mechanics and proper cueing.*
- *Following skilled instruction, child's mother demonstrated ability to position child properly for safe feeding and verbalized understanding of aspiration precautions.*
- *Client was instructed in a home program of therapy putty exercises and precautions. Following instruction, client demonstrated all exercises accurately. Written copy of exercises provided.*

- *Client was instructed in energy conservation for IADLs and provided with written instructions. She demonstrated ability to incorporate these energy-saving techniques during laundry activity.*
- *Client was instructed in use and care of resting hand orthosis and precautions. He demonstrated ability to don/doff orthosis independently and verbalized understanding of wearing schedule and how to check skin. Written instructions provided.*
- *Client able to recall 3/3 total hip precautions when asked. She demonstrated ability to adhere to all hip precautions while dressing lower body using adaptive equipment.*

Be Specific About Assist Levels

Note what specific aspect of the activity the client needed assistance or cues to perform. For example:
- *Veteran doffed night garment with min Ⓐ **to untie strings on back.***
- *Pt. able to sequence steps to prepare cup of tea but required verbal cue **to turn off stove.***
- *Child needed hand-over-hand assist **for accuracy** when cutting with scissors.*
- *Client required two verbal cues **to sit down** in order to doff hosiery.*
- *Consumer able to follow bus schedule with min verbal cues **to identify correct time.***
- *Patient stand → w/c using a standard walker with CGA and min verbal cues **to bring walker completely back to w/c.***
- *Infant able to roll supine to prone with min tactile cues at hip **to initiate movement.***
- *Client required mod Ⓐ **to follow total hip precautions** while using long-handled sponge for washing lower legs and feet.*
- *Student required min verbal cues **to recall the numbers** needed to open combination lock on locker.*

Describe the exact *type* and *amount* of assistance that the client needed. It is essential that you note both the **type** of assistance and **how much** assistance the client needed to perform the activity. Box 8-1 delineates various standard levels of assistance. For example, writing *"Henry required assistance to don upper and lower body garments,"* does not give someone reading your note the full picture. Did the client require minimal assistance, moderate assistance, or maximal assistance? Perhaps the client was able to perform the task but needed contact guard or stand-by assistance for balance or safety. Did the client require hand-over-hand assistance to hold an item or move an extremity to complete the task effectively? Was help needed to line up buttons or manage fastenings? Were verbal cues needed to maintain attention, upright posture, or determine front/back of clothing? Did the client use compensatory methods or any adaptive devices? Were safety concerns or problems apparent with performance skills, client factors, or performance patterns? Also, be sure to indicate that the client **needed** assist rather than labeling the client **as** an assist level. For example, state *"Client **required** min assist for standing balance when shaving at sink,"* rather than *"Client was min assist for standing balance when shaving at sink."*
- *Resident needed max Ⓐ X 2 to stand and pivot when transferring from w/c to bed.*
- *Child required intermittent tactile cues at hip and upper torso to maintain upright posture for 10 minutes when seated at desk.*
- *Toddler required hand-over-hand assist to hold and push toy vacuum with Ⓡ hand.*
- *Client required SBA for balance when standing to pull up and fasten pants.*
- *Patient required mod Ⓐ to stabilize Ⓛ elbow in extended position for Ⓛ UE weight bearing while shaving at sink.*
- *Client required min Ⓐ to place sock on sock aid and then mod Ⓐ to position device properly and pull up sock on Ⓡ LE.*
- *Student needed contact guard assist for dynamic balance when standing up from wheelchair to write on blackboard for 1 minute.*

Box 8-1	
LEVELS OF ASSISTANCE	
Total assistance (TOT)	Individual requires 100% assistance to safely complete task. Individual does not assist at all.
Maximum assistance (MAX)	Individual requires 75% of physical/cognitive assistance to safely complete task. Individual assists 25%.
Moderate assistance (MOD)	Individual requires 50% of physical/cognitive assistance to safely complete task. Individual assists 50%.
Minimal assistance (MIN)	Individual needs no more than 25% physical/cognitive assistance. Individual assists 75%.
Standby assistance (SBA)	Supervision or standby assistance for safe, effective task performance.
Set-up assistance	Individual requires set-up of necessary items to perform tasks.
Independent (IND)	No assistance or supervision is required. Able to perform independently. Safety is demonstrated during tasks.
Reproduced with permission from Jacobs, K., & Simon, L. (Eds.). (2020). *Quick reference dictionary for occupational therapy* (7th ed.). SLACK Incorporated.	

If supervision was needed due to particular safety concerns, mental health issues, or cognitive impairment, you should clearly indicate the reason and level of supervision needed. Did the client require distant supervision within line of sight or, perhaps, just occasional monitoring such as when interacting with peers or completing a self-care or home management activity, worksheet, project, etc.? Maybe, instead, the client required close supervision within arm's length for problem solving, sequencing, or safety when using sharps, hazardous materials or cooking appliances. Did the client require any cues? If so, how many cues and what kind—physical, verbal, auditory, or visual?

- *Student required verbal cues approximately every 30 seconds to attend to task when copying 10 vocabulary words from blackboard.*
- *Client required close supervision for use of sharps during crafts group.*
- *Resident required a visual cue (red line) in order to locate all of the words on the left side of the page.*
- *Student required line-of-sight supervision during recess in order to monitor his tendency to fight with peers.*
- *Resident required three verbal cues for proper hand placement when transferring bed ↔ commode.*
- *Client required five verbal cues in order to verbalize two positive statements about herself.*
- *Patient required close supervision for safe handling of hot foods when cooking.*
- *Client needed a timer in order to take a shower and wash hair in < 15 minutes.*
- *Child required close supervision to avoid putting objects in mouth when making a macaroni necklace.*
- *Child needed three verbal cues to line up buttons correctly when donning shirt.*
- *Charlotte required use of a checklist with pictures to ensure she brought all necessary items back home from school.*

HELPFUL HINT

Chapter 3, Section GG of the *Centers for Medicare & Medicaid Services Long-Term Care Facility Resident Assessment Instrument 3.0 User's Manual: Version 1.17.1* (CMS, 2019) presents an easy-to-understand method of assessing adult clients' functional abilities. The manual can be viewed online and contains many client examples plus clear explanations of what to look for in determining levels of assistance for specific self-care tasks, mobility, and other areas. Although this guide is designed for assessing nursing home residents and documenting applicable codes as part of the mandated Resident Assessment Instrument process, the concepts presented are still very useful to consider while you are learning activity analysis and documentation.

In trying to be concise, sometimes inexperienced OTAs make the mistake of writing an "O" that contains only a list of actions with assist levels. Although this is a common error, it is **incorrect**. Simply writing a list of activities or assist levels does not demonstrate that skilled OT is being provided. Consider this OTA's observation:

Client was seen for 1 hour in the shower room to ↑ activity tolerance and improve balance.

Client OX4.

Client min Ⓐ with verbal cues to sit in w/c to doff hosiery and to dry off LE.

Client spontaneously rinsed soap off hands before gripping grab bar while showering.

Client used walker going to and coming from shower room.

Client tolerated standing Ⓘ during entire shower.

Discussed home showering.

Client will be discharged in 1 week.

Now look at the same observation rewritten in a more useful, professional format to reflect skilled occupational therapy:

Client participated in 1-hour ADL session in the shower room to ↑ activity tolerance and improve balance during showering in order to prepare her for Ⓘ and safe showering after expected discharge in 1 week.

Mobility: *Pt. ambulated to/from shower room Ⓘ and safely with the aid of a standard walker to provide stability in shower room while dressing/undressing.*

Cognition: *Client oriented X 4.*

ADLs: *Client needed min Ⓐ and two verbal cues to sit down in order to doff hosiery and to dry LEs safely. During shower, client spontaneously rinsed soap off hands prior to gripping grab bar without needing verbal cues. Client tolerated standing Ⓘ ~5 minutes during shower without SOB. Skilled instruction provided in safe technique to use in her home shower stall and recommendations given re: grab bar placement.*

Table 8-1 provides suggestions for documenting client transfers accurately and professionally in the "O" part of your SOAP notes. Complete Worksheet 8-2 to practice being specific about assist levels.

Table 8-1	
Documenting Transfers	
Steps for Documenting Transfers	*Examples*
1. Specify the occupational therapy skill provided during the transfer.	Assessment of transfer technique Assessment of DME needs Transfer training Client education Instruction in use of tub bench, commode, etc. Instruction in compensatory techniques Instruction in weightbearing/medical precautions Family/caregiver education Safety training Increase activity tolerance
2. Relate to occupational performance and differentiate from other disciplines, such as physical therapy.	… transfer training in order to bathe ① using tub bench … instruction in compensatory transfer techniques in order to adhere to total hip precautions when toileting … instruction in safe techniques for car transfers
3. Specify the surface from which the client began the transfer.	**From:** Standing position Toilet (high or low) Standing with walker (type) Commode Edge of bed Stool Wheelchair (type) Chair (with or without arms, low or high, wheeled) Geri chair Therapy mat Sofa Tub bench Floor Shower chair Car Bathtub Classroom desk Shower stall
4. Specify the surface to which the client transferred.	**To:** (same as above)
5. List any assistive devices, adaptive techniques, or environmental modifications utilized.	**Using:** Bed rails Rolling walker Trapeze Quad cane Grab bar Cane Raised toilet seat Sliding board Commode frame over toilet Mechanical lift Standard walker Holding onto furniture, counter, sink, etc.
6. List the type and amount of physical and verbal assistance required.	Level of physical assist (e.g., mod, max) Number of persons assisting (x1, x2) Amount of verbal, visual, or tactile cues
7. List the part of the task that required assistance.	… to lock w/c brakes … for redirection to task … to remove lap tray … to scoot to the edge of the bed, w/c, etc. … to adhere to total hip precautions … for balance … to promote weight shift … to flex trunk/lean forward … to prevent knee from buckling … to position lower extremities … to stabilize lower extremity … to position walker, sliding board, etc. … to push up from sitting … for hand placement … to control pacing when returning to sit … for sequence of steps … to manage IV pole … to manage catheter bag
8. Other considerations, if not already noted	Stable versus unstable surface Vital signs/medical considerations such as oxygen level, blood pressure, pulse, telemetry, IV lines, catheter bag, etc. Cognition (e.g., attention, problem solving) Specific safety concerns/ impulsivity Ability to remember and adhere to weight bearing or other precautions Fear or anxiety Endurance/shortness of breath Understanding of process Demonstration required Carryover of technique Number of trials

Worksheet 8-2
Being Specific About Assist Levels

When noting assist levels in your observation, it is not enough to note only the level of assistance required. You must also note the **specific aspect** of the task that required assistance and the **type and amount** of assistance provided. For example:

- *Resident donned pants* **with min Ⓐ to pull up over hips.**
- *Student will be able to operate joystick on power wheelchair Ⓘ* **using 2-lb wrist weight to minimize Ⓡ UE tremors.**
- *When observed for proper technique, foster parent required* **four verbal cues to feed infant more slowly** *in order to promote better swallowing of puréed foods.*
- *Client propelled w/c from hospital room to OT clinic but required* **mod verbal cues to avoid bumping into other clients.**

Rewrite the statements below to indicate a **part** of the task that required assistance. Since you have not seen the client, you cannot really know what part actually required assistance. In the usual world of professional behavior, fabricating information is fraud, so please realize that the client you are about to imagine is just a creative exercise for learning purposes. For this exercise, you will create a client in your mind and imagine that client performing the task. As you watch your client in your mind, note what aspect of the task required assistance and modify the statements below accordingly to make them more specific.

1. Client supine → sit with min Ⓐ; bed → w/c with mod Ⓐ.

2. Client required SBA in transferring w/c ↔ toilet.

3. Client retrieved garments from low drawers with min Ⓐ.

4. Brushing hair required max Ⓐ.

5. Client completed dressing, toileting, and hygiene with min assist.

Use Standardized Terminology to Describe and Grade Your Treatment Activities

It is very important to qualify and quantify the complexity level of the activities that your clients engage in. Consider the various activity demands to determine and document how your interventions are graded and adapted. Often, even a very basic task has gradable components. For example, when putting on footwear, the activity requirements are easier for donning slip-on shoes rather than tall boots or shoes that require tying laces or fastening buckles. Or, perhaps, the client uses shoes with adaptations such as hook and loop closures or elastic laces instead. Pants with elastic waistbands are generally easier to don than tight leggings or pants that have buttons and zippers to fasten. For upper body garments, note if the client is donning a short or long-sleeved button-down shirt or a pullover shirt. For bras, indicate front closure, back closure, or pullover style. In your documentation, try to be as specific as possible with the activity demands of the task you are addressing. For an observation noted as *Client required assistance to don upper and lower body garments,* it would be better to further clarify and say:

While sitting on EOB, client required min Ⓐ and three verbal cues to place elastic waist pants over weak lower extremity with use of reacher. Client donned slip-on shoes with supervision and verbal cue for task initiation. CGA required for balance to stand, pull up pants, then sit back down. Client donned front closure bra with min Ⓐ to fasten, then donned pullover sweater with verbal cue needed to identify front/back of sweater.

As another example, consider a home management task such as preparing lunch. Instead of saying, *Client SBA in preparing lunch,* it would be much better to describe the type or complexity of lunch that the client prepared, such as:

Meal preparation skills assessed. Client required SBA to prepare a simple one-step microwave frozen meal. Client able to read and follow package directions, open package, and program time correctly but required two verbal cues to use potholder for safe handling of hot food.

Table 8-2 presents some suggestions and examples for grading and describing levels of meal preparation tasks for documentation. Depending on the situation, you may come up with other categories or methods of grading. OTs and OTAs use professional reasoning to assesses how a specific activity's requirements relate to a particular individual's condition and circumstances. For example, cooking bacon can be challenging for a client with a hand injury due to the physical requirements involved (i.e., opening the package, separating and placing slices in pan) yet challenging in a very different way for an individual with intellectual disability (i.e., safety concerns for cooking at stove, problem-solving what to do with grease, time management). For each meal preparation task that your client performs, use activity analysis to think about all the activity demands involved, such as sequence and number of steps required, overall level of complexity, specific performance skills and client factors needed. Note if the task involves safety considerations (such as open flames or heat, use of electric appliances or sharp objects); sequencing, problem-solving, and organizational skills; reading directions or interpreting pictures or diagrams; opening packages; measuring; using specific cooking utensils or appliances; clean up and time management; etc.

Table 8-2

Examples of Graded Meal Preparation Tasks (Easier to Harder)

- Obtain a snack (granola bar, chips/crackers from upper/lower cabinet, get yogurt, precut cheese or fruit from refrigerator)
- Simple cold meal preparation (cereal and milk, bologna sandwich)
- Cold meal preparation involving safety/small appliance use (blender, electric can opener) or sharp utensils (knives, grater, peeler) and note number of steps (simple salad, smoothie, canned tuna)
- Task using heat appliances such as toaster, air fryer, toaster oven, or microwave (toast, frozen entree, pizza, waffles, or fries). Note number of steps.
- Simple stovetop task/one to two steps (tea, heat can of soup). Note electric or gas stove.
- Min complex stovetop task with simple, multiple steps (grilled cheese, pudding, scrambled eggs). Note electric or gas stove.
- Mod complex stovetop task/follow multi-step directions (tacos, macaroni and cheese). Note electric or gas stove and relevant objects/methods used.
- Complex meal preparation (following a recipe; two-, three-, four-course meal). Note appliances, methods, and relevant objects used.

You can apply these principles to other activities/occupations, such as home management tasks. Consider the activity demands of light household chores (folding towels, wiping a table, dusting) vs. heavy household chores (mopping a floor, washing windows, changing sheets). Also, if the client uses an ambulation device or wheelchair for mobility or safety during functional tasks, the specific type of mobility aid should be noted. While not an all-inclusive list, various types of mobility devices include:

- Crutches
- Single-point cane
- Quad cane (small/narrow base or large/wide base)
- Hemi-walker
- Standard walker
- Wheeled walker
- Rollator
- Platform walker
- Standard wheelchair
- Power wheelchair
- Bariatric wheelchair
- Sip and puff wheelchair
- Power mobility scooter
- Power mobility chair

Remember that as an OTA, you are not issuing ambulation devices or simply instructing the client in ambulation or gait training. That is most likely considered physical therapy and would be duplication of services or possibly beyond your scope of practice. Rather, in occupational therapy, your focus is on **safe functional mobility for specific occupational tasks**. You might say:

- *Resident required min Ⓐ to get clothes out of closet while standing with wheeled walker.*
- *Using crutches, student required min verbal cues and CGA to stand and use reacher to obtain items on bottom of locker.*
- *Child was able to safely use platform walker to navigate in bathroom, transfer on/off toilet, and stand to manage clothing for toilet hygiene.*
- *Client needed CGA for balance to stand with small-base quad cane and load dishwasher.*
- *To perform job as a discount store greeter, client demonstrates ability to navigate all public areas of store Ⓘ using power wheelchair with joystick and tilt-in-space-feature.*

Document Use of Physical Agent Modalities Properly

OTs and OTAs often use PAMs as a means to improve client factors and conditions for occupational participation. When used appropriately, PAMs can aid in decreasing pain and edema, increasing passive and active ROM, and promoting wound healing. However, the American Occupational Therapy Association (AOTA) asserts that a PAM is not considered to be occupational therapy unless linked specifically to occupational performance and incorporated into a more comprehensive intervention program (AOTA, 2018). Therefore, it is important to document how **the PAM prepares or enables the client to perform specific functional tasks**. In addition, since another OT or OTA might be treating the client in your absence, it is necessary to document the proper parameters for the modality to ensure accuracy, safety, and consistent follow through. The OT determines which PAMs are appropriate for the client's intervention plan and supervises any modalities that the OTA administers (AOTA, 2018). It is important to realize that various states may have strict rules or restrictions regarding the use of PAMs by OTs or OTAs. It is essential that occupational therapy practitioners who supervise or administer PAMs have service competency, follow ethical guidelines, and always adhere to state and federal regulations (AOTA, 2018). Use Table 8-3 as a guide when documenting the use of PAMs.

Table 8-3
Documenting Physical Agent Modalities
Physical Agent Modality Checklist for Documentation
Part and place: Indicate where modality was applied on the body (e.g., right shoulder, left dorsal wrist). **Parameters:** Note settings such as time, temperature, intensity, etc. **Positioning considerations:** Note any special position of client or extremity (e.g., limb placed in a stretched position, digits wrapped in flexion, active exercise while modality applied) **Purpose/preparation:** Specify the client factor, condition, or therapeutic goal that is being addressed (e.g., pain relief, ROM, wound healing, scar or edema management). **Performance of activities/occupations**: Relate use of the PAM to occupational participation. **Problems/progress:** Describe client tolerance/response to the intervention, any modifications required, and any progress or problems pertaining to the modality.

Here are some examples for recording the use of PAMs:

- *Hot pack applied 20 minutes to Ⓡ wrist to ↓ pain and stiffness to enable performance of kitchen tasks (i.e., lifting pots, cutting vegetables). Wrist placed in flexed position for stretch and client's skin checked at 5 minutes and upon removal of hot pack with no problems noted. Client stated that her wrist "feels much looser after the heat." Client was instructed in use of an ergonomic knife to chop vegetables. She demonstrated ability to lift and carry a small pan containing 2 cups of water for a distance of 6 feet without report of pain.*

- *US applied to Ⓛ shoulder to reduce pain and ↑ AROM to enable return to work. Continuous ultrasound applied 5 minutes at 1 MHz and 1.5 W/cm² with client supine. Pt. then stood and worked on pulleys and job simulation task of stacking 1- and 2-lb. cans on shelves with Ⓛ UE. Pt. demonstrated ability to flex Ⓛ shoulder 158° and stack 30 cans without report of pain. Pt. also demonstrated ability to lift and carry 10-lb grocery bag 10 feet X 4.*

- *Fluidotherapy applied 110° for 15 minutes to Ⓛ wrist and hand to ↑ grasp and release for precision tool use. During Fluidotherapy treatment client performed wrist and hand AROM exercises. Client then worked on job-related tasks and successfully used needle nose pliers with Ⓛ hand to bend 18 gauge wire and also place 10 nails in wood for hammering.*

HELPFUL HINT

Good documentation is based on accurate observation, which is based on knowing what to look for. For an experienced professional, this becomes second nature. For an OTA student, it is helpful to review the lists in this manual and to check your observations against what your supervising OT or OTA observed during the intervention session to be sure you are noticing the items that matter most.

Conclusion

Tables 8-4 and 8-5 present many suggestions for documenting dressing and bathing interventions. Using these Tables as a guide, complete Learning Activity 8-1 to practice your clinical reasoning and documentation skills for the "O" part of your note. In the "O" section, it is extremely important that you focus on function, de-emphasize the treatment media, and make it clear that skilled occupational therapy services were provided. Observe and determine the client's performance skills, patterns, and client factors without judging the individual. Succinctly and accurately describe the complexity level and specific activity demands that your interventions entail, along with the amount and type of assistance needed. The next chapter will address the third section of the SOAP note: the assessment.

Table 8-4	
Documenting Dressing Interventions	
Steps for Documenting Dressing	*Examples*
1. Specify the occupational therapy skill provided during the dressing activity/occupation.	Assessment of dressing skills Self-care training ADL reeducation Family/caregiver education Provide recommendations to teacher/teacher's aide Instruction in use of adaptive equipment/DME Instruction in compensatory dressing techniques Instruction in medical precautions (i.e., due to ventricular assist device, hip replacement surgery, lower extremity weight-bearing status, external fixator, catheter) Establish a routine for dressing Instruction in one-handed dressing techniques Safety training/improve safety awareness Increase activity tolerance for ADL Instruction in proper pacing and breathing
2. Relate to occupational performance and differentiate from other disciplines, such as nursing.	… in order to manage clothing during toileting … in order to doff clothing for bathing … in order to change for gym class … in order to don outerwear for recess … in order to adhere to total hip precautions when donning lower body garments … in order to protect ventricular assist drive line when getting dressed … in order to don uniform for work … to reestablish a dressing routine … to choose clothing appropriate for work/social occasions/leisure … for safe positioning of infant during dressing
3. Specify the particular garments donned/doffed and note specific type of fastenings if applicable (i.e., buttons, snaps, zipper, Velcro closure, laces, buckles). Include size and number of fastenings as appropriate (i.e., six ½ inch buttons on shirt, 12-inch zipper on back of dress).	Type of shirt (i.e., long-sleeve button-down dress shirt, pullover sweater, turtleneck sweater, short-sleeve polo shirt, tank top) Pants (i.e., jeans, slacks, elastic waist pants, sweatpants, shorts, leggings, sports pants with leg snaps, etc.) Bra (i.e., front closure, back closure, pullover) Underwear (i.e., boxers, briefs, panties, undershirt, tank top, girdle, body shaper, slip, camisole, onesie) Dress/skirt (i.e., mini, maxi) Sleepwear (i.e., long/short nightgown, long/short pajamas, footed pajamas, long/short bathrobe) Hosiery (i.e., anti-embolism stockings, athletic socks, pantyhose/stockings, knee-high socks) Footwear (i.e., loafers/slip-on shoes, dress shoes with laces or buckles, boots, sneakers [with or without laces, Velcro closure], clogs, sandals, slippers, cleats, ballet shoes) Blazer, sports coat, jacket, cardigan sweater Outerwear (i.e., raincoat, sweatshirt/hoodie, winter coat, fleece jacket, shawl, gloves, mittens, scarf, hat) Accessories (i.e., tie, bowtie, suspenders, belt, hat, apron, scarf, shawl, vest, sash, hat, visor) Work/school uniform or lab coat Sports uniform/equipment (i.e., athletic supporter, helmet, padding, karate belt, bathing suit, ice skates) Cultural considerations (i.e., sari, turban, veil, prayer shawl, fringes, hijab, yarmulke, burqa, robe)

(continued)

	Table 8-4 (continued) # Documenting Dressing Interventions	
Steps for Documenting Dressing	*Examples*	
4. Specify the surface from which the client is performing the dressing activity.	While seated on … While standing (using walker, cane, holding onto counter, etc.) Sitting on edge of bed Lying in bed (supine or degrees the head of bed is raised) Sitting in wheelchair (type) Sitting on a chair (with/without arms) Sitting on commode/toilet (high or low) Sitting on tub bench/shower chair Sitting on therapy mat Sitting on locker room bench	
5. List any assistive devices or adaptive techniques utilized.	**Using:** Reacher Button hook Long-handle shoehorn Dressing stick Sock aid Leg lifter Elastic laces Zipper pull	Over-the-head method to don coat One-handed dressing techniques One-handed shoe-tying technique Velcro closures One size bigger clothing Loops inside pants Rolling side to side Weight shifting while seated in wheelchair
6. Include any mobility devices, postural supports, or environmental modifications needed to stand and adjust clothing.	Holding onto grab bar Holding onto commode frame over toilet Holding onto furniture, counter, sink, wheelchair, pole, wall, etc.	Using standard walker Using wheeled walker Using quad cane Using single point cane Using crutches
7. List the type and amount of physical and verbal assistance required.	Level of physical assist (e.g., mod, max) Number of persons assisting (x1, x2) Amount of verbal, visual, or tactile cues Set-up needed	
8. List the part of the task that required assistance.	… to stand and pull up clothing … to place affected arm in sleeve … to bring shirt/coat around back … to pull up boots or socks … to fasten buckle on sandals … to line up buttons … to begin zipper on jacket … to place underwear and slacks over feet … to place sock on sock aid … to manage fastenings … to flex trunk/lean forward … to position lower extremities … to position walker, cane, etc. … to adhere to total hip precautions … to avoid range of motion of affected shoulder post-surgery … to avoid kinking of ventricular assist drive line … to avoid pulling on nasogastric tube … to avoid tension on catheter or IV line … to manage IV pole	

(continued)

Table 8-4 (continued)	
Documenting Dressing Interventions	
Steps for Documenting Dressing	*Examples*
	… to manage catheter bag
	… to reapply sling/orthosis
	… to initiate getting dressed
	… for sequence of steps
	… for redirection to task
	… to orient garment properly
	… to differentiate front/back of garment
	… to turn clothing right side out
	… to choose clothing appropriate for weather/occasion/activity
	… to differentiate right/left sock, slipper, or shoe
	… to incorporate proper breathing techniques
	… to control pacing
	… to promote weight shift
	… to prevent knee from buckling
	… to stabilize lower extremity
	… to push up from sitting
	… to maintain sitting/standing balance
9. Other considerations if not already noted	Stable versus unstable surface
	Cognition (e.g., attention, sequencing, problem solving)
	Specific safety concerns/impulsivity
	Ability to remember and adhere to weight-bearing or other precautions
	Vital signs/medical considerations, such as oxygen level, blood pressure, pulse, telemetry, IV lines, catheter, etc.
	Fear or anxiety
	Endurance/shortness of breath
	Understanding of process
	Demonstration required
	Carryover of technique
	Number of trials
	Time management

Table 8-5
Documenting Bathing Interventions

Steps for Documenting Bathing	Examples
1. Specify the occupational therapy skill provided during the bathing activity/occupation.	Assessment of bathing skills Self-care training ADL reeducation Improve hygiene skills Teach basic hygiene skills Family/caregiver education Instruction in use of adaptive equipment/DME Instruction in compensatory techniques for lower body bathing Instruction in medical precautions (i.e., due to ventricular assist device, hip replacement surgery, lower extremity weight-bearing status, external fixator, catheter) Instruction in one-handed bathing techniques Improve safety awareness/safety training Instruction in grab bar placement Increase activity tolerance for ADL Instruction in proper pacing and breathing during self-care/bathing Improve time management/organizational skills for self-care/bathing
2. Relate to occupational performance and differentiate from other disciplines such as nursing.	… in order to bathe independently using … (tub bench, shower chair, roll-in shower commode, etc.) … in order to adhere to total hip precautions when bathing lower body … instruction in safety for showering … in order to protect ventricular assist drive line when bathing … to improve time management when showering in locker room … to improve organizational skills when gathering items needed for bathing … to increase activity tolerance for bathing … to develop/reestablish a bathing routine … to develop/improve hygiene skills needed for work/school/interacting with peers … to position infant/child safely for bathing
3. Specify the surface from which the client is performing bathing/showering/sponge-bathing. Indicate shower stall or tub (height), shower curtain, shower doors, built in shower seat, etc.	Standing at sink Seated in chair/wheelchair at sink Seated on edge of bed using bedside table Sitting in bed using bedside table Seated in wheelchair (type) Seated on tub bench Sitting on shower chair Seated on roll-in shower commode/chair Sitting in bathtub Standing in shower stall Seated on commode/toilet

(continued)

Table 8-5 (continued)	
Documenting Bathing Interventions	
Steps for Documenting Bathing	*Examples*
4. List methods and any assistive devices, DME, or adaptive techniques utilized.	**Using:** Washcloth/loofah/shower puff Bar of soap/soap-on-a-rope/shower gel Grab bar Non-slip tub mat Transfer tub bench Shower chair (with or without back) Roll-in shower chair/commode Commode frame over toilet Mobility devices used for transfer (i.e., wheeled walker, cane, sliding board) Long-handle sponge Wash mitt Hand-held shower hose Soap/shampoo dispenser Leg lifter One-handed compensatory bathing techniques Timer Thermometer to check water temperature Reacher
5. List the type and amount of physical and verbal assistance required.	Level of physical assist (e.g., mod, max) Number of persons assisting (x1, x2) Amount of verbal, visual, or tactile cues Set-up needed
6. List the part of the task that required assistance.	… to lock w/c brakes before transfer … to position walker, cane, etc. … to hold onto grab bar … to open/close shower curtain/doors … to open/close faucet … to hold onto shower hose … to operate controls on shower hose … to regulate water temperature … to open shampoo bottle … to apply proper amount of shampoo/shower gel/etc. … to rinse hair/body thoroughly … to wash/dry back and/or feet … to bring towel around back … to flex trunk/lean forward … to lift lower extremities over edge of tub … to wash perineal area … to adhere to total hip precautions … to avoid range of motion of affected shoulder post-surgery … to avoid kinking of ventricular assist drive line … to avoid getting a particular body part/device wet (sutures, wound covering, cast, external fixator, etc.) … to cover cast/incision with a plastic bag … for sequence of steps … to wash body part (i.e., back, feet, left side of face/trunk) … for redirection to task … for thoroughness

(continued)

Table 8-5 (continued) Documenting Bathing Interventions	
Steps for Documenting Bathing	*Examples*
	… to incorporate proper breathing techniques … to control pacing … to complete showering within 10 minutes … to promote weight shift … to push up from sitting … to gather items needed for bathing … to place towel within reach … to maintain sitting balance
7. Other considerations if not already noted	Cognition (e.g., attention, sequencing, problem solving) Specific safety concerns/impulsivity Ability to remember and adhere to weight-bearing or other precautions Vital signs/medical considerations, such as oxygen level, blood pressure, pulse, telemetry, IV lines, catheter, etc. Fear or anxiety Endurance/shortness of breath Understanding of process Demonstration required Carryover of technique Number of trials Time management

Learning Activity 8-1: Documenting Feeding Interventions

This exercise will give you the opportunity to practice your clinical reasoning and documentation skills. Fill in the right-side column below with a variety of possible answers related to feeding. Examples are provided for each category.

Steps for Documenting Feeding	List Possible Skilled Interventions and Observations
1. Specify the occupational therapy skill provided during the feeding activity/ occupation.	**Skilled service provided:** • *ADL retraining* 1. 6. 2. 7. 3. 8. 4. 9. 5. 10.
2. Relate to occupational performance and differentiate from other disciplines such as nursing.	**Relate why:** • *… in order to feed self with modified independence using adaptive equipment* 1. 6. 2. 7. 3. 8. 4. 9. 5. 10.
3. Specify the position and surface from which the client is performing feeding.	**Where:** • *Sitting in bed with head of bed fully raised* 1. 6. 2. 7. 3. 8. 4. 9. 5. 10.
4. List methods and any assistive devices or adaptive techniques utilized.	**Using:** • *Universal cuff* 1. 6. 2. 7. 3. 8. 4. 9. 5. 10.

Steps for Documenting Feeding	List Possible Skilled Interventions and Observations	
5. List the type and amount of physical and verbal assistance required.	**Level of assist needed:** • *Level of physical assist* • *Amount of verbal, visual, or tactile cues* • *Type of set-up needed*	
	1.	6.
	2.	7.
	3.	8.
	4.	9.
	5.	10.
6. List the part of the task that required assistance.	**Aspect of task:** • *... to scoop food onto spoon*	
	1.	6.
	2.	7.
	3.	8.
	4.	9.
	5.	10.
7. Other considerations if not already noted	**Other considerations:** • *Cognition (e.g., attention, sequencing, problem solving)*	
	1.	6.
	2.	7.
	3.	8.
	4.	9.
	5.	10.

References

American Occupational Therapy Association. (2018). Physical agents and mechanical modalities. *American Journal of Occupational Therapy, 72*(Suppl. 2), 7212410055. https://doi.org/ 10.5014/ajot.2018.72S220

Centers for Medicare & Medicaid Services. (2019). *Long-Term Care Facility Resident Assessment Instrument 3.0 user's manual: Version 1.17.1* (Chapter 3). Retrieved October 21, 2021 from https://downloads.cms.gov/files/mds-3.0-rai-manual-v1.17.1_october_2019.pdf

Fairchild, S. L., O'Shea, R. K., & Washington, R. D. (2018). *Pierson and Fairchild's principles & techniques of patient care* (6th ed.). Elsevier.

Jacobs, K., & Simon, L. (Eds.). (2020). *Quick reference dictionary for occupational therapy* (7th ed.). SLACK Incorporated.

Scott, R. W. (2013). *Legal, ethical, and practical aspects of patient care documentation: A guide for rehabilitation professionals* (4th ed.). Jones & Bartlett Learning.

Chapter 9

Writing the "A"—Assessment

The third part of the note is the **ASSESSMENT**. This section consists of the occupational therapy practitioner's skilled appraisal of the client's progress, functional limitations, pertinent issues, and expected gains from rehabilitation. In the assessment section of the note, you will use your professional judgment to discern the meaning of the data you have presented in the "S" and "O" sections. You will also relate how this data will impact on the client's ability to benefit from occupational therapy and engage in meaningful occupations.

For example, during the intervention session, you may have observed that the client does not attend to the left side. Perhaps you observed that they only ate food on the right side of the meal tray and couldn't find the toothpaste tube or brush on the bathroom counter. You will note both the problem (left neglect) and the areas of occupation in which it is a problem (ADL tasks). In your assessment, to address the impact of this deficit, you might write:

Left neglect interferes with client's ability to perform ADLs.

In the assessment section of the note, the OTA will remark on the **3 P's: problems, progress**, and rehab **potential**. The OTA might also identify and explain inconsistencies, discuss emotional components, deliberate contexts or new issues, or present the reason that something was not implemented or achieved as planned.

Assessing the Data

To assess the data, go **sentence by sentence** through the data presented in the "S" and the "O." For each component, consider the implications for the client's engagement in meaningful occupations and role performance. Note what problems, progress, or rehabilitation potential you surmise. Consider the following possibilities.

Problems May Include the Following

Safety Risks

- *Safety concerns noted when child attempted to stand without locking brakes on w/c.*
- *Poor problem solving when using the stove raises safety concerns.*
- *Client's poor short-term memory limits ability to adhere to THR precautions.*
- *Client's limited coping strategies for dealing with stress raise concerns for continuing the use of opioids.*

Morreale, M. J. *The OTA's Guide to Documentation: Writing SOAP Notes, Fifth Edition* (pp. 151-161). © 2023 Taylor & Francis Group.

Inconsistencies Between Client Report and Objective Findings

- *Although client reports anticipating no difficulty in returning to driving, her left-side neglect and visual field deficit would cause significant safety risks.*
- *Although the client expresses a willingness to perform ADLs, her sequencing and motor planning problems create barriers to tasks.*
- *Although the client expresses a desire to regain skills for return to work, he has not followed through with his home exercise program and has missed several OT appointments.*
- *Client verbalizes a desire to progress to the next level of responsibility but shows ↓ behavioral control when reward incentives are unavailable.*
- *Although student expresses a desire to improve handwriting, student has not followed through with use of thumb stabilization orthosis and built-up pen.*

Factors Not Within Functional Limits That Can Be Influenced by Occupational Therapy Intervention

- *Left-side weakness interferes with standing balance in tub.*
- *Unilateral neglect necessitates verbal cues to attend to left side during ADL tasks.*
- *Continued verbal threats toward other clients indicate a need for anger management techniques.*
- *Right hand pain limits client's ability to perform heavy household chores.*
- *Lack of spatial orientation to identify letter shapes interferes with ability to learn to read.*
- *Increased tone in Ⓡ upper limb hinders infant's ability to maintain prone on elbows Ⓘ.*

Progress Remarks May Indicate One or More of the Following

Verification That the Treatment Being Provided Is Effective

- *Weighted utensils decrease intention tremors by ~50% when eating.*
- *Spouse demonstrates good carryover in ability to transfer client safely.*
- *Gains in fine motor skills this week now enable child to manage finger foods Ⓘ.*
- *Patient has shown progress since the beginning of the week by demonstrating the ability to follow one-step commands 80% of the time during ADL tasks.*
- *Client's spontaneous participation in group discussion shows good progress in developing social interaction skills.*
- *Infant's trunk strength is increasing as demonstrated by ability to sit unsupported for 60 seconds.*
- *Child's progress from 70% to 90% accuracy in shape recognition indicates good recall.*
- *Pt. demonstrates good carryover in care and use of orthotic device.*

Statements That Previous Goals Have Been Met or Changed

- *STG #2 (Transfer to toilet with min assist) met this week.*
- *STG #3 upgraded to "Stand at sink for 10 minutes to perform grooming tasks with SBA."*
- *STG #4 changed to "Initiate conversation with peer during craft group."*

Reasons for the Lack of Progress

- *Student has become more dependent in transfers this week 2° medication change resulting in ↑ tone in Ⓑ LEs.*
- *Patient has become more dependent in ADL tasks this week due to acute respiratory infection.*
- *Client has been unable to follow through with home program due to death of spouse.*
- *Resident has had increased difficulty self-feeding this week 2° recent wound in dominant hand.*

Potential for Success in Rehabilitation

- *Resident's intact sensation and presence of voluntary movement demonstrate good rehabilitation potential.*
- *Client's ability to recognize stressors shows good potential to change maladaptive coping strategies.*
- *Student's improvement from 50% to 60% accuracy with typing words using mouthstick indicates good potential to meet goals stated in IEP.*
- *Patient's ability to recall and demonstrate 3/3 total hip precautions shows good potential to follow hip precautions after discharge.*

HELPFUL HINT

The assessment section demonstrates your clinical reasoning as an OTA and is the heart of your note. Based on thoughtful appraisal of data obtained from the "S" and "O," the assessment section communicates succinctly how the client's problems, progress, or rehabilitation potential impact that person's ability to benefit from therapy and engage in meaningful occupations.

Assessing Factors Not Within Functional Limits

Every note does not necessarily reflect **progress** and/or rehabilitation **potential**. However, most notes do indicate **problem** areas. This is because the problems are what limit occupational performance and necessitate client intervention. The most common problem area that the OTA assesses is the impact of an underlying limiting factor such as a performance skill or client factor that is deficient. Of course, other areas delineated in the *OTPF-4* can also hinder the client's occupational performance, such as context and environment, performance patterns, and activity demands (American Occupational Therapy Association [AOTA], 2020; Gateley & Borcherding, 2017). When OTA students and new practitioners are first learning to write SOAP notes, they may find it difficult to distinguish observations from assessments. This may also result in notes that are redundant. There is a helpful formula to address a problem area that is not within functional limits. This will ensure that you are actually writing an assessment rather than an observation. State the limiting factor, skill, or circumstance at the beginning of the sentence, and then describe or relate how that factor impacts a client's functional ability in a particular area of occupation.

| Underlying Limiting Factor ———————▶Functional Impact ———————▶Ability to Engage in Occupation |

Look at the examples that follow and note how **the subject of the sentence** reflects a particular aspect of the occupational therapy domain that is not within functional limits (Gateley & Borcherding, 2017). What follows next is the negative influence it has on a specific area of occupation. This method is useful when you are first learning, but do realize there can be other ways to write assessment statements.

- Client factors:
  - ℝ *shoulder pain* interferes with client's ability to perform sliding board transfers.
  - *Lymphedema* in right arm hinders client's ability to reach into upper kitchen cabinets.
  - *Excessive tone in left upper extremity* interferes with infant's ability to crawl.
  - *Lack of voluntary wrist and finger extension* limits child's ability to engage in developmental play activities.
- Context and environment:
  - *The sound of sirens* triggers flashbacks of client's accident and interferes with task completion at work.
  - *Lack of elevator access* impedes client's ability to enter his office.
  - *Unavailability of public transportation* limits client's ability to obtain groceries.
  - *Poor parental supervision* creates a concern for toddler's safety in the home.

- Performance patterns:
  - ○ Student's **routine of eating pizza and milkshakes every day for lunch** contributes to his weight gain, which hinders gym class participation.
  - ○ Client's **compulsive habit of checking locks excessively in the morning** interferes with getting to work on time.
  - ○ Client's **dialysis schedule** is a barrier to full-time employment.
  - ○ Client's **habit of purging after meals** creates significant tension in her relationship with spouse.
- Performance skills:
  - ○ **Inability to self-regulate alcoholic intake** results in difficulty maintaining employment.
  - ○ **Deficits in attention span** create safety concerns for riding a bicycle.
  - ○ **Decreased oral-motor control** interferes with child's ability to manage solid foods.
  - ○ **Deficits in problem solving** create a need for maximum verbal cues to perform kitchen tasks safely.
- Activity demands:
  - ○ **Inability to tolerate closed spaces** interferes with client's ability to use the bus.
  - ○ Client's **fear of germs** interferes with money handling tasks at his fast food job.
  - ○ Child's **tactile defensiveness** is a barrier to completing projects in school that require glue.
  - ○ Client's **heat intolerance** hinders ability to return to his outdoor construction job during the summer months.

Writing the Assessment

As you carefully and systematically review the material in your "S" and "O", you might find it helpful to create a quick list of things to discuss in the "A" section of your note. For example, consider the following "S" and "O":

S: *Client stated his dominant right hand "feels clumsy." He also reported difficulty with managing clothing fastenings.*

O: *Client participated in 30-minute session in OT clinic for remediation of fine motor skills and hand strength for ADLs. Client worked on right three-point and lateral pinch using graded clothespins with 1 lb. resistance. He was issued lightly resistive therapy putty and instructed in home exercise program. Written copy of exercises also provided and client demonstrated all exercises accurately. Client was issued a buttonhook with built-up handle. He demonstrated ability to use buttonhook to fasten and unfasten six ½ inch buttons on button board ① following skilled instruction. Client expressed willingness to continue use of buttonhook and putty at home.*

The following areas of problems/progress/potential can be identified:

- **Problems**
  - ○ Client is concerned regarding deficits in hand function.
  - ○ Client is still unable to manage fastenings independently.

- **Progress**
  - ○ Client is able to understand and integrate therapy tasks.
  - ○ Client is able to use adaptive equipment to compensate for ADL deficits.
  - ○ Client is willing to follow through with home program.

- **Potential**
  - ○ By using professional judgment, the OTA would consider the client's progress shown thus far a good indicator of rehabilitation potential. The assessment of the data can then be written as follows:

    A: *Client's ability to accurately demonstrate exercises and use buttonhook indicates good rehab potential for managing fastenings and dressing ①. Client is actively engaged in therapy program and able to follow through with home program.*

Justifying Continued Treatment

One very useful way of justifying continued OT intervention for your client is to end the "A" with the statement, *"Client would benefit from ..."* Then, based on your observations and assessment, complete the sentence with a justification of continued intervention that requires the skill of an occupational therapy practitioner rather than another discipline such as a nurse, physical therapist, or aide. Not every OT or OTA ends the "A" in this fashion, but for purposes of learning, we will end the "A" with this method. This helps to make certain that justification for continued intervention is present in the note, and is a good way to set up the plan. As you become more proficient in writing notes and are confident that your note justifies continued intervention, you may choose to cover this material in the plan instead.

The following examples of "A" statements show justification for further skilled occupational therapy:

- *Resident would benefit from visual cues to orient him to environment.*
- *Child would benefit from assistive technology to perform classroom tasks.*
- *Parent would benefit from further instruction in positioning child for feeding.*
- *Consumer would benefit from continued instruction in problem-solving and anger management techniques needed for successful personal and social relationships.*
- *Client would benefit from continued skilled OT to improve decision-making skills and time management to ↓ maladaptive behaviors.*
- *Client would benefit from instruction in self-ranging exercises to increase left shoulder AROM for work tasks.*
- *Client would benefit from further instruction in total hip precautions in order to manage IADLs safely.*
- *Infant would benefit from activities that encourage trunk rotation to facilitate rolling over.*
- *Client would benefit from use of a reacher, sock aid, and long-handled shoe horn to minimize low back pain when performing lower body dressing.*
- *Resident would benefit from skilled instruction in sequencing of tasks to increase safety while performing toilet hygiene and bathing tasks.*
- *Client would benefit from instruction in energy conservation and work simplification techniques to perform meal preparation and clean up.*

Review the criteria for skilled occupational therapy in Chapter 3 along with the list of specialized services that occupational therapy practitioners provide. For each of your clients you will collaborate with the OT to consider any safety concerns, risks for secondary complications, and determine what specific interventions can facilitate the client's health and occupational performance. Use your professional reasoning to communicate and document *ethically* the principles and strategies used during an intervention session to justify the skilled occupational therapy implemented and the need for continued services if appropriate. Also, if you state that the client will benefit from further specific occupational therapy interventions, you must be prepared to follow through with this. Remember that the justification for continued occupational therapy must be reasonable and necessary for the client's condition and support the frequency, duration, and outcomes delineated in the intervention plan. If the last sentence of your "A" reads, *"Client would benefit from information on energy conservation techniques,"* do not expect the payer to approve more than one additional intervention session unless you indicate that functional training and practice is required for implementation.

If this is the client's last session, complete the sentence with the OT's discharge plan for which you might have contributed to. For example:

- *Client would benefit from continued PROM provided by caregiver.*
- *Client has been instructed in home safety modifications and would benefit from the installation of bathroom grab bars.*
- *Client would benefit from Meals on Wheels to eliminate need for grocery shopping.*
- *Student would benefit from continued participation in peer support group.*
- *Client would benefit from continued use of home paraffin and TENS unit PRN for pain relief.*
- *Client would benefit from a personal emergency response system at home for safety.*
- *Child would benefit from continued participation in recreational tennis and swimming to improve upper body strength and endurance.*

Ending the Assessment

Now we can finish the assessment section of the note we began earlier:

S: *Client stated his dominant right hand "feels clumsy." He also reported difficulty with managing clothing fastenings.*

O: *Client participated in 30-minute session in OT clinic for remediation of fine motor skills and hand strength for ADLs. Client worked on right three-point and lateral pinch using graded clothespins with 1 lb. resistance. He was issued lightly resistive therapy putty and instructed in home exercise program. Written copy of exercises also provided and client demonstrated all exercises accurately. Client was issued a buttonhook with built-up handle. He demonstrated ability to use buttonhook to fasten and unfasten six ½ inch buttons on button board Ⓘ following skilled instruction. Client expressed willingness to continue use of buttonhook and putty at home.*

A: *Client's ability to accurately demonstrate exercises and use buttonhook indicates good rehab potential for managing fastenings and dressing Ⓘ. Client is actively engaged in therapy program and able to follow through with home program.* **Client would benefit from** *further instruction in adaptive equipment, compensatory techniques, and remediation of fine motor skills in order to regain Ⓘ in all ADLs.*

Here are some more examples of what the completed assessment section of your note might look like for other practice settings:

A: *Client is beginning to regain some of the independent living skills she had prior to her recent psychotic episode. Fear, isolation, and ↓ activity tolerance slow her progress and are the focus of current intervention. Client would benefit from continued skilled instruction in self-care skills as well as ↑ socialization and ↑ physical activity.*

A: *Child's poor attention span and inability to tolerate auditory stimuli limit her ability to control her classroom behavior. She would benefit from more activities to ↑ tolerance of auditory stimuli and strategies to manage self-control.*

HELPFUL HINT

The assessment section is not the place to introduce new information. Do not put anything in your "A" that has not already been discussed in the "S" or "O." If you find yourself wanting to make a statement in the "A" that is not supported by the data in your "S" or "O," ask yourself what you might have observed to support the assessment statement. Then decide whether you need to add it to your "S" or "O."

Use Professional Reasoning

Now you can try to integrate the information in this chapter and practice writing the "A." Review the following occupational therapy note:

S: *Client stated she has difficulty moving Ⓡ UE, although she does not know why it will not move. She reported, "It really doesn't hurt. It's just tight."*

O: *Client participated in 30-minute OT session in hospital room to ↑ AROM and strength in Ⓡ shoulder, ↑ activity tolerance and dynamic standing balance in order to ↑ independence in ADL activities.*

ADLs: Client was instructed on safety techniques and adaptive equipment use for toileting. Client required use of bilateral grab bars in bathroom to sit → stand safely. Client first attempted to stand while pulling on walker and one grab bar. Client was instructed on proper procedures for safe transfers and the use of bilateral grab bars.

Performance skills: Client sit → stand CGA for balance. Client worked on activity tolerance, dynamic standing balance, and ↑ AROM in right shoulder by moving personal hygiene items from bathroom counter to medicine cabinet for 5 minutes before needing to sit and rest 2 minutes. She then participated in activities to ↑ dynamic standing balance by pouring liquid from a pitcher while standing CGA for balance. After a 1-minute rest, client continued activities to ↑ dynamic standing balance and safety in ADL activities by pushing wheeled walker with CGA while picking up objects from the floor with a reacher.

Client factors: AROM in right shoulder abduction < 90°. PROM right shoulder abduction WNL.

Think about how you would assess this information in the "S" and "O." Review the suggestions given earlier in the chapter, and then organize your thoughts by identifying the problems, progress, and rehabilitation potential you see in this client's intervention session today. What **problems** and safety risks can you identify? Are there performance skills and client factors not within functional limits that occupational therapy might impact? Do you see any evidence of **progress** or rehab **potential**? What would this client benefit from? Identify problems, progress, and rehab potential using Worksheet 9-1. Then compare your ideas with the suggested assessment that follows.

Worksheet 9-1
Organizing Your Thoughts for Assessment

Problems

Progress

Potential

Now write the assessment part of this note:

© 2023 Taylor & Francis Group.
Morreale, M. J. (2023). *The OTA's guide to documentation: Writing SOAP notes* (5th ed.). SLACK Incorporated.

In preparing an assessment of the data in this note, two main **problem** areas can be determined: the safety of transferring to and from the toilet and the client factors that were not within functional limits. The OTA should be particularly concerned about the safety issues, and those should be addressed first. Also, the OTA should note the rehabilitation **potential** that would help a reviewer to decide whether the client's progress is sufficient to warrant the expense of treatment.

Safety concerns (impulsivity, ↓ dynamic standing balance) noted when client attempts to transfer sit → stand during toileting. Client verbalized an understanding of safety instructions and has potential to progress to independence.

Next, the OTA should note the clinical reasoning behind devoting time to addressing client factors, considering the client's rehabilitation potential.

Safety concerns (impulsivity, ↓ dynamic standing balance) noted when client attempts to transfer sit → stand during toileting. Client verbalized an understanding of safety instructions and has potential to progress to independence. **Client's ↓ AROM in right shoulder, ↓ activity tolerance, and ↓ dynamic standing balance all interfere with ability to complete ADL tasks safely and independently.**

Finally, the OTA can then complete the assessment by justifying continued intervention as shown in the example that follows.

A: *Safety concerns (impulsivity, ↓ dynamic standing balance) noted when client attempts to transfer sit → stand during toileting. Client verbalized an understanding of safety instructions and has potential to progress to independence. Client's ↓ AROM in right shoulder, ↓ activity tolerance, and ↓ dynamic standing balance all interfere with ability to complete ADL tasks safely and independently.* **Client would benefit from Ⓡ UE AROM and strengthening exercises along with continued skilled instruction on safety and energy conservation techniques.**

In this case, the OTA can address client factors in two different ways, both by working on ↑ AROM, strength, and activity tolerance and by teaching some energy conservation strategies.

Third-party payers often deny ongoing treatment of range of motion and strength unless significant functional gains are evident. Occupational therapy practitioners must consider the expected improvement in function versus the costs of continuing intervention. Clinical decisions must be made to determine if a home exercise program could accomplish the same results or if skilled services remain appropriate and necessary. In Chapter 10, you will see how an OTA can cost-effectively provide the proper interventions to benefit this client.

Worksheet 9-2
Justifying Continued Treatment

Indicate which of the following require the skill of an OTA. Note that OTA tasks are performed under the OT's supervision so, of course, an OT would be able to perform these tasks also.

1. ___ Administering paraffin irrelevant to occupational performance
2. ___ Instructing the client in leisure skills for stress management
3. ___ Having a client watch a video on assertiveness training without further instruction or without role-playing the techniques
4. ___ Analyzing and modifying functional tasks/activities through the provision of adaptive equipment or techniques
5. ___ Determining that the modified task is safe and effective
6. ___ Carrying out a routine maintenance program
7. ___ Upgrading the intervention plan
8. ___ Teaching the client to use the breathing techniques he has learned while performing his ADL activities
9. ___ Interpreting initial evaluation results and establishing the intervention plan
10. ___ Providing individualized instruction to the client, family, or caregiver
11. ___ Giving the client a replacement piece of hook and loop fastener
12. ___ Making the decision to discharge a client from occupational therapy
13. ___ Writing out a home exercise program and instructing the client
14. ___ Teaching compensatory skills
15. ___ Gait training with goal of increasing ambulation distance
16. ___ Making recommendations to a parent for a child's positioning and feeding
17. ___ Educating clients to eliminate safety hazards
18. ___ Teaching adaptive techniques such as one-handed shoe tying
19. ___ Helping a client in the bathroom
20. ___ Telling a client about a new computer app

Morreale, M. J. (2023). *The OTA's guide to documentation: Writing SOAP notes* (5th ed.). SLACK Incorporated.

Worksheet 9-3
Assessing Factors Not Within Functional Limits

Use the following formula to rewrite the assessment statements and make them more effective.

Underlying Limiting Factor ────────▶	Functional Impact ────────▶	Ability to Engage in Occupation

For example, this statement is an observation:

> *Client's activity tolerance for standing at the stove was < 4 minutes 2° inability to tolerate prosthesis.*

It tells you the client behavior and measurable factors the OTA can observe while providing intervention. To make it into an assessment statement, you would need to change the emphasis by turning your sentence around and by adding the impact the client's standing tolerance has on their independence in cooking. Using the formula above, you might write:

> *Client's activity tolerance for standing with prosthesis for < 4 min limits performance of kitchen tasks.*

Rewrite the following statements using the formula given above.

1. Child wrote poorly due to immature pencil grasp and difficulty with spatial orientation of letters.

2. Client demonstrated difficulty with balancing her checkbook due to memory and sequencing deficits.

3. Client problem solved poorly while performing lower body dressing as evidenced by multiple attempts to button shirt and don socks.

4. Client was unable to hang clothes in closet or place dishes in upper kitchen cabinets due to P/AROM shoulder flexion/abduction limited to 105°.

Morreale, M. J. (2023). *The OTA's guide to documentation: Writing SOAP notes* (5th ed.). SLACK Incorporated.

Worksheet 9-4
Social Skills Worksheet

Your client is a middle-aged woman presently diagnosed with bipolar disorder. In a prior admission, however, she was diagnosed with schizophrenia. One of her goals is to talk to the mental health center staff about her problems rather than acting out her feelings. Today she participated in an occupational therapy social skills group with five other clients who also need help with relationship issues.

S: *Client reports that she understands the purpose of social skills group. She expressed a desire to attend all of the groups, saying that they are "fun."*

O: *Client participated in an OT group session on friendship in order to improve interpersonal skills and coping mechanisms. Client appeared unkempt, with hair not combed and shirt rumpled. Client engaged in conversation with the other clients and the facilitator, but interrupted others on five occasions. Client spontaneously verbalized her experiences with past friendships and her ideas of useful ways to make new friendships, but had to be redirected to the topic twice during discussion.*

1.   What **problems** are evident in the above "S" and "O"?

2.   What **areas of occupation** are affected by these problems?

3.   What evidence of **progress** and/or **potential** do you see?

Write your assessment below.
A:

Morreale, M. J. (2023). *The OTA's guide to documentation: Writing SOAP notes* (5th ed.). SLACK Incorporated.

References

American Occupational Therapy Association. (2020). Occupational therapy practice framework: Domain and process (4th ed.). *American Journal of Occupational Therapy, 74*(Suppl. 2), 7412410010. https://doi.org: 10.5014/ajot.2020.74S2001

Gateley, C. A., & Borcherding, S. (2017). *Documentation manual for occupational therapy: Writing SOAP notes* (4th ed.). SLACK Incorporated.

Chapter 10

Writing the "P"—Plan

The final section of a SOAP note is the **PLAN**. In this section, you determine and set forth the specific interventions that will be used to achieve the occupational therapy goals. You will record what follow-up is required, such as what you plan to do in the client's next occupational therapy session, near future, or what must be addressed immediately. The plan might also be a recommendation that you want the client, family, or caregiver to follow through with, such as attend a support group, install grab bars, wear an orthotic device for work, communicate with the doctor about a particular concern, try out a home exercise program, or use a piece of adaptive equipment. The plan in your SOAP note must follow the OT's intervention plan (containing long- and short-term goals, frequency and estimated duration of treatment) that was established from the initial evaluation. It should also relate to the information that you just presented in the "O" and the "A," and to your skilled assessment of what the client would benefit from.

The plan will inform the reader of your priorities regarding intervention strategies. In a contact note or a progress note, you will address any part of the plan that has not been covered in the last sentence of your assessment, "*Client would benefit from....*" You will address how often the client will be treated, how long intervention will continue, and your priorities for what you will work on next or follow up with.

Consumer will continue prevocational program 5 days/wk. in order to ↑ task behaviors for work such as correct use of timecard and time management during breaks.

Some facilities require that occupational therapy practitioners include goals in the "P" section. Those goals follow the OT's intervention plan and may depict the incremental steps to the established long- or short-term goals. In a practice setting such as a school system where monthly notes are written, your goal in the "P" might be what you hope to accomplish in the next month. In a skilled nursing facility, it might be your goal for the next week. In an acute care setting, it might be your goal for tomorrow.

- *Continue 1-hour daily sessions for 2 weeks to improve motor planning skills for dressing. By the end of next session, veteran will demonstrate the ability to identify front and back of shirt with one verbal cue.*

- *Client will continue to participate in values clarification groups 3x/wk for 2 weeks to address low self-esteem and alcohol use. Client will demonstrate awareness of self-help strategies by verbalizing three alternatives to handle stress rather than drinking, within two group sessions.*

- *Continue OT for 30-minute sessions daily until discharge to facilitate improved function of affected limb for ADLs. By end of next treatment session, client will demonstrate Ⓘ in donning/doffing of orthosis and positioning of Ⓡ UE to minimize edema.*

- *Student will continue OT 3x weekly in order to ↑ perceptual and fine motor skills for better classroom performance. Student will be able to use loop scissors to cut a straight dotted line Ⓘ within ¼ inch 3/4 opportunities by the end of next month.*

Morreale, M. J. *The OTA's Guide to Documentation: Writing SOAP Notes, Fifth Edition* (pp. 163-169). © 2023 Taylor & Francis Group.

Many facilities do not include goals in the "P" section and may only update and include goals in progress notes or reevaluation notes. You will learn how to write goals in Chapter 15. For the purpose of completing your SOAP notes at this time, we will not end the plan with a goal. Once you are proficient in goal writing, it is easy to simply add a goal statement to your plan if your facility requires it.

HELPFUL HINT

If for some reason you are not able to see your client as scheduled, the "P" section of your note should allow another occupational therapy practitioner to continue intervention uninterrupted.

Determining the Plan

Now let us determine the plan for the note that we assessed in the last chapter. As you recall from Chapter 9, this client has deficits in safety and standing balance.

S: *Client stated she has difficulty moving Ⓡ UE, although she does not know why it will not move. She reported, "It really doesn't hurt. It's just tight."*

O: *Client participated in 30-minute OT session in hospital room to ↑ AROM and strength in Ⓡ shoulder, ↑ activity tolerance and dynamic standing balance in order to ↑ independence in ADL activities.*

ADLs: Client was instructed on safety techniques and adaptive equipment use for toileting. Client required use of bilateral grab bars in bathroom to sit → stand safely. Client first attempted to stand while pulling on walker and one grab bar. Client was instructed on proper procedures for safe transfers and the use of bilateral grab bars.

Performance Skills: Client sit → stand CGA for balance. Client worked on activity tolerance, dynamic standing balance, and ↑ AROM in right shoulder by moving personal hygiene items from bathroom counter to medicine cabinet for 5 minutes before needing to sit and rest 2 minutes. She then participated in activities to ↑ dynamic standing balance by pouring liquid from a pitcher while standing CGA for balance. After a 1-minute rest, client continued activities to ↑ dynamic standing balance and safety in ADL activities by pushing wheeled walker with CGA while picking up objects from the floor with a reacher.

Client Factors: AROM in right shoulder abduction < 90°. PROM right shoulder abduction WNL.

A: *Safety concerns (impulsivity, ↓ dynamic standing balance) noted when client attempts to transfer sit → stand during toileting. Client verbalized an understanding of safety instructions and has potential to progress to independence. Client's ↓ AROM in right shoulder, ↓ activity tolerance, and ↓ dynamic standing balance all interfere with ability to complete ADL tasks safely and independently. Client would benefit from Ⓡ UE AROM and strengthening exercises along with continued skilled instruction on safety and energy conservation techniques.*

Use Worksheet 10-1 to write your plan for this client. Begin with a statement about how often (once or twice daily, 2x/wk, etc.) and for how long (for 3 days, for 2 weeks, for 1 month, etc.) she will receive occupational therapy. Look at the items indicated above that she would benefit from, and set your priorities.

Worksheet 10-1
Determining the Plan

Frequency:

Duration:

What would client benefit from?

What are the client's priorities for the near future?

Now write the "P" below.
P:

Completing the Plan

In assessing the data, the OTA has set up the plan for this note. The OTA has already justified the main intention and indicated the client's rehabilitation potential. Now the OTA needs to be specific about how often the client will be treated and for what length of time. This will reflect the frequency and duration of treatment that the OT initially established in the intervention plan. Some facilities do not restate the frequency and duration in every subsequent treatment note, but we will write the plan this way:

P: *Continue OT 5X wk for 1 week …*

The OTA might also decide to indicate the length of the treatment sessions (i.e., for 1 hr. sessions) in this note, although that information does not always need to be included in this section. Next, the OTA specifies how the treatment time will be used:

P: *Continue OT 5X wk for 1 week **for skilled instruction in safe transfers and toileting.***

Because discharge is anticipated in 1 week, the OTA must prioritize treatment time in order to implement the OT's intervention plan. As the OT has delegated treatment of this client to the OTA, the OTA might choose in this case to work on balance and energy conservation as a part of functional mobility and ADL activities. Because the OTA has already written that the client would benefit from additional AROM and strengthening exercises, there now needs to be a specific note of how these needs will be addressed:

P: *Continue OT 5X wk for 1 week for skilled instruction in safe transfers and toileting. **Home program for AROM and strengthening exercises for Ⓡ shoulder will be taught.***

This OTA has also shown professional reasoning in planning for discharge in advance of the discharge date. When providing feedback to the OT and recording later notes, the OTA will indicate the client's progress in learning the home program. Simply handing the client a set of printed exercises is not considered a billable service. The client's progress in learning the home program will also confirm the OTA's assessment that the client's rehabilitation potential was on target. This note is now finally complete. Here is another example of how the plan might be written for the same client.

P: *Continue OT for 1 hour 5X wk until anticipated discharge in 1 week. Client will work on safe transfers, toileting, and improving activity tolerance. Client will also be instructed in HEP to improve* ®️ *shoulder AROM and strength.*

Remember that **the time frames in the "P" section should be consistent with those established in the OT's intervention plan.** While there are often standards or norms for time frames based on the type of practice area and diagnosis, time frames also vary based on payment source, facility requirements, and the client's specific circumstances (Gateley & Borcherding, 2017). When establishing the intervention plan, the OT takes those factors into account along with the physician's orders and client's past history, present status, and anticipated needs. For example, in an acute care setting, a client might be seen for just one or two occupational therapy sessions (such as for an orthotic device, home exercise program, or equipment recommendations) or could receive therapy daily until discharge from the facility if the situation warrants it (Gateley & Borcherding, 2017). Even the length of sessions can vary from only a few minutes (such as for a client in the ICU) to 15 or 30 minutes or longer for clients who are more medically stable; whereas, clients in an inpatient rehabilitation center usually receive therapy once or twice daily for a total of 60 to 90 minutes (Gateley & Borcherding, 2017). In other settings, such as home care and outpatient clinics, the amount of therapy will vary quite a bit depending on the individual's condition, situation, and payer. Therapy in these settings can range from only one or two sessions in total or, possibly, therapy for one to three times weekly for several weeks or months, with each session typically lasting approximately 30 to 60 minutes. Clients in a school setting receive occupational therapy according to what is delineated in the annual IEP, such as a monthly session or, perhaps, one or two times weekly. As you can see, each setting is different. Follow the specific requirements for your facility regarding what aspects of the OT's intervention plan to include in the "P" part of your note.

Worksheet 10-2
Completing the Social Skills Plan

As you recall from Chapter 9, your client is a middle-aged woman diagnosed with bipolar disorder. In a prior admission, however, she was diagnosed with schizophrenia. One of her goals is to talk to the mental health center staff about her problems rather than acting out her feelings. Today she participated in an occupational therapy social skills group with five other clients who also need help with relationship issues. The assessment's last sentence indicates some areas of intervention that might benefit this client. Now fill in the specifics of the plan.

S: *Client reports that she understands the purpose of social skills group. She expressed a desire to attend all of the groups, saying that they are "fun."*

O: *Client participated in an OT group session on friendship in order to improve interpersonal skills and coping mechanisms. Client appeared unkempt, with hair not combed and shirt rumpled. Client engaged in conversation with the other clients and the facilitator but interrupted others on five occasions. Client spontaneously verbalized her experiences with past friendships and her ideas of useful ways to make new friendships but had to be redirected to the topic twice during discussion.*

A: *Client's unkempt appearance, interrupting behaviors, and need for redirection to topic of conversation interfere with her ability to engage in social participation with peers. Her expressed interest in groups and her willingness to engage in conversation and share her ideas show good potential to develop relationships and to express herself verbally in place of acting out. Client would benefit from participating in groups where conversational skills are stressed along with further facilitation of attention to social cues, and from assistance with ADL activities stressing hygiene and appearance.*

P:

Morreale, M. J. (2023). *The OTA's guide to documentation: Writing SOAP notes* (5th ed.). SLACK Incorporated.

Worksheet 10-3
Completing the Plan—Additional Practice

Now finish the plan section for the following note. Think about what you would need to follow up with. Also consider what other specific interventions or adaptive equipment might help this client.

S: *Client stated his dominant right hand "feels clumsy." He also reported difficulty with managing clothing fastenings.*

O: *Client participated in 30-minute session in OT clinic for remediation of fine motor skills and hand strength for ADLs. Client worked on right three-point and lateral pinch using graded clothespins with 1 lb. resistance. He was issued lightly resistive therapy putty and instructed in home exercise program. Written copy of exercises also provided and client demonstrated all exercises accurately. Client was issued a buttonhook with built-up handle. He demonstrated ability to use buttonhook to fasten and unfasten six ½ inch buttons on button board Ⓘ following skilled instruction. Client expressed willingness to continue use of buttonhook and putty at home.*

A: *Client's ability to demonstrate exercises accurately and use buttonhook indicates good rehab potential for managing fastenings and Ⓘ dressing. Client is actively engaged in therapy program and able to follow through with home program. Client would benefit from further instruction in adaptive equipment, compensatory techniques, and remediation of fine motor skills in order to regain Ⓘ in all ADLs.*

P:

Morreale, M. J. (2023). *The OTA's guide to documentation: Writing SOAP notes* (5th ed.). SLACK Incorporated.

Reference

Gateley, C. A., & Borcherding, S. (2017). *Documentation manual for occupational therapy: Writing SOAP notes* (4th ed.). SLACK Incorporated.

Chapter 11

Documenting Special Situations

OTAs may encounter special situations that require documentation, even if the client was not seen face to face or did not receive a complete occupational therapy session. Sessions sometimes get canceled for various reasons or may involve unusual circumstances, such as mishaps or unexpected events. Besides recording these types of situations and notifying the supervising OT, you should carefully document any pertinent communication and relevant follow-up actions. The note must also be dated and signed. Certain types of events may necessitate alerting designated personnel and completing a separate incident report in accordance with facility policy. Proper documentation and adherence to established policies and procedures will ensure coordination of care and also help protect you should any legal issues arise later on (Fremgen, 2020). The following are some examples of notations for various special situations.

Refusals and Cancellations

Sometimes occupational therapy services might be refused or canceled by the client for just a particular session or, perhaps, entirely. Always document the refusal or cancellation and indicate the reason why whenever possible. Note any attempts to reschedule if applicable.

- _Client refused OT today because he felt "dizzy and nauseous." Nursing was notified and OT session scheduled for tomorrow morning._
- _Student went on class trip and, therefore, was unable to receive OT today. OT to resume next week._
- _Client called to cancel OT appointment because his car broke down. Appointment was rescheduled for tomorrow._
- _Patient called and canceled his OT initial evaluation. He stated he does not want any therapy. Patient was educated regarding the reason for referral and benefits of OT, but he still refused services. MD notified._
- _Attempted to see client today, but client was unavailable due to medical test procedures (X-ray and MRI). Will attempt to see client again tomorrow._
- _Father called to cancel child's appointment today because child has a stomach virus. Session rescheduled to 5/21/22._
- _Client called crying and stated she was canceling OT today because of her agoraphobia. She reported having a "severe anxiety attack" earlier this morning and was fearful of leaving her home. She also reported her medication made her "feel worse." Attempted to reassure client and advised her to contact her psychiatrist to discuss her anxiety and medication concerns. Encouraged client to attend next OT session scheduled in 2 days._

Morreale, M. J. _The OTA's Guide to Documentation:_
Writing SOAP Notes, Fifth Edition (pp. 171-174).
© 2023 Taylor & Francis Group.

No-Shows

Sometimes clients have a scheduled OT appointment and simply do not show up.

- *Pt. did not show up for appointment. Call made to pt.'s home. Pt. stated he forgot appointment. OT rescheduled for tomorrow.*
- *No-show. Attempted to call pt. but no one answered the phone.*
- *Child did not show up for appointment. When parent was contacted by phone, she stated she could not get the time off from work today to bring child to OT. Appointment was confirmed for next OT session in 2 days.*
- *Client did not show up for appointment. Call made to client's home. Client stated he could not "get motivated" to get out of bed and get dressed due to "very depressed mood." Client did not express suicidal ideation and stated he was adhering to his medication regime. Client also stated that he realizes OT is important for his recovery and will ask his sister to bring him to tomorrow's OT session. Notified OT and social worker (Emmet Empathy, MSW) by phone regarding client's absence.*
- *Resident did not arrive for scheduled OT session. Called nurse's station and was informed by RN that resident had vomited twice this morning and was now sleeping. Will attempt to see resident again this afternoon.*

Treatment Interruptions

Sometimes you are about to start an OT session or, perhaps, get interrupted while in the midst of treating a client and cannot complete the session for various reasons. Any intervention provided should be documented along with the reason for the therapy interruption.

- *Client transferred from bed to w/c with min assist. Client then stated she did not feel well and vomited. Changed client's soiled shirt and notified nursing staff.*
- *Child seen in dining room for instruction in feeding skills. Five minutes into session, the physician came to take child for medical evaluation. Will attempt OT session again tomorrow for further skilled instruction in feeding.*
- *Upon arrival to OT clinic, resident stated she needed to have a bowel movement. Resident was transported back to her room and nursing staff was notified.*
- *Pt. arrived at OT room tremulous and tearful. She stated, "I can't go on. I really feel like killing myself." Attempted to calm pt. and contacted social worker (Hilda Helpful, MSW), who requested that pt. be brought to her office. Pt. was then transported immediately to social worker's office. OT also notified by phone.*

Medical Hold

Sometimes the client's medical condition or circumstances warrant that therapy be put on hold for a period of time. In some instances, this is formally indicated in the physician's orders or mandated by facility policy for certain situations. There may be other circumstances, such as a sudden change in the client's health or temporary side effects from a recent medical intervention, for which a therapy hold is recommended by nursing staff or determined by the occupational therapy practitioner's clinical judgment. The occupational therapy practitioner should document why scheduled therapy was not implemented and any relevant follow up needed.

- *As per MD orders, client is on hold for therapy today due to possible blood clots in Ⓛ LE.*
- *Nursing requested that OT be deferred today due to pt.'s side effects from chemotherapy.*
- *Upon pt.'s arrival at OT clinic, pt. stated she fell yesterday on her affected Ⓡ UE. Right hand is now moderately edematous with ecchymosis present on dorsum of hand and along dorsal thumb, index, and long fingers. Pt. also reports hand pain as "throbbing." OT immediately notified and referring hand surgeon contacted. Surgeon requested OT be put on hold until surgeon evaluates Ⓡ UE status. Therapy deferred and pt. advised to follow up with her surgeon ASAP.*
- *OT deferred today due to child having surgery for insertion of feeding tube.*

- *Pt. called to report he was hospitalized for two nights 2° pneumonia. OT deferred until physician's orders are received to resume OT.*
- *MD orders state client on hold 2° to psychotic episode.*

Incidents

Sometimes accidents or incidents happen no matter how careful a health practitioner may try to be. Each facility or agency should have specific policies and procedures in place regarding how to document and handle incidents involving staff, clients, visitors, or volunteers. For example, a hospital visitor might tell you they just fell in the parking lot, an assisted living resident may accidentally get cut by a piece of therapy equipment, an outpatient client may have a sudden heart attack during a therapy session, or a toddler you are working with might bite you. Protocols are normally in place to deal with various problems that may arise regarding safety, security, and health. Workers must know and follow proper emergency procedures; use standard precautions appropriately; notify superiors and other personnel as necessary; be cognizant of liability issues; and follow-up accordingly. *Clinical* information related to a client incident should be recorded in that client's health record. In addition, separate **incident report** forms are typically filled out that include additional *administrative* information, such as why the incident occurred (i.e., a wet floor or broken equipment) interviews with staff members, or witnesses to the occurrence (Scott, 2013). The incident report is not mentioned or included in the health record (Scott, 2013). If an accident or incident happens to a visitor, staff, or volunteer (such as falling, passing out, or getting hurt), usually an incident report must be filled out. Even if the individual involved does not appear to have suffered any harm from the error or incident, the report must still be completed because it will alert staff to potential problem areas and maintain facts should that person develop any problems later or a lawsuit happens (Fremgen, 2020; Scott, 2013). Facility policy will specify who is responsible for completing the incident report. Only report the actual facts. Do not embellish, guess, or make assumptions about what occurred when you are noting the incident. **Learn the exact policies and procedures in your facility so you are prepared to handle any incidents promptly and properly.**

- *Upon OTA's arrival at pt.'s hospital room, pt. was found lying on floor awake, alert, and crying. Unit nurse (Helen Helper, RN) was immediately notified and Dr. Seth Oscope was contacted by phone.*
- *Client sustained a ¼" superficial cut to left small finger distal phalanx while cutting vegetables during IADL session. Wound cleansed with soap and water and bandage applied. OT and home care nurse notified by phone.*
- *When child was told he must stay seated in his chair he yelled several profane words and bit OTA's hand. Child was then sent to principal's office to address inappropriate behavior.*

Phone Calls and Electronic Communication

Document pertinent communications from emails, text messages, and phone calls regarding the client, such as problems reported by the client or family/caregiver and any instructions, follow-up, or education you provided. Include the date, time, and describe relevant content of the communication. Always adhere to HIPAA guidelines and ensure the client has given permission for the health team to communicate with those other individuals, if applicable.

- *Client called to report she lost her orthotic device 3 days ago when trying on clothes at the mall. Appointment scheduled tomorrow for fabrication of replacement device.*
- *Client called today to ask about possible local support groups he could attend. Following phone conversation, client was sent information by email today regarding 3 local support groups for people with multiple sclerosis*
- *Email received from client at 3:10pm requesting another copy of written instructions for her orthotic device because she "can't find" the instructions given to her this morning. Copy of these instructions was emailed to client at 4:25pm.*
- *Spoke with case manager (Nick Nerz, RN) telephonically to discuss client's need for a tub seat and grab bars in order to shower safely. Informed RN that client's daughter agreed to obtain this equipment and arrange for grab bar installation.*
- *Client called to clarify procedure for exercise #3 of home exercise program. Client reinstructed in proper method telephonically and he verbalized understanding. Client advised to discontinue exercises if increased pain or swelling occur. Confirmed follow-up appointment for 5/10/2022.*

Photos and Videos

Do not use your personal smart phone, tablet, or camera to take any photos or videos of children, clients on your caseload, or other people at a facility or school. While it may be tempting during fieldwork or clinical practice to take pictures of cute/funny children or those older adult clients you have grown fond of, the taking of client photos or videos is normally prohibited to protect client confidentiality. In certain situations, if allowed by the facility or agency, some providers do utilize photos and videos in clinical documentation such as to track wounds or assess posture (Fremgen, 2020; Scott, 2013). These images become part of the health record and are considered protected health information. **HIPAA guidelines and facility policies must always be followed**. Do not take any pictures or videos of clients without their permission and use only approved facility devices that meet mandated security and privacy requirements. Also, ensure that no other clients are in the photo or video. Any images taken or used for professional articles or public relations purposes (such as posters or brochures), also require written client permission and must adhere to proper protocols for that facility; for example, going through the public relations department.

Conclusion

Cancellations, refusals, no-shows, deferred, or interrupted sessions should be noted in the record. Document pertinent phone conversations and electronic communications regarding the client but do not take personal photos or videos of clients. When special situations or unusual circumstances arise, an OTA must always use good clinical judgment, maintain professional demeanor, and keep the supervising OT and other pertinent staff informed as appropriate. It is essential that practitioners understand relevant laws and implement best practices in occupational therapy when dealing with unexpected circumstances and emergency situations. Always follow facility or agency policies/procedures and adhere to privacy laws. Document in a timely manner, avoid speculation, and report the facts carefully and accurately.

References

Fremgen, B. F. (2020). *Medical law and ethics* (6th ed.). Pearson Education.

Scott, R. W. (2013). *Legal, ethical, and practical aspects of patient care documentation: A guide for professionals* (4th ed.). Jones & Bartlett Learning.

Chapter 12

Improving Observation Skills and Refining Your Note

Effective documentation requires that you hone your observation skills, organize data, and record information accurately and professionally. OT practitioners make numerous skilled observations during an intervention session and use professional reasoning to assess the client's responses, behavior, performance skills, and other factors related to the client's condition. These skilled observations are documented such that someone else reading the note will get a clear mental picture of the client's situation and what transpired during the intervention session. As you gain clinical proficiency and develop your own repertoire of professional terminology, recording your observations quickly and accurately will become easier over time.

Tips for Improving Observation Skills

Here are some additional questions and tips to consider during client interventions. Use these suggestions to improve your observation skills and help organize information for your therapy notes.

WHO Is Involved in the Intervention Session?

- Are family members/significant others, caregivers, or other staff present or involved in the intervention session?
- Is this a group activity?
- Is your client interacting with other clients? (Remember, do not include the other clients' names in your note.)

WHEN Did the Intervention Session Take Place?

- Did you treat the client during a specific mealtime, during morning self-care, after dinner, during a classroom activity, group session, etc.?
- What did the client do just before your intervention session and will this impact the client's performance in occupational therapy? For example, perhaps the client just underwent a strenuous medical treatment or completed a rigorous physical therapy session, which is the reason why the client is now tired, doesn't feel well, or performs poorly.

WHERE Did the Intervention Session Take Place?

- Did you work with the client bedside, in the emergency department, OT clinic, ICU, rehab gym, classroom, outdoors, in a group session, at the client's home or worksite, or in the community?
- Did the client perform ADLs/IADLs in the kitchen, bedroom, bathroom, dining room, or other area?
- Did client transfer or ambulate from one place to another and, if so, did the client require any adaptive equipment/durable medical equipment such as grab bars, a trapeze, mechanical lift, sliding board, or mobility aid?

Morreale, M. J. *The OTA's Guide to Documentation: Writing SOAP Notes, Fifth Edition* (pp. 175-188). © 2023 Taylor & Francis Group.

- Did the client remain in bed, in a wheelchair, Geri chair, or regular chair the entire session?
- Did the chair have a back support and/or armrests and was the chair stable or on wheels?
- Were any positioning devices used such as, a lap tray, arm rest, lateral supports, or cushions?
- If client was in a hospital bed, how far was the head of the bed raised, if at all? Were bedrails up, down, or used to assist with balance or mobility?
- Did the client sit or stand at a desk, kitchen table, stove, bathroom counter, computer workstation, shower stall, or other area?
- Was the client sitting on a stable surface or, perhaps, an unstable one such as edge of bed or therapy ball?
- Did the client sit or lie on a scooter board, mat, bed, floor, bolster, or other surface? Did the client sit on a tub bench/seat, commode, stool, bicycle, or swing?
- If lying down, was the client positioned in prone, supine, or sidelying?

WHAT Happened During the Intervention Session?

- What did the client, caregiver, family, or staff members say or ask?
- What interventions to support occupations did the client participate in?
- What activities and occupations did the client engage in?
- What skilled services were implemented to address the client's occupational therapy goals?
- What client factors or performance skills were specifically addressed?
- What tasks, methods, equipment, or occupational modifications were used, provided, or taught (such as adaptive equipment, weights, therapy putty, worksheets, games, orthotic devices, or physical agent modalities)?
- Were any measurements taken or specific skills assessed/reassessed during this intervention session?
- What specific instruction or reinstruction did you provide to the client, family, caregiver, or staff? What was the client's response to the instruction given?
- What abilities, limitations, problems, safety concerns, or progress were evident during the therapy tasks?
- What follow up is needed?

WHY Is the Particular Intervention Important?

- Why is this specific treatment relevant to the client's intervention plan and goals?
- Why is the implemented task, method, or activity a skilled service that requires the expertise of an occupational therapy practitioner?
- Why did the client have a particular outcome during this session?

HOW Did the Client Perform or Participate in the Task?

- How does the intervention plan need to be modified as based on this session? (The OT is responsible for updating the intervention plan but the OTA can contribute to this process; American Occupational Therapy Association [AOTA], 2021)
- How were problems or issues handled?
- How is the client progressing or not progressing?
- How did the client, family, caregiver, or staff respond, react, or perform during this intervention?
- How well is the client, family, caregiver, or staff carrying through with therapy recommendations or home programs?

Documenting Observations Accurately

Descriptive words and clinical jargon facilitate understanding of the client's specific traits, behavior, or environment and help create a clear picture in the reader's mind. However, you must always choose professional language carefully and avoid judgmental words and personal opinions. The "O" section of your note is where you will note the pertinent, specific behaviors, factors, performance skills, or contextual conditions you observed. Your "A" will then summarize those items as indicators of something in particular, such as a concern or an asset. For example, if you are assessing and describing a home environment, you would indicate specific hazards or problems in the "O" part of the note, such as exposed electrical wires, mold, raw sewage, piles of garbage, presence of mice, etc. The "A" would then indicate how the "unsafe home environment" or a particular "unsanitary" or "hazardous condition" impacts the client's life or needs to be addressed. If the home does not meet your own personal standards for cleanliness, do not express that value judgment in your note. Simply state what you observed if that observation is relevant and needs to be communicated in the record: *"Pet waste was evident on three areas of kitchen floor. Kitchen garbage pail was overflowing with approximately two dozen pieces of trash next to it on the floor. Six uncovered dishes containing half-eaten food were on counter with flies on them."*

Use the "O" to describe specific behaviors pertinent to the client's condition or situation. For example, for a client diagnosed with bipolar disorder, you might note frequency of drug use, careless driving acts (i.e., number of accidents or tickets), altercations at bars, or other dangerous acts. Your "A" will then professionally assess the negative impact the "risk-taking" behaviors have on the client's life, such as relationships or ability to engage in meaningful occupations. Again, be careful to avoid judgmental terms. For example, a client *you* might perceive as aggressive might perceive his own behavior as self-protective. The act of hitting someone, however, is an *observable* clear fact, not a perception. Also, be careful not to use a *diagnostic* term, such as "depression," as a *descriptive* term. Describe the actual behaviors you observe instead (for example, avoids eye contact, identifies own mood as intense sadness, movements slower than typical) and how those behaviors impact occupation. The performance skills list in the *OTPF-4* (AOTA, 2020) is especially useful to review as it describes the kinds of observable behaviors occupational therapy practitioners look for and document relating to a client's occupational performance. Refer to Table 12-1 for additional documentation suggestions. Realize this is not an all-inclusive list but merely some suggestions. Not everything will fit neatly into these categories, but it will give you a good idea of the types of things to consider.

Table 12-1		
Documenting Observations Accurately		
Areas to Consider	*"O"—What are your professional observations of client factors, performance skills, and environment?* *Provide objective data from your intervention session and avoid value judgments. Consider some of the following suggestions relevant to your client's situation that you might elaborate upon and document with specificity:*	*"A"—What professional phrases summarize your relevant observations for the assessment?* *Describe why those specific observations matter for your client and relate to intervention plan. Realize the statements below are merely examples of some of the many possible indicators of problems, progress, or rehabilitation potential.*
Appearance	• Hair combed/styled/clean or not? • Make-up well-applied or not (e.g., lipstick extends to ear)? • Clean-shaven/trimmed facial hair (or typical for context)? • Teeth/face unclean (e.g., food particles, nasal discharge)? • Teeth missing, dentures in place, glasses, hearing aids? • Clothes wrinkled or neatly pressed? • Clothing torn, dirty, or ill-fitting (e.g., sleeve/pant leg nearly detached, clothing size too small for fastenings to close, multiple stains on front of shirt)? *** Realize that certain clothing features may be the current fashion trend (e.g., muddy jeans, ripped denim). • Clothing disordered/incorrect on body (e.g., only one arm in sleeve, underwear over pants, wearing only one sock, bra not fastened)? • Clothing appropriate for situation and weather? • Fastenings closed or open (e.g., due to lack of attention, poor prehension/sensation, clothing size)? • Wearing sling, cast, orthotic/prosthetic device, bandage? • Visible dirt on skin/hands, are nails clean and groomed? • Presence of skin lesions, cuts, needle marks, thick callous?	• Client's neat/well-groomed appearance this past week may indicate … (e.g., improved mood, better understanding of appropriate attire for social situations/work, improved time management skills) • Lack of attention to personal hygiene may be a sign that … (e.g., client is not adhering to his medication regimen, client is preoccupied with her spouse's illness) • Client's poor hygiene and unclean clothing raise concerns regarding … (e.g., possible changes in mood, caregiver's ability to care for client)
Level of Alertness, Orientation, and Activity Tolerance	• Eyes open or closed? • Can client wake up (stays awake how long)? • Appears groggy, drowsy, listless, or slow-moving? • Does client exhibit confusion (describe statements/actions)? • Awareness of person, place, time, situation? • Type of stimuli needed for responsiveness? • Ability to follow/respond to specific auditory, visual or tactile stimuli, questions or motor commands?	• Recurrent _____ (e.g., syncope, vertigo) when out of bed hinders client's ability to … (e.g., care for child, shower safely, go out into the community) • Client's difficulty with _____ (e.g., staying awake during the day, sustained attention) impedes his ability to … (e.g., perform job duties safely, drive)

(continued)

Table 12-1 (continued)		
Documenting Observations Accurately		
Areas to Consider	*"O"—What are your professional observations of client factors, performance skills, and environment?* *Provide objective data from your intervention session and avoid value judgments. Consider some of the following suggestions relevant to your client's situation that you might elaborate upon and document with specificity:*	*"A"—What professional phrases summarize your relevant observations for the assessment?* *Describe why those specific observations matter for your client and relate to intervention plan. Realize the statements below are merely examples of some of the many possible indicators of problems, progress, or rehabilitation potential.*
Level of Alertness, Orientation, and Activity Tolerance	• Rest and sleep patterns (sleep-wake cycle, insomnia, hypersomnia)? • Ability to attend and for how long? • Current vs. past performance patterns (sedentary or active behavior), any concerns, and typical or not? • Is client's behavior related to recent anesthesia/medical procedures/medication? • Ability and amount of time needed for task completion? • Uses oxygen (e.g., nasal cannula, number of liters, ventilator)? • Measurement of blood oxygen levels/heart rate/blood pressure at rest and/or activity? • Pacing, timing, any rest periods needed (quantify/describe)? • Is client pale, diaphoretic, short of breath, perspiring profusely, or reports fatigue, dizziness, vertigo, nausea?	• Client's poor activity tolerance is a barrier to … (e.g., returning to work, functional mobility at school, carrying out homemaker role) • Client's ability to complete _____ (e.g., showering, dressing) without shortness of breath or rest periods demonstrates… (e.g., good gains in endurance since initial evaluation, good potential to return to independent living)
Affect/ Demeanor, Behavior, and Task Skills	• Eye contact or avoidant, downward gaze? • Does client move erratically, toss/turn, are postures typical? • Client's stated mood/feelings (e.g., anhedonia, expresses intense feelings of sadness, guilt, shame, anger)? • Nonverbal communication/facial expression? • Client tearful/crying and for how long (how consoled)? • What did client do and say (specific positive or negative statements expressed)? • Expresses harmful thoughts regarding self or others (e.g., suicidal ideation, threats of bodily harm)? • What is client's stated opinion/outlook regarding present situation/future circumstances, response to intervention? • Examples of problem solving, decision making, judgment? • Safety awareness/emergency preparedness (give examples)? • Approach to new or difficult situations? • Attention to detail? • Is client easily frustrated (statements made/actions taken)? • Does client engage in risk-taking behaviors (e.g., physical altercations, excessive speeding, promiscuity)? • Expresses awareness of deficits or consequences of actions, willingness to learn from mistakes, and change behavior? • Client's assessment of own abilities, appearance, etc.? • Eating behaviors (e.g., healthy diet, avoids eating, binges, purges)? • Does client adhere to/comply/follow through with prescribed medications, diet, orthosis use, exercises, etc.? • Demonstrates ability to complete task within acceptable standards/time frames? • Kinds of relationships, social supports, interpersonal skills? • Is encouragement needed to initiate or complete tasks? • Does client engage easily with others (e.g., peers, family, authority figures) alone/or in group situations? • Describe how client reacts in new situations, adapts to new routines, or shows preference for highly structured tasks? • Does client use profane language, yell or scream inappropriately (describe situations)? • Does client express fears/worries (realistic or unrealistic)? • Specific avoidance behaviors exhibited? • Describe client's coping strategies/behaviors for managing anger, stress, anxiety, etc.? • Does client exhibit behaviors such as spitting, hitting, kicking, hurting others, destroying objects? • Exhibits self-injurious behaviors (e.g., head banging, scratching, hitting) or self-mutilation (e.g., cutting)?	• Client's _____ (e.g., good frustration tolerance, careful approach to completing projects in task group) is an asset for … • Client's ability this week to _____ (e.g., describe several things she is good at) is an indicator of improved … (e.g., self-confidence, self-esteem) • Client's tendency to _____ (e.g., engage in risk-taking behaviors without considering consequences) is a concern for his … (e.g., safety, health, financial stability, maintaining steady employment) • Client's good _____ (e.g., organizational and decision-making skills) are strengths for … (e.g., getting her own apartment, sticking to a budget) • Client's tendency to avoid _____ (e.g., eating, initiating conversations, driving over bridges) is a barrier to … • Client's intense fear of _____ (e.g., germs, dying, social encounters, closed spaces) prevents her from … (e.g., leaving the home, seeking employment, performing necessary childcare tasks) • Client's preference for _____ (e.g., expressing feelings using actions rather than words, eating fast food instead of healthier choices) creates problems with … • Client's poor follow through with _____ (e.g., attending AA meetings, taking prescribed medications, eating a healthier diet, HEP) impedes his ability to … (e.g., abstain from alcohol, manage diabetes/weight/stress)

(continued)

Table 12-1 (continued)		
Documenting Observations Accurately		
Areas to Consider	*"O"—What are your professional observations of client factors, performance skills, and environment?* *Provide objective data from your intervention session and avoid value judgments. Consider some of the following suggestions relevant to your client's situation that you might elaborate upon and document with specificity:*	*"A"—What professional phrases summarize your relevant observations for the assessment?* *Describe why those specific observations matter for your client and relate to intervention plan. Realize the statements below are merely examples of some of the many possible indicators of problems, progress, or rehabilitation potential.*
Affect/ Demeanor, Behavior, and Task Skills	• Does client exhibit psychomotor activity/self-stimulation behavior (e.g., rocking, rubbing, pacing, restlessness)? • Exhibits repetitive thoughts/behaviors/rituals? • Client's stated attitude and behavior toward task at hand? • Is client easily persuaded or sticks to an opinion/decision, has fixed ideas (describe pertinent situations)?	• Client's preoccupation with _____ (e.g., own weight, checking door locks, son's illness) hinders ability to …
Motor Function and Factors	• Uses mobility device (e.g., wheelchair, walker, cane)? • Joint mobility and range within normal/functional parameters? • Relevant stiffness/tightness/restrictions/contractures/capsular patterns/hypermobility/crepitation? • Joint stability and alignment concerns (subluxation, joint deformity, scoliosis, kyphosis, lordosis)? • Postural alignment/position at rest/sitting/standing or during an activity (e.g., decorticate/decerebrate posture, symmetry/asymmetry, midline orientation, tendency to lean to side/forward/backward, forward head posture, posterior/anterior pelvic tilt)? • Does client have functional reach, grasp/release and prehension (grasp/pinch patterns used, dexterity)? • Does client have isolated, voluntary movement? • Quality, symmetry, timing of movement (e.g., gross- and fine-motor coordination skills, praxis, agility)? • Are involuntary/extraneous movements or tremors evident at rest or upon AROM (e.g., intention tremors, ataxia, muscle twitching, tics, spasms, clonus)? • Substitution or compensatory motions evident? • Are muscles well-defined or atrophied? • Muscle grades, evidence of weakness/paresis? • Excessive, low, or abnormal tone evident (e.g., spasticity, rigidity, hypertonicity, hypotonicity, flaccidity)? • Balance seated/standing and risk of falling? • Unsteady or shuffling gait? • Wide base of support needed? • Reciprocal motion when ambulating? • Ability to weight-shift in different directions/positions? • Muscle tension/pain reported or not (quantify/describe)?	• Client's _____ (e.g., fair balance, unsteady gait) create safety concerns for … (e.g., using stove, showering, living alone at home due to fall risk) • Client's gains in _____ (e.g., left shoulder flexion P/AROM from 95 to 125 degrees since last week) indicate good progress toward goal of … • Client's ability to now _____ (e.g., maintain upright posture seated on EOB 10 minutes, stand without assistance) demonstrates potential for … (e.g., self-care independence) • Client's _____ (e.g., limited AROM Ⓡ elbow, poor hand strength, Ⓛ hip pain) prevents him from … (e.g., returning to work, performing yard chores, working on his car) • Student's ability to now _____ (e.g., use Ⓡ hand as a functional assist) indicates good potential for … (e.g., independently managing clothing during toileting at school)
Physical Environment	• Type and level of dirt/grime/unsanitary conditions (e.g., feces smeared on walls, spilled carton of milk on kitchen floor, piles of dirty dishes in bedroom)? • Items in appropriate places or not (e.g., purse in oven)? • Can client or others locate items easily? • Noise level and types of auditory/visual distractions (e.g., proximity to construction site, train station)? • Specific fall hazards? • Sharps hazards? • Fire hazards? • Childproofing needed? • Presence/quantity of insects or rodents? • Mold present/amount? • Presence of lead, peeling paint? • Rotting food or open containers? • Raw sewage/pet waste? • Exposed electrical wires? • Garbage not in proper containers? • Areas inaccessible due to piles of … (e.g., clothes, garbage, food containers, boxes)? • Is ambient temperature inadequate (e.g., lack of heat)? • Specific physical or architectural barriers?	• Client's inability to _____ (e.g., get adequate sleep due to firehouse sirens, train station noise) shows need for … (e.g., night-time use of ear plugs/white noise machine) • Client's recent efforts with _____ (e.g., improving cleanliness in the home) demonstrate … (e.g., willingness to comply with plan for getting her child back) • Hazardous/unsafe/unsanitary conditions of _____ (e.g., peeling lead paint, mold, broken steps) in the home raise concern regarding … (e.g., child staying there, client falling/getting sick/injured, client's ability to live alone safely) • Lack of w/c accessibility for _____ (e.g., entering client's home) creates need for … (e.g., ramp, alternate living arrangement) *(continued)*

	Table 12-1 (continued) **Documenting Observations Accurately**	
Areas to Consider	*"O"—What are your professional observations of client factors, performance skills, and environment?* *Provide objective data from your intervention session and avoid value judgments. Consider some of the following suggestions relevant to your client's situation that you might elaborate upon and document with specificity:*	*"A"—What professional phrases summarize your relevant observations for the assessment?* *Describe why those specific observations matter for your client and relate to intervention plan. Realize the statements below are merely examples of some of the many possible indicators of problems, progress, or rehabilitation potential.*
Communication/ Speech	• What is the client's primary language? • Does the client speak or understand English? • Is client able to hear, speak, read, or write? • Does client have a speech impediment/specific difficulties with verbal communication (e.g., expressive aphasia, receptive aphasia, slurred speech, oral apraxia, word-finding difficulties, lisp, stutter)? • Does the client just grunt or make other types of noises? • Is client willing to speak or is client uncommunicative? • Can you hear/understand what client is saying (clear, coherent, or unintelligible)? • Is speech monotone or does client modulate speech and tone of voice? • Speech cadence, quality of speech, and flow (e.g., fluent, halting)? • Difficulty recalling words? • Does the client's speech make sense? • Can client answer verbal/written questions, respond to commands, and express ideas effectively? • Does infant babble? • Is speech age-appropriate or is language delay evident? • Is communication relevant to the situation? • Does client repeat things over and over (perseverate) or exhibit echolalia? • Profanity or words that might be perceived by others as threatening exhibited? • Length of responses/conversation? • Oral-motor weakness or difficulty forming words? • Pain or loose/missing teeth causing difficulty? • Social interaction skills? • Amount of time needed to initiate or complete response when asked a question (typical or not)? • Are responses direct and accurate? • Does client demonstrate interrupting behaviors, talk about unrelated topics, or need redirection?	• Client's communication difficulties raise concerns regarding … (e.g., ability to use telephone in emergency situations, ability to stay in contact with distant relatives) • Client's ability to make needs known and ask for help when needed is a strength for … • Client's _____ (e.g., difficulty with interpreting social cues, need for frequent redirection to topic) is a barrier to … (e.g., passing a job interview, attending medical appointments independently) • Client's continued _____ (e.g., expression of words that might be perceived as threatening by others) … (e.g., creates potential for being fired, hinders ability to establish positive peer relationships, demonstrates poor judgment) • Client's _____ (e.g., interrupting behaviors, inability to answer questions in a timely manner, speech impediment) is a challenge for … (e.g., obtaining a client-facing job, ordering goods/ services by phone)

Complete Worksheets 12-1 and 12-2 to review the mechanics of documentation and terminology that you learned in Chapters 2, 4, and 5. Then, complete Learning Activities 12-1, 12-2, and 12-3 to help you integrate the suggestions in this chapter with information you learned in the previous chapters. The worksheets will help you to start making professional observations and use clinical reasoning skills for writing your own original SOAP notes. You may practice writing SOAP notes using Figures 2-2 and 2-3 in Chapter 2 of this book.

A Quick Checklist for Evaluating Your Note

Use the following two summary charts as a quick reference guide to ensure that your note contains all of the essential elements.

	S: Subjective	
☐	1.	Use something significant the client says about their treatment or condition.
	O: Objective	
☐	1.	Begin this section with:
☐		○ Indication of active client engagement/participation
☐		○ Length of session
☐		○ Setting
☐		○ Purpose of session
☐	2.	Report your observations succinctly and accurately, either chronologically or using categories.
☐	3.	Remember to do the following:
☐		○ De-emphasize the treatment media
☐		○ Specify what part of the task required assistance
☐		○ Specify the exact type and amount of assistance needed
☐		○ Use professional language and standard abbreviations
☐		○ Show skilled occupational therapy happening
☐		○ Leave yourself out
☐		○ Focus on the client's response
☐		○ Avoid being judgmental
	A: Assessment	
☐	1.	Look at the data in your "S" and "O" sentence by sentence, asking yourself what problems, progress, and rehab potential you see.
☐	2.	Ask yourself, "So what? Why is this important in the client's life?" For each underlying factor not within functional limits, identify the impact it will have on an area of occupation.
☐	3.	End the "A" with *"Client would benefit from …"*
☐		○ Justify continued skilled occupational therapy
☐		○ Set up the plan
☐	4.	Be sure the timelines and interventions you are putting in your plan match the skilled OT you indicate your client needs.
	P: Plan	
☐	1.	Specify the frequency and duration of occupational therapy intervention.
☐	2.	Tell what you will be working on during that time to address the client's needs.
☐	3.	Relate to a performance skill/area of occupation and client's OT goals.
☐	4.	Indicate any other pertinent follow-up needed for the client's present situation.
	Remember to:	
☐	Include the client's identifying information, delineate OT department and type of note.	
☐	Correct errors properly, do not erase or use correction fluid, and do not leave blank spaces.	
☐	Make certain engagement in occupation is integral to the note.	
☐	Sign and date your note.	

Morreale, M. J. (2023). *The OTA's guide to documentation: Writing SOAP notes* (5th ed.). SLACK Incorporated.

S: Subjective
- ☐ Use something **significant** the client says about their **treatment** or **condition**.
- ☐ If there is nothing significant, ask yourself whether you are using your interview skills to elicit the proper information about how the client sees things.

O: Objective
- ☐ Begin this section with length of session, where the intervention took place, and for what purpose. Make sure you indicate active client participation. For example,
  Client participated in 30-minute OT session in hospital room for instruction in compensatory dressing techniques.
- ☐ Summarize what you observe, either chronologically or using categories.
- ☐ Focus on performance skills and de-emphasize the treatment media. For example,
  Client worked on three-point pinch using pegs.
- ☐ Relate methods/tasks (i.e., ROM, physical agent modalities) to occupational performance.
  Client worked on three-point pinch using pegs in order to manage buttons on clothing.
- ☐ Specify the **part** of the task needing assistance and the exact **type** and **amount** of assistance provided.
  Client required five verbal cues for correct hand placement during w/c ↔ toilet transfers.
- ☐ Indicate that the client **needed** assistance rather than labeling the client as an assist level.
  "Client required min assist ..." rather than *"Client is min assist ..."*
- ☐ Use standardized terminology to grade and describe interventions and client performance.
- ☐ Show skilled occupational therapy happening—make it clear that you were not just a passive observer. For example, do not just list all of the assist levels and think that is enough.
- ☐ Write from the client's point of view, leaving yourself out.
  "Client was repositioned in w/c ..." rather than *"COTA repositioned client in w/c ..."*
- ☐ Focus on the client's response rather than on what you did.
  Client able to don socks using sock aid after demonstration.
- ☐ Avoid judging the client. For example,
  Say client *"... didn't complete the activity."* Don't add *"... because he was stubborn."*

A: Assessment
- ☐ Look at the data in your "S" and "O" sentence by sentence, identifying problems, progress, and rehab potential. Ask yourself what each statement means for the client's occupational performance. Consider the following formula:

Underlying Limiting Factor ⟶ Functional Impact ⟶ Ability to Engage in Occupation

  For example, if in your "O" you noted that client falls to the left when sitting unsupported, what do you think this means they will be unable to do for themselves? For example,
  Client unable to sit EOB unsupported to don clothing.
- ☐ Make sure you have not introduced any new information.
- ☐ End the "A" with *"Client would benefit from ..."*
- ☐ Justify continued skilled occupational therapy.
  Client would benefit from skilled instruction in use of adaptive devices and compensatory techniques for performing IADL tasks one-handed.
- ☐ Set up the plan and match time lines in your plan to the skilled OT you document that your client needs. For example, if you justify skilled OT by saying only, *"Client would benefit from skilled instruction in energy conservation techniques,"* then do not say that you plan to treat client twice a day for 2 weeks. Skilled instruction in energy conservation should generally take only one session or, at most, two sessions.

P: Plan
- ☐ Specify the frequency, duration of treatment, and specific OT interventions that will be implemented.
- ☐ Identify the performance skills and occupations that will be addressed during that time.
  Continue OT 1 hour daily for 2 weeks for upper body strengthening and instruction in adaptive devices needed for safe and ① transfers to bed, toilet, and tub.

Morreale, M. J. (2023). *The OTA's guide to documentation: Writing SOAP notes* (5th ed.). SLACK Incorporated.

Worksheet 12-1
Mechanics of Documentation

Certain basic elements must be present in all documentation formats. Look at the following handwritten contact note and determine the elements that are incorrect or missing. Realize that this note reflects a "special situation" and, therefore, does not need to include the complete, structured S, O, A, and P format.

XYZ School District

Albany, NY

Stewart Stoodant

6/01/22 Upon arrival at therapy room, student reported he had a headache, felt nauseous, and stated he was "burning up." OT session defered and student excorted to ~~teach~~ nurse's office.

C. Caring, COTA

1.

2.

3.

4.

5.

6.

7.

8.

9.

10.

11.

12.

Morreale, M. J. (2023). *The OTA's guide to documentation: Writing SOAP notes* (5th ed.). SLACK Incorporated.

Worksheet 12-2
Documentation Basics

For each of the following SOAP note sentences, correct any errors in spelling, grammar, abbreviations, and basic mechanics of documentation.

1. The client used compensitory techniques to donn his shoes and socks.

2. The client preformed bed mobility Ⓘ, then sat on SOB with SBA to doff his shirt.

3. Child was seen for 20 minutes in classroom to help her put her coat on.

4. Client stated he will "not wear his orthosis to work."

5. The CVA pt. demonstrated ability to transfer bed ↔ commode with SBA and VC.

6. The child demonstrated progress by using her bad hand to stabilize the paper when writing.

7. During her Occupational Therapy session, the pt. worked on ↑ Ⓛ neglect and ↓ safety to perform ADLs.

8. I instructed the client in arom exercises to improve her ability to braid her two daughter's hair.

9. While eating her pudding desert, the client performed self-feeding with modified assistance.

10. The THR client's Ⓛ hip is sore because the PT made her walk too long.

11. The student was mod assist to write his name.

12. The child had a rash around her naval which she kept itching.

Morreale, M. J. (2023). *The OTA's guide to documentation: Writing SOAP notes* (5th ed.). SLACK Incorporated.

LEARNING ACTIVITY 12-1: IMPROVING OBSERVATION SKILLS

Try a creative role-playing exercise with a partner to practice your observation and documentation skills. Imagine your partner has had a stroke and cannot use the dominant upper extremity. Pick an ADL or IADL to work on (e.g., putting on a shoe or jacket, making a sandwich) and teach your partner compensatory techniques, just as you would a client. Then, using the suggestions in this chapter as a guide, list your observations for the "intervention session."

WHO

WHAT

WHERE

WHEN

WHY

HOW

Using this information, write an organized and professional SOAP note regarding your partner's "intervention session" on a separate page.

Learning Activity 12-2: Improving Observation Skills—More Practice

Now try another creative role-playing exercise with a partner to practice your observation and documentation skills. Imagine your partner has a diagnosis of arthritis or COPD and has decreased upper extremity AROM and difficulty performing daily activities. Pick one ADL or IADL to work on (e.g., cooking, grooming, managing fastenings) and teach joint protection, energy conservation, or compensatory techniques. Also, teach your partner some exercises to improve AROM. Then, use the suggestions in this chapter to list your observations for the "intervention session."

WHO

WHAT

WHERE

WHEN

WHY

HOW

Using this information, write an organized and professional SOAP note regarding your partner's "intervention session" on a separate page.

LEARNING ACTIVITY 12-3: VIDEO OBSERVATION SKILLS

Using an internet search engine, find a video of an OT intervention session or a video that demonstrates use of an adaptive device or technique. Consider the suggestions in this chapter as you carefully watch and analyze the video. Write down your observations of the client and situation shown in the video. Realize this is simply a creative writing exercise to practice your observation and documentation skills.

WHO

WHAT

WHERE

WHEN

WHY

HOW

Using this information, now write an organized and professional SOAP note regarding this client's "intervention session" on a separate page.

LEARNING ACTIVITY 12-4: DOCUMENTING PROFESSIONAL OBSERVATIONS

List 15 to 20 words that can be used to document professional observations of skin or lesions (relating to appearance, turgor, temperature, and descriptions of wounds).
Examples: Pale, rash

References

American Occupational Therapy Association. (2020). Occupational therapy practice framework: Domain and process (4th ed.). *American Journal of Occupational Therapy, 74*(Suppl. 2), 7412410010. https://doi.org: 10.5014/ajot.2020.74S2001

American Occupational Therapy Association. (2021). Standards of practice for occupational therapy. *American Journal of Occupational Therapy, 75*(Suppl. 3), 7513410030. https://doi.org/10.5014/ajot.2021.75S3004

Chapter 13

Making Good Notes Even Better

This chapter will help you review the four sections of the SOAP note. Complete the worksheets to practice what you have learned and to improve your skills.

Writing the "S"—Subjective

This section includes anything significant the client says regarding their intervention, condition or situation. When you are working with a young child or a client who is confused or unable to communicate, you may report on nonverbal communication or state what the primary caregiver says. Complete Learning Activity 13-1 to practice interviewing a client who is nonverbal.

Sometimes inexperienced OTAs will simply list anything the client had to say about their condition, but that is not always appropriate. Professional reasoning is used to determine what information is relevant enough to include in the note. Worksheet 13-1 will test your understanding of the different sections of the SOAP note. In Worksheet 13-2 you will find that all of the information presented is relevant but does not form a coherent whole. You will have the opportunity to practice condensing and organizing the information to make the "S" more concise.

LEARNING ACTIVITY 13-1: NONVERBAL COMMUNICATION

Your adult client has hemiparesis, is nonverbal, but nods yes or no appropriately when asked a question. This client was issued an orthosis 2 days ago for positioning hand and wrist properly and returned to OT today for scheduled follow-up. List the questions you might ask this client regarding the orthotic device.

You are working in a school setting with Logan, a 6-year-old with autism who is uncommunicative. Two of the goals in Logan's Individualized Education Program (IEP) include the ability to verbalize a one to two word response when asked a question and independence in managing clothing for recess and toileting. You plan to work with Logan in his classroom today. List the questions you might ask him at the beginning of the session.

Morreale, M. J. *The OTA's Guide to Documentation: Writing SOAP Notes, Fifth Edition* (pp. 189-200). © 2023 Taylor & Francis Group.

Worksheet 13-1
SOAPing Your Note

Indicate which section of the SOAP note you would place each of the following statements.

1. ___ Client supine → sit in bed Ⓘ.
2. ___ Client moved kitchen items from counter to cabinet Ⓘ using Ⓛ hand.
3. ___ Parent reports child's handwriting has improved significantly within the past month.
4. ___ Problems include decreased coordination, strength, sensation, and proprioception in left hand, which create safety risks in home management tasks.
5. ___ Client reports that his fingers are stiff this morning and that he is having trouble handling small items like buttons.
6. ___ By the end of next intervention session, client will demonstrate ability to don/doff orthosis Ⓘ.
7. ___ Increase of 15 minutes in activity tolerance for UE activities permits her to prepare a light meal Ⓘ.
8. ___ Child participated in 30-minute OT session to promote development of FM skills for ADLs.
9. ___ Deficits in proprioception and motor planning limit client's ability to dress herself.
10. ___ Continue ROM and retrograde massage to Ⓡ hand for edema control and to enable grasp of objects needed for ADLs.
11. ___ Consumer will be seen 2X weekly to improve attention to task in order to obtain a job.
12. ___ Client reports that she cannot remember her hip precautions.
13. ___ Client would benefit from further instruction to incorporate total hip precautions into lower body dressing, bathing, and toilet hygiene.
14. ___ Learning was evident by client's ability to improve with repetition.
15. ___ Client's request to take rest breaks demonstrates knowledge of her limitations in endurance.
16. ___ Client required three verbal prompts to interact with peers in OT social group.
17. ___ Fair plus muscle grade in Ⓡ wrist extensors this week shows good progress toward goals.
18. ___ Poor temporal organization interferes with getting to work on time.
19. ___ Next session, instruct parent in proper positioning of infant for bottle feeding.
20. ___ Client demonstrated ability to perform sliding board transfer w/c ↔ mat with min assist to position board properly.

Morreale, M. J. (2023). *The OTA's guide to documentation: Writing SOAP notes* (5th ed.). SLACK Incorporated.

Worksheet 13-2
Writing the "S"—Subjective

Try to write a more concise version of the following "S."

Client told OTA she has very bad arthritis in her Ⓡ shoulder and Ⓡ knee.
Client said, "It really hurts a lot to stand on my right leg."
Client described Ⓡ LE pain as 7/10 when weightbearing.
When client was told she would be working on sliding board transfers today, client stated, "It [sliding board] needs to be moved further up on the seat."
When asked how she felt at start of session, client said, "I'm just tired."
Client said, "This is the hardest transfer for me."
Client stated she prefers to approach transfers from her Ⓡ side.

S:

Morreale, M. J. (2023). *The OTA's guide to documentation: Writing SOAP notes* (5th ed.). SLACK Incorporated.

Writing the "O"—Objective

Your professional, skilled observations are summarized and recorded in this section, either chronologically or in categories. Start with a statement indicating active client participation, where the intervention took place, length of session, and purpose. The "O" focuses on the client's response to the intervention provided. Remember to de-emphasize the treatment media and describe assist levels accurately. Try to show your professional skill in the first sentence but keep the focus on the client, not the OTA. Consider this example of a male client whose limited mobility is compromising his positioning. Rather than saying, *"Client seen for positioning,"* a better choice of an opening sentence would be:

Client and spouse participated in 25-minute session in home for education on positioning to prevent skin breakdown.
Client participated in 30-minute session in rehab gym for assessment of w/c positioning to improve sitting posture for mealtimes.
Pt. participated in 40-minute session bedside for positioning strategies to minimize risk of falling out of w/c.

Complete Worksheet 13-3 to practice writing good opening lines in the "O" part of the note.

Worksheet 13-3
Making Opening Lines Better

Rewrite the following opening sentences to show how your skill as an OTA is important in each situation.

1.   **Old opening sentence:** *Client practiced laundry tasks for 45 minutes.*
     Additional information:
     - Client has total hip precautions, which raise safety concerns during functional mobility, especially during performance of household chores.
     - Adaptive equipment is available if needed.
     New opening sentence:

2.   **Old opening sentence:** *Consumer seen at workshop for 1 hour to improve job skills.*
     Additional information:
     - Deficits in time management skills ↓ his ability to work Ⓘ.
     - Bilateral coordination problems interfere with client completing an essential job function of opening/closing boxes.
     - ↓ tolerance to auditory stimuli contribute to client's high distractibility during task completion.
     New opening sentence:

3.   **Old opening sentence:** *Client seen in his hospital room bedside for 30 minutes for feeding.*
     Additional information:
     - Client has Ⓛ neglect.
     - Client's dominant hand is flaccid.
     - Adaptive equipment is available.
     New opening sentence:

4.   **Old opening sentence:** *Worked with client in kitchen for 1 hour to ↑ Ⓘ in cooking.*
     Additional information:
     - Client's problems include decreased tolerance for standing and inattention of affected left upper extremity, which raise safety concerns.
     New opening sentence:

Be Specific About Assist Levels

Remember that in addition to reporting the level of assistance needed, you also must be specific about the **part of the task** that required assistance.

Not specific enough:

> *Resident supine → sit with max Ⓐ, sit → stand mod Ⓐ.*

Specific:

> *Resident supine → sit with max Ⓐ to lift legs over EOB, sit → stand with mod Ⓐ for balance and to maintain toe-touch weight-bearing precautions with use of walker.*

There is a difference between telling **why** the assist was needed, for example:

> *Client needed mod verbal cues to eat lunch due to perceptual deficits.*

… and **the part of the task** that required assistance:

> *Client needed mod verbal cues to locate utensils and food on Ⓛ side of meal tray.*

It is helpful to list both the part of the task that needed assistance and the observable reason for why the assist was needed:

> *Client needed mod verbal cues to locate utensils and food on Ⓛ side of meal tray due to unilateral inattention.*
> *—or—*
> *Due to his Ⓛ neglect, mod verbal cues were needed for client to locate all items on Ⓛ side of meal tray.*

Make the "O" Complete and Concise

In the objective section of your note, you record your observations of the intervention session concisely. As you become more proficient, it becomes easier to determine what to include and what to omit. Below is an observation of an intervention session that is very concise and could use some improvement.

Client was seen in hospital room for ADLs and transfer activities.

ADLs

> *Client donned robe Ⓘ with set-up.*
> *Client donned/doffed socks Ⓘ with set-up.*

Mobility

> *Bed → chair with CGA*
> *Supine → sit Ⓘ*

What problems are evident with this "O"?

This note is *too* concise and omits pertinent information. It lacks an indication that skilled occupational therapy was provided. This note could begin with an opening sentence that shows why your skill as an OTA is needed in this situation. As it stands, it is apparent that someone observed the client dress and transfer and recorded assist levels, but nursing staff or a rehabilitation aide could simply have done this.

Secondly, the activities documented in this note do not appear to require much time, so the session could be very short. If this is a 1-hour therapy session, was anything else done? Was education or special instruction provided? If the client was slow to do the things recorded above, what caused so few activities to take such a long time? Is there a cognitive or perceptual problem? Is there a problem with coordination, safety, or motor planning? Did the client use compensatory techniques or adaptive equipment to be independent?

Third, as this note indicates the client is independent, there is nothing else in this note to justify that additional occupational therapy is necessary. Unless this is the final intervention session, there needs to be information provided that will justify continued therapy.

Worksheet 13-4
Writing the "O"—Objective

Now it is your turn to practice. Read the observation below and consider what this note needs to make it better. Instead of rewriting the entire note, just write suggestions to improve the note in the space below:

Toilet transfers:　　mod Ⓐ
Toileting:　　min Ⓐ with SBA 2° inability to support self with Ⓛ arm and to dress
UE dressing:　　min Ⓐ, verbal cues, set up, Ⓘ in pulling shirt over head
LE dressing:　　used dressing stick
　　min Ⓐ pants to hips
　　max Ⓐ pants to waist
　　modified Ⓘ to don Ⓛ shoe (elastic shoelaces)
　　modified Ⓘ to don Ⓡ shoe (elastic shoelaces)
Ⓡ hand status:　　Ⓡ fingers: small has spasticity (index finger greatest amount)
　　Thumb: CMC joint painful in abduction
　　Ⓡ wrist: flaccid

Suggestions to improve this note:

1.

2.

3.

4.

Writing Effective Assessment Statements

It is sometimes difficult for a student or inexperienced OTA to differentiate an observation from an assessment. An observation is anything you see a client **do,** whereas your assessment is how that behavior **impacts** an area of occupation. The assessment is your professional opinion about the meaning of what you have just observed in the intervention session. As you analyze the information you gathered, you will look for evidence of problems, progress (or lack of progress), and rehab potential. Problems may include any aspect of the occupational therapy domain that is not within functional limits or creates a concern (Gateley & Borcherding, 2017). The assessment is not the place to include any new information and it should end with a statement of what the client would benefit from. For example, for a client who has hip precautions and for whom you have observed some problem areas, you might say:

A: *Client's inability to remember hip precautions without verbal cues during IADLs puts her at risk for re-injury. Supportive daughter and ability to use adaptive equipment properly after instruction indicate a good potential for reaching stated goals. Client would benefit from further skilled instruction in maintaining hip precautions during IADL tasks, sit ↔ stand, and transitional living skills.*

In Chapter 9 you learned a useful formula to assess the underlying factors that are not within functional limits. While not the only correct way to write assessments, this formula will help you to include all of the necessary components in your assessment.

Underlying Limiting Factor ⟶ Functional Impact ⟶ Ability to Engage in Occupation

There are several steps needed to assess an underlying factor that is not within functional limits:

1. First determine what the basic deficit or problem is (such as *poor muscle strength, inability to attend to task, an environmental barrier,* or *a challenging aspect of the activity*).

2. Make the problem or deficit the subject of your statement for emphasis.

3. Determine whether the area of difficulty you have observed today is an indicator of a broader area of occupation. For example, is the decreased strength you observed causing grooming difficulties also creating problems in other basic ADL tasks? Will the client's intense worry, fear of falling or poor attention impede work tasks? Will the problems you observed today create any safety concerns or affect the ability to return home?

4. Your assessment statement must relate how the problem areas impact the client's ability to engage in meaningful occupation. After each problem you note (e.g., limited strength, poor attention, intense worry, fear of falling), ask yourself, "So what?" So the client is unable to do that—how does this impact his or her life? The answer to your "so what" question becomes your assessment of the situation.

5. Relate how the client would benefit from further occupational therapy. If no further occupational therapy is warranted or other recommendations are appropriate at this time, indicate why.

Let us now compare some observation and assessment statements.

Suppose you are working with a female client who plans to return home to live alone in her apartment. Your intervention has included teaching her hip precautions following her total hip replacement, but she forgets to incorporate these when practicing home management tasks. What is this client's basic or core problem? Why does it matter or why is it important?

The following statement is an objective **observation** of the client's behavior:

Pt. was unable to adhere to hip precautions during laundry task due to memory deficit.

However, when phrased differently, it demonstrates the OTA's clinical reasoning and becomes an **assessment** of what was observed:

Memory deficit interferes with client's ability to adhere to total hip precautions, which limits her ability to safely perform self-care and IADL tasks needed to return to prior Ⓘ living situation.

The OTA has determined in the assessment that this client's basic problem is the inability to retain instructions. The OTA should then address this problem with a recommendation to use compensatory techniques (memory cues) of some kind. The safety concerns that impact the client's ability to return home should be considered. Otherwise, why should a third-party payer continue to pay for instruction that will not be remembered? According to the formula, rather than repeat what was observed, the assessment begins with the underlying problem, expands the scope of the area of occupation to include related tasks, (in this case IADLs and self-care tasks), and answers the question, "So what? Why does this matter in this client's life or why is it important?"

Sweeping Assessment Statements

Due to a busy schedule and time constraints, it can be tempting for an OTA to make brief and sweeping assessment statements such as:

A: *Deficits in upper body strength, fine motor skills, and feeding limit Jordan's ability to be Ⓘ in home and classroom activities.*

Although accurate, this statement is limited and would benefit from some elaboration. A better way to assess Jordan's information would be to say:

A: *Deficits in upper body strength limit Jordan's Ⓘ in eating, functional mobility, and dressing. Decreased fine motor skills impede typical classroom activities such as holding a pencil/crayon, manipulating small items, as well as age-appropriate IADL tasks in which Jordan is beginning to show an emerging interest. Jordan would benefit from continued upper body strengthening, reach-grasp-release tasks, and skilled feeding activities to move Jordan more expediently through typical developmental milestones.*

The assessment demonstrates your clinical reasoning as an OTA and enables others reading your note to better understand the client's situation.

Worksheet 13-5
Differentiating Between Observations and Assessments

Identify which of the statements below are observations and which are assessments.

1. _____ Client is unable to don Ⓛ LE prosthesis for functional mobility.

2. _____ Inability to don Ⓛ LE prosthesis Ⓘ prevents client from performing safe functional mobility around the house to live alone.

3. _____ Decreased tolerance to auditory stimuli limits the student's ability to attend to classroom tasks.

4. _____ Student required three verbal cues to stay on task due to decreased tolerance to auditory stimuli.

5. _____ Client was unable to incorporate relaxation and stress reduction techniques, requiring several verbal prompts to complete task.

6. _____ Inability to incorporate relaxation and stress reduction techniques when interacting with sales clerk limits client's ability to manage shopping tasks Ⓘ after discharge.

Reword the following observations to make them **assessments**.

1. Client required five verbal cues to attend to and sequence task of balancing checkbook due to memory deficits.

2. Client needed moderate assistance to complete grooming and laundry tasks due to Ⓛ neglect, impulsive behavior, and decreased attention to task.

3. After the use of behavior modification techniques, child demonstrated ability to remain seated at his desk for the remainder of the treatment session.

Morreale, M. J. (2023). *The OTA's guide to documentation: Writing SOAP notes* (5th ed.). SLACK Incorporated.

Worksheet 13-6
Problems, Progress, and Rehab Potential

For the following observation, note the problems or underlying factors not within functional limits for this male client recovering from a Ⓛ CVA. Then, list the information that indicates potential for progress.

O: *Client participated in 30-minute session in OT clinic to work on improving functional movements of Ⓡ UE, dynamic sitting balance, and cognitive skills needed for ADL performance. Client needed mod Ⓐ in shifting weight to get to edge of w/c and max verbal cues to use correct posture and shift feet during standing pivot transfer w/c → mat. Client required max verbal cues to initiate grasp of bag in beanbag activity. Client required mod Ⓐ to initiate reaching with Ⓡ UE but demonstrated ability to complete Ⓡ UE shoulder flexion required to toss bag appropriately 2 feet with max verbal cues. Client demonstrated cognitive understanding of activity with mod verbal cues by stating desired goal to be achieved by accurate aim.*

Problems:

Progress/Rehab Potential:

Assessment: How do the problems and progress you noted impact the client's ability to engage in meaningful occupation (such as safety concerns or ability to care for self)? What would the client benefit from? What skilled OT intervention is indicated? Integrate this information to write the "A" part of this note.

A:

Plan: Your plan contains a statement of how often and for how long you will be seeing the client and your treatment priorities toward the client's goals. Here is an example for a client recovering from hip surgery:

P: *Continue OT 3 x wk for 1 wk to work on incorporating hip precautions into ADL tasks.*

While this plan states what intervention is necessary, it is not very specific. The plan should reflect your clinical reasoning and clarify what specific ADL or problem is a priority to address with the client. For example, it would be better to say:

P: *Continue OT 3 x wk for 1 wk to work on incorporating hip precautions into ADL tasks. Next session, instruct client in use of adaptive equipment for lower body dressing.*

Now finish the note with the plan for the male client with Ⓛ CVA.

P:

Morreale, M. J. (2023). *The OTA's guide to documentation: Writing SOAP notes* (5th ed.). SLACK Incorporated.

Worksheet 13-7
The "Almost" Note

Now it is your turn to integrate all you have learned. This note is **almost** good enough. In fact, it appears to be quite good on the surface, but actually has major flaws in organization and clinical reasoning. This client is a 78-year-old woman who sustained a Ⓛ CVA and has Ⓡ hemiparesis. Her OTA wrote the contact note below. How can this note be improved? There is no need to try to rewrite the entire note. For this worksheet, simply make suggestions about what this note needs to be more effective.

S: *Client reports stiffness in Ⓡ hip, but improvement from previous pain. She states a preference for transferring to her left. Client states that she is willing to do "whatever it takes to get out of the hospital."*

O: *Client seen in room to work on dressing and functional mobility.*

Transfer:	*Client SBA for standing pivot transfer bed → w/c to the left*
	Client is min Ⓐ with transfers w/c → toilet using grab bar
Mobility:	*Client SBA with VCs to flex trunk when rolling from supine to Ⓡ side*
	Client SBA supine → sit; min Ⓐ sit → stand
	Client Ⓘ in w/c mobility
Dressing:	*Client Ⓘ in donning shirt*
	Client is min Ⓐ with VCs to don bra while standing
	Client Ⓘ in donning socks and shoes
	Client min Ⓐ with walker and VCs in donning underwear and pants
	Client needs setup for dressing activities
UE ROM:	*Ⓛ UE—WFL*
	Ⓡ UE—↓ range in shoulder flexion
Static standing:	*Client SBA with walker*
Dynamic standing:	*Client SBA with walker for balance*

A: *Deficits noted in Ⓡ UE coordination, Ⓑ UE strength, and dynamic standing balance. Client Ⓘ in dressing EOB, but is min Ⓐ in dressing when standing with a walker. Ⓛ UE AROM is WFL, but Ⓡ UE has deficits noted in shoulder flexion. Client is SBA in bed mobility when rolling to unaffected side and min Ⓐ sit → stand 2° ↓ UE strength. Client is SBA for transfer to unaffected side in pivot transfer bed → w/c and min Ⓐ w/c → toilet. Client would benefit from skilled OT to continue UE strengthening and coordination exercises and to ↑ dynamic standing balance using walker in order to ↑ Ⓘ in ADLs.*

P: *Client to be seen twice daily for 30-minute sessions to continue to work on dynamic standing balance.*

Suggestions for improving the Almost Note:

© 2023 Taylor & Francis Group.

Morreale, M. J. (2023). *The OTA's guide to documentation: Writing SOAP notes* (5th ed.). SLACK Incorporated.

Reference

Gateley, C. A., & Borcherding, S. (2017). *Documentation manual for occupational therapy: Writing SOAP notes* (4th ed.). SLACK Incorporated.

Chapter 14

Evaluation and Intervention Planning

Referral Process

As discussed in Chapter 1, occupational therapy practitioners write different kinds of notes for different stages of the intervention process. The process begins when a client is referred to occupational therapy, typically by a physician (or approved nonphysician practitioner [NPP] in that state). In medical settings, this referral might also be called _doctor's orders_, _medical orders_, _prescription_, or _script_. The OT is responsible for responding to the new referral (American Occupational Therapy Association [AOTA], 2021). It is important to realize that occupational therapy practice acts (licensure) may differ in key aspects from state to state. For example, practice acts delineate whether a prescription is required for evaluation and/or treatment and specify which health care professionals can legally write a referral for occupational therapy in that state (such as a physician, optometrist, nurse practitioner, or physician's assistant). States may also differ regarding continuing competency requirements or scope of practice delineating what the occupational therapy practitioner legally is allowed to do or may be prohibited from doing in that particular state. For example, some states mandate additional training in order for occupational therapy practitioners to administer physical agent modalities [PAMs] and might not allow OTAs to use certain PAMs such as ultrasound or electrical stimulation with clients. It is essential that you know the requirements for practicing occupational therapy in the specific state in which you want to work.

Each facility will have specific policies and procedures in place to facilitate the referral process according to the type of practice setting, licensure laws, other legal and payer requirements. This chapter presents some examples of the referral process. The unique documentation requirements for different practice settings are explained in Chapter 17.

Inpatient Setting and Home Health

For an inpatient setting (hospital, inpatient rehabilitation facility, or skilled nursing facility) or clients receiving home health services, a referral for occupational therapy is typically established in the health record by the physician (or other appropriate NPP). In certain instances, verbal orders may be received but must always be followed up with a written and signed copy. Guidelines will be in place for which disciplines may legally accept and document the verbal order in the record. The occupational therapy referral could be initiated when the client is first admitted to the facility/agency or might be established later as the need for occupational therapy arises. For example, a physical therapist or nurse working with the client might determine that the client is having difficulty with ADLs and recommend that the physician refer the client to occupational therapy. The occupational therapy department is then

Morreale, M. J. _The OTA's Guide to Documentation:_
Writing SOAP Notes, Fifth Edition (pp. 201-217).
© 2023 Taylor & Francis Group.

notified of the order by procedures established by the facility or agency, such as electronic communication and/or a call from the unit secretary or agency personnel. The client is then evaluated by the OT as soon as possible according to established guidelines for evaluation time frames, for example, within 24 or 48 hours.

Outpatient Setting

In an outpatient setting, when a new client calls, emails, or stops by to schedule an appointment, the occupational therapy department will consider the medical urgency of the appointment (such as if the client must be seen immediately for post-surgical care or a protective orthosis) and schedule it according to the client's needs and OT's schedule. The client's diagnosis, referral information, health insurance, and contact information are usually verified during that initial contact.

School-Based Setting

In a school-based setting, the request for special services or occupational therapy might be initiated by a parent, teacher, or other staff. The request is considered by the Child Study Team and the child is evaluated as appropriate by the necessary disciplines. An Individualized Education Program (IEP) is then established to determine what specific services will be provided if indicated.

We will now look at each step of the occupational therapy evaluation process.

Overview of the Occupational Therapy Process

Very early in the process, an **intake note** may be written by the OT acknowledging the referral and stating a plan to evaluate. Next, the OT writes a **screening report** or **evaluation report** that contains the client's occupational profile, current concerns and priorities, as well as the assessment results. A screening differs from an evaluation in that it is only a brief assessment to determine initially whether an occupational therapy evaluation is warranted or if referral to another service is better suited for the client's situation (AOTA, 2018). For example, an OT working in a school district might be asked to take a look at each kindergartener to determine whether there are obvious developmental challenges that OT might be able to help with, or a hospital might have an OT screen each client with a diagnosis of stroke who comes through the emergency room. When clients are referred to occupational therapy for an evaluation, the OT performs this as soon as the direct encounter with the client can be scheduled. From this evaluation comes the **intervention plan**, technically the part of the evaluation report that outlines the specific areas of occupation to be addressed, the outcomes expected, and the specific services that will be provided in occupational therapy. An OTA can contribute to this screening and evaluation process by performing delegated assessments and providing feedback and documentation to the OT (AOTA, 2021).

Facilities vary in the type, format, and frequency of **contact** or **progress notes** required. Some settings require a **contact note** (also called a *treatment note* or *visit note*) for each visit. Others may only require a progress note every week, 2 weeks, 30 days, or more frequently for new referrals or for a change in status. Contact notes and progress notes are written by the OT or OTA (under the supervision of the OT) and often use the SOAP format you have learned in this manual. The requirements for type and frequency of notes (and which personnel are allowed to write them) are usually a function of the practice setting, payment source, and the accrediting agency. Sometimes a **reassessment note** is required at regular intervals. When a client is transferred from one setting to another within the same service delivery system, a **transition plan** may be written. Most facilities require a **discharge** or **discontinuation report** at the end of occupational therapy treatment. This report makes recommendations, summarizes the occupational therapy services provided, and notes changes in a client's ability to engage in meaningful occupation as a result of occupational therapy intervention (AOTA, 2018). Reevaluation, transition, and discharge or discontinuation reports are the responsibility of the OT. However, the OTA may contribute to these stages of treatment by performing delegated assessments and providing feedback and documentation to the OT (AOTA, 2021).

In actual practice, you will probably find that contact, progress, and reassessment notes have some overlap. For example, in outpatient settings, the contact notes often include the client's progress from session to session. Contact notes in practice settings where the client's status may change quickly, such as acute care, may seem much like progress notes. In some ways, progress notes reassess the client's status and may sound much like reassessment notes. Notes could possibly be named differently in some settings, but there are still basic guidelines for each kind of note. Review the fundamentals of documentation in Chapter 2 (e.g., client and facility identifying information, standards of signature, error correction). It would also be useful to review the description of skilled and unskilled services in Chapter 3. These criteria are applicable to all types of occupational therapy notes.

In *Guidelines for Documentation of Occupational Therapy* (AOTA, 2018), criteria for notes in four process areas are described: screening, evaluation, intervention, and outcomes. Evaluation reports, along with reevaluation reports, are considered **evaluations**. The **intervention process** consists of the intervention plan, contact notes, progress reports, and transition plans. Discontinuation or discharge notes record professional activity in the area of **outcomes**. We will now look at documentation for evaluation and intervention planning.

Initial Evaluation Reports

The Evaluation Process

From the moment the referral is received, intervention planning begins in the mind of the OT. The client's name, age, and reason for referral will allow an OT to begin thinking about the particular occupations needing assessment, areas of deficits likely to be found, and possible interventions the OT might want to use. Each client is different, of course, and there will be many variations, as well as some surprises as the assessment begins. The mental preparation for *"Andrew Smith, age 68, Ⓛ CVA, evaluate and treat"* takes a therapist on a mental journey along one road of thought, whereas *"Ava Steed, age 4, ADHD,"* takes the therapist mentally down a different pathway. From day one, a good practitioner also begins discharge planning based on the client's occupational profile, prior functional level, and probable discharge placement.

One of the first steps is a review of the client's record if available. This allows the OT to better understand the client's condition, determine the direction of the interview, and decide what assessments to administer. Information obtained from the health record might include the following:

- Primary and secondary diagnoses/reason for admission/hospitalization
- Medical orders—in addition to actual orders for therapy, these might include pertinent issues such as weight-bearing status, type of diet (e.g., pureed, clear liquid, NPO, low salt), orthopedic or cardiac precautions, oxygen or MET levels, permission to get out of bed, etc.
- Medications
- Procedures or surgery implemented or pending
- Past medical history
- Test results such as X-rays, lab tests, and MRIs or neurological, developmental, or psychological tests
- Living situation and expected discharge plan
- Information from other disciplines such as physical or speech therapy evaluation results and goals

Data are also obtained from the client, family/caregiver, and other pertinent sources. Sometimes it is necessary for occupational therapy practitioners to talk to the nursing staff or contact the physician directly to clarify orders or discuss the client's condition or precautions before the client is seen. In early intervention and school settings, the therapist will review the child's available information and collaborate as needed with the parents, teachers, and other appropriate disciplines, such as social work, speech therapy, or psychology. The OT determines what information is needed for the client's occupational profile. This includes focusing on the client's occupational history, determining what that client needs and wants from occupational therapy, as well as what factors impact engagement in occupation (AOTA, 2018, 2020). The OT selects and administers any standardized tests or survey instruments that will help determine more exactly what underlying factors support or hinder participation in occupations. The therapist might delegate some aspects of the chart review, interview, specific assessments, or other functions to the OTA.

If the client is verbal and oriented, an interview is top on the agenda. If the client is unable to provide information, the family or other caregiver may be able to provide the necessary information instead. The occupational therapy practitioner must ask questions to determine the client's occupational profile and find out what roles are important to this client. What areas of life present the most problems? What does the client hope to gain from treatment? What results are desired by the family or teacher? What was the client able to do prior to this injury, illness, or hospitalization? What personal, family, or community supports are available to facilitate the desired outcomes?

Often, much information is gleaned from simply watching the client enter into the treatment area, classroom, or other venue. Does the client guard for pain? Is a supportive family member accompanying the client? What is the quality of mobility, posture, and upper extremity motion or function that is evident? Are there apparent cognitive or perceptual problems? Are obvious social, behavioral, or interpersonal concerns evident? Formal and informal assessments will then be administered based on the client's condition, practice setting, and influenced by what third-party payers are looking for. In addition to the reporting of mandated quality measures, assessments might include instruments relating to areas of occupation such as the Canadian Occupational Performance Measure (COPM); Functional Independence Measure (FIM); a leisure inventory; functional observations (e.g., ADLs, play, classroom performance); or various standardized or informal tests (i.e., cognitive, perceptual, motor, sensory, developmental) to assess specific performance skills or client factors.

Considering the initial evaluation findings, the OT will identify and prioritize the areas of occupation and underlying factors that require attention, and develop an intervention plan. Most facilities and electronic documentation programs provide specific formats for an initial evaluation report. The assessment results are recorded along with pertinent observations and comments. Some specific assessments might be recorded on a separate form or EMR template designated for that particular test (e.g., goniometry, manual muscle testing) but are still included as part of the evaluation report. Facilities sometimes use the same form for reevaluation and discharge reports so that the evaluation material does not have to be rewritten or reentered. An example of an initial evaluation form from Capitol Region Medical Center in Jefferson City, Missouri (Figure 14-1) is presented in this chapter so that you can see what might be included on a good facility form. Note that this form emphasizes some areas of occupation (ADLs) over others (such as social participation or play) based on the type of practice setting. You can use an internet search engine to find other examples of forms and compare different formats.

If an initial evaluation is written as a SOAP note, this is the way information would be categorized:

S: The interview material, background information, and occupational profile
O: The tests, results, and clinical observations
A: The OT's professional assessment of the data presented in the S and the O (often written as a problem list)
P: Frequency and duration of planned interventions and the long- and short-term goals

You will find that facilities and EMRs vary in how they organize and present the information. Forms may include checklists, grids, fill-in-the-blanks, or spaces for narrative reports. Several different formats are used in this manual to make it clear that there is not one correct organizational strategy.

The *Guidelines for Documentation of Occupational Therapy* (AOTA, 2018) recommends the following criteria for the content of an evaluation report:

Evaluation Report—Documents the referral source and data gathered through the occupational therapy evaluation process.

  a. *Referral information*—Date and source of referral, services requested, and reason for referral.

  b. *Client information*—Description of client's occupational history, experiences, and performance; health status and previous services required and accessed; and applicable medical, educational, and developmental diagnoses, precautions, and contraindications.

  c. *Occupational profile*—Client's reason for seeking occupational therapy services; areas of occupation in which the client is successful and challenged; contexts and environments that support and hinder occupational performance; medical, educational, and work history; occupational and psychosocial history (e.g., patterns of living, interest, values); client's priorities; and targeted goals (AOTA, 2017).

  d. *Assessments used and results*—Types of assessments used (e.g., interviews, record reviews, observations, standardized or nonstandardized assessments) and description of results.

  e. *Analysis of occupational performance*—Analysis of occupational performance and identification of factors that support and hinder performance and participation (objective and measurable identification of performance skills, performance patterns, contexts and environments, activity demands, outcomes from standardized measures or nonstandardized assessments, and client factors).

  f. *Summary and analysis*—Interpretation and summary of the occupational profile and and occupational performance issues, identification of targeted areas of occupation and occupational performance to be addressed, and expected outcomes.

Reproduced with permission from American Occupational Therapy Association. (2018). Guidelines for documentation of occupational therapy. *American Journal of Occupational Therapy, 72*(Suppl. 2), 7212410010.https://doi.org/10.5014/ajot.2018.72S03

The *Guidelines for Documentation of Occupational Therapy* (AOTA, 2018) also delineates that the evaluation report summary and analysis should indicate complexity level of the evaluation (low, moderate, or high) as required for CPT code reporting.

Recommendations are also presented in the evaluation report, based on the OT's judgement regarding the need for skilled occupational therapy or other services (AOTA, 2018).

CAPITAL REGION MEDICAL CENTER
OCCUPATIONAL THERAPY
❑ **INITIAL EVALUATION** ❑ **DISCHARGE SUMMARY**

DIAGNOSIS _____ ONSET: _____

MED. HX: _____

_____ CODE STATUS: _____

RELEVANT SURG. PROC.: _____

REFERRAL DATE: _____ DATE: _____

REFERRING PHYSICIAN: _____ MEDICARE #: _____

ACTIVITIES OF DAILY LIVING   REHAB POTENTIAL: _____

DRESSING Put on & remove the following	INDEP	SBA	MIN. ASSIST	MOD. ASSIST	MAX. ASSIST	ADAPT. EQUIP.	COMMENTS/ADAPTIVE EQUIPMENT ISSUED
front opening shirt							
pull on shirt							
underwear							
bra							
pants/slacks							
socks/hose							
shoes							
manage fasteners							
braces/splints/prosthesis							
GROOMING/HYGIENE							
sponge bath							
tub/shower bath							
shave							
comb hair							
brushing teeth							
opens jars/bottles							
make-up							
EATING							
drink from cup/glass							
feeds self							
cuts meat							

ROM   **UPPER EXTREMITY ROM & STRENGTH**

ACTIVE LEFT	PASSIVE LEFT	ACTIVE RIGHT	PASSIVE RIGHT		STRENGTH L	R
				SHOULDER: Elevation		
				Flexion		
				Abduction		
				Horizontal Abduction		
				Horizontal Adduction		
				Internal Rotation		
				External Rotation		
				ELBOW: Flexion		
				Extension		
				Supination		
				Pronation		
				WRIST: Flexion		
				Shoulder Subluxation L R		
				UE Edema L R		
				Pain L R		

PERTINENT FINDINGS

Wears glasses _____ Dentures _____ Hearing _____

MUSCLE TONE/UPPER EXTREMITIES

Hypotonic _____ Normal _____ Hypertonic _____
Comments _____

UPPER EXTREMITY SENSATION

SENSATION	Intact	Impaired	Absent
Light touch			
Sharp/Dull			
Temperature			
Proprioception			
Stereognosis			

COORDINATION/UPPER EXTREMITIES

Tremors _____ Apraxia _____ Ataxic _____

	Impaired	WNL
Gross Motor		
Fine Motor		
9 Hole Peg Test	L	R
Grip Strength	L	R
Lateral Pinch	L	R
Tripod Pinch	L	R
Hand Dominance	L	R

ORIENTED TO:

Person _____ Place _____
Time: Month _____ Day _____ Year _____
Situation _____

COMMUNICATION/COGNITION

	YES	NO
Verbal		
Understandable		
Appropriate		
Perseveration		
Follows Simple Commands		
Reads		
Writes		

2,605,003 (9/99) INIT EVAL/DISCHG SUM (FRONT)

PERCEPTION

		Impaired	WNL
A.	R/L Neglect _____		
B.	Body Schema		
C.	Discrimination		
	Shape		
	Size		
	Color		
D.	Visual Perception		

Overall Endurance   WFL _____
    Fair _____
    Poor _____

SURVIVAL SKILLS	Indep.	Min. Assist	Mod. Assist	Max. Assist
Phone Book Usage				
Money Mngmt.				
Situational Problem Solving				
Homemaking				

Figure 14-1A. Occupational therapy initial evaluation and discharge report form (page 1). (Reproduced with permission from Capital Region Medical Center, Jefferson City, Missouri.)

HOME SITUATION:_____

LIVING ARRANGEMENTS: (PT ADDRESS) _____

HOME TYPE:_____

PRIOR FUNCTIONAL INDEP.: _____

_____

_____

LEISURE INTERESTS: _____

ADAPTIVE EQUIP.: _____

COMMENTS: _____

_____

_____

_____

PATIENT / FAMILY GOALS:_____

❏ INITIAL ASSESSMENT (PROBLEMS / STRENGTHS)   ❏ DISCHARGE STATUS OF SHORT / LONG TERM GOALS

_____

_____

_____

_____

_____

PLAN:_____

SHORT-TERM GOALS - ESTIMATED TIME TO ACHIEVE: _____

_____

_____

_____

_____

❏ LONG-TERM GOALS - ESTIMATED TIME TO ACHIEVE: ❏ RECOMMENDATIONS:

_____

_____

_____

_____

_____

❏ Yes   ❏ No   **Patient has participated in evaluation process and agrees with treatment plan as stated above.**

Therapist _____ Date_____

I have reviewed and agree with the treatment plan as stated above.

Physician Signature _____ Date_____

2,605,003 (9/99) OT INITIAL EVALUATION/DISCHARGE SUMMARY (BACK)

Figure 14-1B. Occupational therapy initial evaluation and discharge report form (page 2). (Reproduced with permission from Capital Region Medical Center, Jefferson City, Missouri.)

In an evaluation, the "S" may contain all or part of the occupational profile. Based on the previous guidelines, specific areas to consider could include these (and/or others):

- The client's living situation—type of dwelling, architectural barriers, who resides with the client, access to family or community services
- Client's responsibility for caring for children, pets, or others
- Roles, responsibilities, and ability to care for self
- Performance patterns—typical day, limiting behaviors
- Cultural and religious considerations—dietary factors, personal values, customs/beliefs
- Educational considerations—level of education, literacy, special skills, goals
- Work—type of occupation, paid or volunteer work, is client working now, did injury occur on the job, desire to return to work, work capabilities
- Play/leisure—opportunity and barriers regarding leisure, hobbies/interests, sedentary versus active leisure interests
- Community mobility—methods of transportation, barriers to mobility
- Community support systems
- Virtual—access, competency, barriers
- Social—type and level of participation, clubs/organizations, successful relationships, opportunities and barriers

Here are two examples of the "S" in a paragraph format.

Client reports that she was admitted after a fall that resulted in confusion and left-sided weakness. Prior to admission, she was living alone in a one-story home and was Ⓘ in all activities of daily living. She reports that she is a retired librarian, widowed for 10 years. Client states she values her independence and fully intends to return to her own home. She reports that her activities are primarily sedentary, including sewing, reading, and playing cards with friends. She states her daughter lives two blocks away and provides transportation when needed.

The client talked about his current symptoms and the events leading up to his hospitalization. He reports losing his job with a construction company after not reporting for work for 2 weeks due to depression, having an argument with his wife, and taking an overdose. He states that he has always "worked construction" and does "not know how to do anything else." He reports concern that his former employer will not give him "a decent reference." He expresses he really has no leisure interests except going out "drinking with the guys after work" and sometimes going hunting in the fall.

Review the following example of an initial evaluation report and intervention plan for a client diagnosed with CVA. The occupational profile contained in this note is organized into categories rather than written as a paragraph. Note that the detailed intervention plan for this client is presented separately later in this chapter.

Healthy Hospital
Occupational Therapy Department
Initial Evaluation Report

Name: Payshent, Polly   **Medical Record #:** 12345   **Insurance:** Medicare
DOB: 11/10/1953   **Age:** 68   **Gender:** F
Physician: Will Heelue, MD
Date of onset: 5/1/22   **Date of admission:** 5/2/22
Referral Date: Client referred 5/3/22 by Dr. Heelue for evaluation and treatment.
Primary Dx: Ⓡ CVA r/o OBS   **Secondary Dx:** Type 2 diabetes
Date of evaluation: 5/3/22   **Time:** 10:00 am
Occupational Profile:
History of present condition: Client was admitted from the ER after a fall at home on 5/1/2022, resulting in confusion and left-sided weakness. CT scan and MRI both positive for Ⓡ CVA.
Past medical history: Left CTR 2005, Type 2 diabetes diagnosed in 2010 (insulin dependent since 2015)
Prior level of function: Prior to admission, client was Ⓘ in all activities of daily living.
Living situation: Client lives alone in a one-story home with three steps to enter. Spouse deceased 10 years. Daughter works for United Wickets, lives two blocks away, and is willing to visit daily and assist with transportation but cannot provide supervision.

Work: Client worked as a school librarian and retired 4 years ago.

Social/leisure: Hobbies include mostly sedentary activities such as sewing, reading, and playing cards with friends.

Client's goals: Client states she values her independence and fully intends to return to her own home.

S: Client stated, "I'm doing this so I can be independent and go home."

O: Client participated in 70-minute OT session bedside and in shower room for Mini-Mental State Exam, evaluation of ADL tasks (toileting, dressing ↔ undressing, and showering) functional mobility, and underlying factors (manual muscle test, AROM)

Bathing: Upper body: min Ⓐ to sequence task; Lower body: min Ⓐ for sequencing except max Ⓐ to reach perineal area and feet

Dressing: Seated in chair with arms, min Ⓐ to maintain dynamic balance when bending, mod Ⓐ to initiate donning bra, and max Ⓐ to reach feet. Verbal cues needed for sequencing and environmental orientation

Toileting: Verbal cues to flush, min Ⓐ to obtain tissue and manage clothing

Transfers: CGA with verbal cues for safety/proper arm placement sit to stand; min Ⓐ from low surfaces

Bed Mobility: Rolls & supine ↔ sit SBA for safety

Standing Balance: static: CGA

Activity Tolerance: Fair (3) (1-5 scale) < 10 min tolerance to any activity with physical/mental challenges

Motor Planning/Perception: WFL

Cognition: Score of 17/30 on Mini-Mental State Exam. Sequencing problems during dressing tasks noted. Client could not attach bra in back and required verbal cues to attach in front.

UE AROM: WFL for all Ⓑ UE movements except: abd, int/ext. rotation of Ⓛ shoulder lack ¼ range

UE Strength: Grip: Ⓡ 42#.; Ⓛ 21#. Pinch: Ⓡ palmar 14#; Ⓡ lateral 15#; Ⓛ palmar 6#; Ⓛ lateral 8#

Manual Muscle Test: All movements 4/5 except Ⓛ elbow ext. 3/5, Ⓛ thumb opposition and abduction 3+/5

Sensation: Ⓛ UE: Light touch, pain, temperature intact; stereognosis 3/5; Ⓡ UE all intact

A: Client's poor problem-solving skills (trying to doff pants prior to doffing shoes/socks and inability to initiate an alternative way to don bra) and the need for verbal cues to initiate some ADL tasks limit her ability to manage her basic and instrumental ADL activities Ⓘ. Decreased AROM and strength in the Ⓛ elbow and hand along with slow response to cognitive tasks, decreased ability to sequence tasks, and decreased short-term memory are safety concerns in an independent living situation. Client would benefit from environmental cues to orient her to environment, facilitation of problem solving and sequencing activities, and activities to increase strength in the Ⓛ UE. Rehab potential is good for modified Ⓘ in ADL activities.

P: OT for 45-minute sessions 5 X wk for 2 wks for sequencing during ADL tasks, problem-solving strategies, transfer training, activities to increase activity tolerance & strength in Ⓛ UE for ADL performance. Put calendar in client's room to increase orientation to month, day, and season. Evaluate ability to handle emergency situations.

Alice Altruism, OTR/L

Intervention Planning

The "A," or assessment, is a summary of deficits or problems that the OT determines from the initial evaluation. It can be in a narrative (paragraph) format but is often written as a numbered list of problems (called a *problem list*). Problems are defined as areas of occupation that are not within functional limits that will be addressed in treatment. Problem statements should include an underlying factor (performance skill, client factor, contextual limitation, etc.) and a related area of occupation. The best problem statements give a way of measuring the extent of the problem (such as "needs max assist" or "needs verbal cues"). Also remember that those who use occupational therapy services are more than an assist level, so documentation should reflect what the client is **unable to do or needs assistance in doing** rather than saying that the client **is** a particular assist level. Instead of a narrative format as shown in the evaluation for Polly Payshent, the assessment can be written as a problem list.

Problem List

1. Client needs min to max physical assist and verbal cues to dress and bathe self due to ↓ AROM, ↓ activity tolerance, and inability to sequence the task.
2. Client's lack of orientation to environment and inability to problem solve create safety concerns with ADL and home management.
3. Client needs CGA to min assist with functional mobility and transfers 2° decreased dynamic standing balance and decreased cognitive functions.
4. Fair activity tolerance limits ability to manage ADLs and home management tasks.
5. Moderately decreased left hand strength limits grip and prehension for grooming and hygiene tasks.
6. Min AROM deficits in left shoulder limit client's ability to fasten bra and wash her back.

Now that the functional problems have been identified, the detailed intervention plan for this client is presented a little later in this chapter.

LEARNING ACTIVITY 14-1: DETERMINING FUNCTIONAL PROBLEMS

Imagine you had surgery recently to repair a lacerated flexor tendon in your dominant hand, which is now immobilized in a protective hand orthosis. Choose an ADL and an IADL that you do in a typical day. Create a list of 10 specific activity demands for each that you would have difficulty performing one handedly.

Example:

IADL—Laundry: Carrying a laundry basket, folding clothes, etc.

ADL: _____	IADL: _____
Activity Demands:	Activity Demands:
1.	1.
2.	2.
3.	3.
4.	4.
5.	5.
6.	6.
7.	7.
8.	8.
9.	9.
10.	10.

Worksheet 14-1
Initial Evaluation Report

Use this worksheet to help you compare the initial evaluation in this chapter to AOTA's recommended criteria in the *Guidelines for Documentation of Occupational Therapy* (AOTA, 2018). You can also use this worksheet to compare a "real" evaluation report to AOTA's criteria.

Background Data

Criteria	How Does the Evaluation Comply With the Criteria?
Are all of the following present: name, date of birth, gender? Are all applicable diagnoses and health information listed along with applicable case number?	
Is it clear who referred the client to occupational therapy, on what date, and what services were requested?	
Is the funding source listed for this client?	
Is anticipated length of stay indicated for this client?	
Why is the client seeking occupational therapy services?	
Are there any secondary problems, preexisting conditions, contraindications, or precautions that will impact therapy?	

Occupational History and Profile

Is there an occupational history/profile? Is it adequate?	
Which areas of occupation are currently successful and which are problematic?	
What factors hinder the client's performance in areas of occupation? What factors support performance in areas of occupation?	
What are the client's priorities? What does the client hope to gain from occupational therapy?	
What areas of occupation will be targeted for intervention? Do these match the client's priorities?	
What are the targeted outcomes?	

Results of the Assessment

What types of assessments were used?	
What were the results of the assessments?	
What client factors, performance skills, patterns, contextual aspects, and activity demands are identified as needing attention?	
What factors (strengths, supports) facilitate the client's occupational performance?	
Are there other areas that need to be assessed that are not listed?	
Is occupational therapy appropriate for this client? Why or why not?	

Morreale, M. J. (2023). *The OTA's guide to documentation: Writing SOAP notes* (5th ed.). SLACK Incorporated.

The Intervention Plan

Guidelines for Intervention Planning

The assessment is the basis upon which the OT establishes the intervention plan. The therapist collaborates with the client (along with the family or significant other when appropriate) to prioritize the identified problems and establish an intervention plan to achieve desired outcomes. The OT considers what the client's discharge setting and plan will be and the types of follow-up or support that will be needed. According to *Guidelines for Documentation of Occupational Therapy* (AOTA, 2018), the intervention plan should include: appropriate occupation-based long- and short-term goals; the type of approach, methods and interventions to achieve those goals; the frequency, intensity, and duration of treatment; service provider and location; and recommendations/referrals for other services or specialized interventions and tools used to measure outcomes. The intervention plan is oriented toward the client's quality of life, desired occupational engagement, health and wellness, occupational justice, and ultimate success in fulfilling life roles (AOTA, 2018, 2020). The intervention plan must show the need for skilled occupational therapy and be realistic; that is, it must have a good chance of success in a reasonable period of time.

Estimating Rehabilitation Potential

Rehabilitation potential is normally stated as good or excellent for the goals the OT establishes. If it is not good or excellent for the client, then a smaller more incremental goal must be selected. There is not much point in setting and working toward goals that do not have a good chance of being accomplished. Estimating rehab potential as guarded, fair, or poor is a red flag to reviewers, and they may be reluctant to set aside health care dollars for someone who is not likely to benefit from occupational therapy services. Rehab potential does not mean independence. It simply means potential to reach the goals the OT and client have set or potential for the client to make significant change. If a client's condition has a poor prognosis, such as cancer or Alzheimer's disease, goals might be established regarding what the caregiver needs to achieve to care for the client, such as ability to implement a home program of PROM, transfer or position the client properly, or safely feed a client who has dysphagia.

Expected Frequency and Duration

The frequency and duration of occupational therapy will vary according to physician orders, diagnosis, individual client needs and circumstances, payment source, and facility guidelines (Gateley & Borcherding, 2017). For example, in acute care, rehabilitation clients recovering from hip surgery, COPD exacerbation, or a CVA might be seen once or twice daily until discharge, but the length of sessions may vary depending on what the client can tolerate. Clients with general medical conditions such as pneumonia or another illness might only require one to two sessions for equipment recommendations or safety instructions prior to discharge home, whereas, in an inpatient rehabilitation center, clients are typically seen once or twice daily for a total of 60 to 90 minutes for several weeks (Gateley & Borcherding, 2017). Outpatients could receive occupational therapy one to three times weekly for 30 to 60 minutes for one or two sessions total or, continue for several weeks or months depending on complexity of the client's condition or situation. The plan of care might also indicate that the frequency of therapy will be tapered as the client progresses, such as this Centers for Medicare & Medicaid Services (CMS) example: *"once daily, 3 times a week tapered to once a week over 6 weeks"* (CMS, 2019).

Children in early intervention or a school system receive occupational therapy based on what is delineated in the Individualized Family Service Plan (IFSP) or Individualized Education Program (IEP). This might entail only a few occupational therapy sessions for consultation or ongoing therapy several times a week or month for the duration of the established time frame or until end of the school year. The plan is individualized to each client but the frequency and duration of skilled care must be medically (or educationally) necessary and include reasonable time frames according to established standards of care.

Selecting Intervention Strategies

Occupational therapy is a dynamic process of creative problem solving with each client for pertinent occupations. What is meaningful to one client may not be to another. Even a very basic task such as dressing may not seem meaningful to some clients. A person with quadriplegia who has a personal attendant, for example, may never need to dress themselves and may consider it an enormous waste of time to be required to learn to do so. However, this same client may be very motivated to learn to hold a mouth stick in order to engage in computer tasks for vocational retraining. Some clients will never need to balance a checkbook, while others may not be able to return to living independently without this skill. The occupational therapy practitioner asks questions like the following:

- What do you want to be able to do?
- What keeps you from being able to do that?
- What are the possible options for making that happen?

The options for intervention strategies may include teaching new performance skills or patterns for occupations; improving client factors (strength, range, endurance, etc.); implementing methods/tasks to support occupations; modifying the environment (context); adapting activities/occupations; providing education, consultation, etc. Occupational therapy practitioners consider doing things in many different or creative ways and try to make interventions meaningful and purposeful to the client.

The treatment media used by occupational therapy is also different from that used by other disciplines. Occupational therapy practitioners often use common household objects to accomplish functional tasks. For example, the client's own clothing is a common treatment media. The clothes may be used for dressing to teach the client to don clothing; for folding in order to be doing a meaningful IADL activity while increasing standing tolerance; for sorting colors for laundry; or for hanging in a closet to increase AROM at the shoulder for occupational participation. The approach would depend upon what the client will need to do in the expected discharge environment. An experienced OT or OTA can creatively find many different uses for common household items. The same net ball that is used to wash dishes may be used for squeezing to develop grip strength, for tactile stimulation, or for throwing to develop UE range of motion. Any methods and tasks that OTs and OTAs use with clients should always support occupational participation. However, *occupation-based* interventions should be implemented whenever feasible. Let us look at the intervention plan for Polly Payshent, which includes the goals and methods to achieve those goals.

Intervention Plan

Problem #1: Client needs min to max physical assist and verbal cues to dress self due to ↓ AROM and strength, ↓ activity tolerance, and inability to sequence the task.

Long-term goal: Client will be able to dress with SBA and < 3 verbal cues after set-up within 2 weeks.

Short-Term Goals:	Interventions:
Client will don bra with min Ⓐ using adaptive technique within 3 days.	• Teach adaptive techniques. • Post picture of how to don bra correctly using adaptive technique. • Reinforce correct responses. • Teach strengthening program for UE.
Client will don shoes and socks with min Ⓐ using adaptive technique and a long shoe horn within 5 days.	• Provide long shoe horn and instruct client in correct use. • Instruct in adaptive techniques for donning shoes and socks. • Post picture of adaptive techniques and long shoe horn being used to don shoes. • Instruct in using affected side as a functional assist in dressing. • Expand exercise program to include AROM.
Client will sequence dressing tasks correctly 3/3 tries within 1 ½ weeks.	• Verbalize steps before beginning to dress. • Verbalize steps while dressing. • Post list of steps for client to follow. • Take rest breaks as needed for activity tolerance.

Problem #2: Client's lack of orientation to environment and inability to problem solve create safety concerns with ADLs and home management.

Long-term goal: When asked, client will correctly use calendar, schedule, clock, and emergency information posted on wall within 2 weeks.

Short-Term Goals:	Interventions:
Client will identify time, date, and situation correctly when asked within 1 week.	• Post calendar, schedule, and emergency information near clock in client's room. • Instruct family, nursing staff, and other therapy staff to ask client date, time, and situation several times daily and to reinforce correct responses.
Client will be able to follow a daily schedule with < 2 verbal cues within 1 to 2 weeks.	• Post daily schedule on wall near clock. • Cue client to look at schedule to determine what she should be doing at any given time.
Client will correctly problem solve responses to emergency situations with 90% accuracy within 2 weeks.	• Provide situations for client to problem solve, progressing from easy to more complex. • Provide telephone directory or other props as needed for problem solving.

Problem #3: Client's fair activity tolerance, decreased dynamic standing balance, and decreased cognitive functions necessitates CGA to min assist for functional mobility and transfers.

Long-term goal: Client will be able to perform functional transfers safely in bedroom and bathroom with modified Ⓘ within 2 wks.

Short-Term Goals:	Interventions:
Client will complete toilet transfers with modified Ⓘ within 2 weeks.	• Instruct client in use of grab bars and raised toilet seat. • Recommend purchase and installation of grab bar and raised toilet seat. • Post list of steps for client to follow and verbalize steps. • Implement grooming activities standing at sink to improve dynamic standing balance and endurance.
Client will perform commode transfers with SBA within 1 week.	• Place commode next to bed. • Recommend a commode be placed next to bed at home for use during the night. • Implement upper body AROM exercises while standing to improve dynamic standing balance and endurance.
Client will perform transfers EOB ↔ standing with modified Ⓘ using bed rail within 1 week.	• Instruct client in bed mobility and transfers. • Post list of steps for client to follow and verbalize steps. • Implement exercise band strengthening program while standing to improve dynamic standing balance and endurance.

Client to participate in OT for 45-minute sessions 5 X wk for 2 wks until anticipated discharge to her home. Will set up meeting with client's daughter to discuss equipment needs for home.

Alice Altruism, OTR/L

Worksheet 14-2
Intervention Plan

Use this worksheet to help you compare the intervention plan in this chapter to AOTA's recommended criteria (AOTA, 2018, 2020). You can also use this worksheet to compare a "real" intervention plan to AOTA's criteria.

Criteria	How Does the Intervention Plan Comply With the Criteria?
Are the intervention goals and objectives measurable and realistic?	
Are the goals and objectives directly related to the client's occupational role performance?	
Are specific occupational therapy interventions identified?	
Are the interventions listed appropriate to work toward the established goals?	
What is the anticipated frequency/duration/intensity of services?	
What is the discontinuation criteria or expected outcomes?	
What is the anticipated discharge location?	
What is the anticipated plan for follow-up care?	
Where will service be provided?	
Will these services meet payer requirements?	
Are there areas of concern that are not addressed in the goals/intervention plan specifically?	

Choosing Activities for Your Intervention Session

As an OTA student or new practitioner, you might experience some anxiety when your supervisor asks you to come up with specific intervention ideas for clients. You might wonder how you can even begin to think of appropriate activities to target the client's needs when the client has so many different issues and challenges. You might be unsure as to what to work on first or how you can achieve all the goals in such a limited time frame. While you will certainly collaborate with your occupational therapy supervisor, you are also expected to think creatively and independently and to use your professional skills as an OTA to select appropriate methods, treatment media or techniques. **The OT's intervention plan is your guide.** It spells out the areas to work on and the approaches to achieve those goals. For example, if a goal states, *"Client will be able to button half-inch buttons with modified Ⓘ using buttonhook,"* then your intervention session would include providing your client with a buttonhook and instructing the client how to use it. You would have the client practice buttoning and unbuttoning ½" buttons with the adaptive device. You could choose to do this on a button board or have the client practice on a shirt. A good occupational therapy activity combines working on several goals at once. If that same client also had the goal, *"Client will demonstrate increased activity tolerance for ADLs by standing 10 minutes at sink during grooming,"* you could have the client stand while practicing use of the buttonhook. Perhaps the client had a third goal, *"Client will increase strength of Ⓡ UE by one muscle grade in order to carry a laundry basket."* You might put a weighted cuff around the client's wrist while the client is standing and using the buttonhook. You have now worked on three goals with one intervention activity. Let us look at another example in Learning Activity 14-2.

LEARNING ACTIVITY 14-2: CHOOSING ACTIVITIES

Suppose the occupational therapy intervention plan had the following goals:

1. *Client will demonstrate improved decision-making skills for IADLs by planning a two-course meal for OT cooking group with min verbal cues within 2 weeks.*

2. *Client will demonstrate organizational skills needed to complete IADLs within appropriate time periods within 3 weeks.*

3. *Client will demonstrate improved social interaction skills by asking a peer for assistance in OT group without prompting within 2 weeks.*

How could you work on all these goals simultaneously? What would you choose as intervention activities? Compare your ideas with the suggestions that follow this Learning Activity.

You might begin by having your client discuss ideas for an appropriate meal that can be completed in the available time frame and possibly look through a cookbook for ideas and recipes. The client might then prepare aspects of the meal by collaborating with others in an occupational therapy cooking group. During this process you, the OTA, would provide verbal cues (i.e., for process, redirection to task, pacing, etc.) or encouragement as needed. You can provide the opportunity for the client to ask others in the group to assist with some of the steps so it can be completed within the allotted time frame. This would integrate all of the goals at the same time and would be a good occupational therapy intervention.

For additional practice in choosing appropriate interventions, complete Worksheet 14-3.

Worksheet 14-3
Choosing Activities—More Practice

Suppose the occupational therapy intervention plan had the following goals:

1. *Student will be able to open all containers and wrappers Ⓘ for his lunch at school.*

2. *In order to perform bimanual classroom tasks, student will use Ⓛ hand spontaneously as a functional assist 5/5 opportunities.*

3. *Student will attend to classroom tasks for 10-minute periods with only one verbal cue for redirection.*

How could you work on these goals simultaneously? What would you choose as intervention activities?

Morreale, M. J. (2023). *The OTA's guide to documentation: Writing SOAP notes* (5th ed.). SLACK Incorporated.

Now that you understand the initial evaluation process, you can begin to choose appropriate, realistic, and meaningful activities and occupations for your clients. Good occupational therapy interventions often combine working on several goals at once to effectively achieve desired outcomes within the shortest time possible.

References

American Occupational Therapy Association. (2017). AOTA occupational profile template. *American Journal of Occupational Therapy, 71*(Suppl. 2), 7112420030. https://doi.org/5014/ajot.2017.716S12

American Occupational Therapy Association. (2018). Guidelines for documentation of occupational therapy. *American Journal of Occupational Therapy, 72*(Suppl. 2), 7212410010. https://doi.org :10.5014/ajot.2018.72S203

American Occupational Therapy Association. (2020). Occupational therapy practice framework: Domain and process (4th ed.). *American Journal of Occupational Therapy, 74*(Suppl. 2), 7412410010. https://doi.org: 10.5014/ajot.2020.74S2001

American Occupational Therapy Association. (2021). Standards of practice for occupational therapy. *American Journal of Occupational Therapy, 75*(Suppl. 3), 7513410030. https://doi.org/10.5014/ajot.2021.75S3004

Centers for Medicare & Medicaid Services. (2019). *Medicare benefit policy manual* (Pub. 100-02: Ch. 15, Section 220.1.2). Retrieved October 14, 2021 from https://www.cms.gov/Regulations-and-Guidance/Guidance/Manuals/Downloads/bp102c15.pdf

Gateley, C. A., & Borcherding, S. (2017). *Documentation manual for occupational therapy: Writing SOAP notes* (4th ed.). SLACK Incorporated.

Chapter 15

Goals and Interventions

Occupational therapy goals must be written in functional, measurable, observable, and action-oriented terms. They must be realistic for the client's condition and circumstances, appropriate for the practice setting, and able to be achieved in a reasonable amount of time. Goals are initially formulated in the OT's intervention plan and reflect outcomes that the client hopes to gain from occupational therapy such as occupational participation, health and well-being, quality of life, and role competence (AOTA, 2020). Although improving underlying client factors or biomechanical components may be necessary components to work on based on the client's condition, those are much less important to a third-party payer than what functional tasks the client can actually do safely. An OTA's primary role is implementing delegated interventions to support occupational participation and help clients achieve the desired outcomes delineated in the intervention plan. What transpires during the intervention session is summarized and recorded in a contact note. As noted in Chapter 10, if a SOAP format is used, the "P" could end with a goal statement, depending on facility or payer requirements, but this is not always needed. Progress notes may also incorporate goals. It is not necessary to repeatedly restate goals that are already written in the initial evaluation. You will be aligning your treatment to the established intervention plan and, with the OT's supervision, might write goals to reflect the steps along the way that your client needs to achieve desired outcomes. Electronic documentation programs often have templates or drop-down menus for standard client goals based on clinical pathways for the diagnosis or the functional problems identified/checked off. Practitioners might pick and choose from these options and indicate appropriate desired assist levels. Depending on the software program, practitioners may be able to customize goals further or create completely new ones. Goals should reflect the individual needs of the client and should not be compromised for convenience or to just fit the specifications of a particular software program.

Goals in an intervention plan are called **long-term goals** (LTG) or *outcomes*. These are usually what the client hopes to accomplish by the time of discharge. The OT will typically create at least one LTG for each problem identified in the occupational therapy evaluation. Time frames for LTGs will vary significantly according to the type of practice setting and the client's circumstances. **Short-term goals** (STG), also called *objectives*, are the incremental goals or sub-steps that are met while progressing toward the long-term or discharge goals. For example, if the LTG is:

In order to perform job without injury, client will be able to move 35 lb objects needed for work from table to counter without ↑ in pain by 10/25/22.

A relevant STG might be:

Client will be able to lift 10 lb objects needed for work without ↑ in pain by 10/4/22.

There may be several STGs (objectives) for each LTG. For example, suppose you are treating a client who is a 49-year-old postal worker who sustained a ® CVA a few days ago and has Ⓛ side hemiplegia. The OT's evaluation states that this client has verbal abilities and intact mental functions. The intervention plan has identified a goal of independent upper body dressing by 8/25/22. This will require skilled instruction and the correct adaptive equipment.

Morreale, M. J. *The OTA's Guide to Documentation:*
Writing SOAP Notes, Fifth Edition (pp. 219-235).
© 2023 Taylor & Francis Group.

A series of short-term goals must be established:

1. *Client will be able to maintain dynamic sitting balance at EOB for >5 minutes while reaching for clothing at arm's length, within three intervention sessions.*

2. *By the sixth intervention session, client will demonstrate increased activity tolerance for >10 minutes of dressing while sitting at edge of bed.*

3. *Client will be able to don shirt sitting EOB using the over-the-head method by 8/15/22.*

4. *Client will be able to button shirt with modified Ⓘ using a buttonhook by 8/18/22.*

5. *While sitting EOB, client will demonstrate independence in upper body dressing by 8/25/22.*

As you can see, each of these STGs is measurable, observable, and client-action oriented. The first four STGs are steps to reach the ultimate LTG (Figure 15-1).

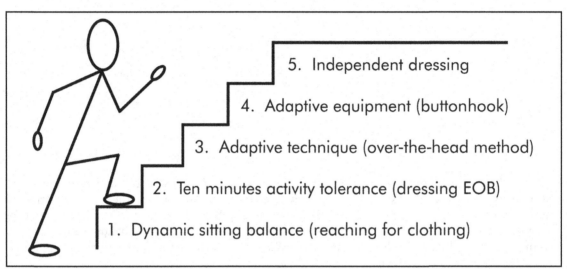

Figure 15-1. Steps to the ultimate LTG.

An intervention plan is always a work in progress, so you and the OT will collaborate to provide the most appropriate care. Unexpected events and conditions can impact the progress your client will be able to make toward their goals. The OT will modify the intervention plan as needed (based upon your feedback), as it is not useful to continue with a plan that is not working. In order to write appropriate goals and objectives in a way that can be measured, the elements to be included are very specific. The COAST format, developed by Gateley and Borcherding (2017) is a useful method as you are learning. The COAST format will help you to include all of the necessary components and can easily be adapted for the specific terminology and criteria used in different practice settings. Sometimes the order of the COAST elements may need to be changed slightly in order for your sentence to make sense. As long as all of the required elements are present, you can begin with any of the COAST elements—the client expectation, functional occupation, assist level, conditions, or timeline (Gateley & Borcherding, 2017).

THE COAST METHOD

C—Client	Client will perform
O—Occupation	What occupation?
A—Assist Level	With what level of assistance/independence?
S—Specific Condition	Under what conditions?
T—Timeline	By when?

Reproduced with permission from Gateley, C. A., & Borcherding, S. (2017). *Documentation manual for occupational therapy: Writing SOAP notes* (4th ed.). SLACK Incorporated.

Now let us look at each of the COAST categories (Gateley & Borcherding, 2017).

C (Client)

When writing goals in occupational therapy, the **client** must be the main focus. The goal statement is **not** the place to tell what the OT or OTA will do. That goes later, under intervention strategies. The occupational therapy practitioner sets the expectation for what the client—not the OT or OTA—will achieve:

- *The client will …*
- *The client will perform transfers w/c ↔ toilet with SBA by 10/4/22.*
- *Child will demonstrate ability to tie her shoes Ⓘ within 3 weeks.*

Use an appropriate action verb such as *demonstrate, complete,* or *perform* to indicate the client expectation (Gateley & Borcherding, 2017). In some instances, the goal might indicate what the parent or caregiver will achieve after your skilled instruction:

- *After skilled instruction, **parent will** demonstrate proper technique to position child for feeding by end of 2nd treatment session.*
- ***Client's spouse will** demonstrate ability to transfer client safely from bed ↔ commode within 1 week.*

O (Occupation)

Goals should pertain to and specify **occupation** and directly relate to a problem that was identified in the occupational therapy intervention plan (Gateley & Borcherding, 2017). The ability to engage in occupation is the heart and core of occupational therapy practice. It should be the **first** thing you think of when writing goals, and it should be the goal statement's prime focus. For example:

- *Client will **don pullover sweater** …*
- *Client will be able to **complete his morning medication regimen** …*
- *The client will **perform a three-step cooking process** …*

If your goal emphasizes a particular client factor or performance skill as an essential part of a desired occupation, be sure to include the area of occupation that this factor or skill will ultimately enable the client to do, such as, "*in order to return to work as a carpenter,*" "*in order to be able to be bathed by his caretakers,*" or "*in order to be able to write his name at school.*" The following is an example:

- ***In order to begin writing her name at school,** student will demonstrate ability to hold pencil with a static tripod grasp by 6/19/22.*

  The occupation may go after the action if you prefer. For example:
- *Student will demonstrate ability to hold pencil with a static tripod grasp when **writing her name at school** by 6/19/22.*

A (Assist Level)

This part of the goal delineates the expected level of assistance that the client will achieve when performing the specific occupation. This includes quantifiable physical assistance levels or verbal, tactile, or visual cues. If your facility uses a specific outcome measure such as the Functional Independence Measure [FIM], it might be appropriate to incorporate those criteria into your goals (Gateley & Borcherding, 2017). Review Chapter 8 for various ways to describe assist levels. The following are some examples:

- *Client will complete shaving **with less than four verbal cues to attend to left side of face** …*
- *Client will don pullover shirt **with min assist to place Ⓛ arm in sleeve** …*
- *To demonstrate increased self-esteem for socialization, client will verbalize three positive attributes about self with **min verbal prompting** within 1 week.*

S (Specific Condition)

This represents additional criteria or conditions under which the client is expected to be able to perform the desired action such a compensatory technique, use of durable medical equipment/adaptive equipment, client position, location, etc. (Gateley & Borcherding, 2017). For example:

- *Client will perform upper and lower body dressing Ⓘ,* ***taking less than three 60-second rest breaks*** *by 6/8/22.*
- *In order to perform dressing, client will maintain static sitting balance Ⓘ on* ***edge of bed for 3 minutes*** *by 6/3/22.*

The conditions make your goal more specific. One of the most common mistakes in goal writing is omission of the conditions under which the activity is expected to be performed. Usually it is helpful to put the condition **after** the skill rather than before it, but sometimes you may want to start with the condition. For example,

- ***While standing at sink for 5 minutes,*** *client will demonstrate ability to wash and dry dishes with SBA by 9/20/2022.*
- ***Using a buttonhook,*** *client will button at least three buttons on her shirt with modified Ⓘ by 7/1/22.*

Using both the "A" and the "S" will help ensure that your goal is measurable and will demonstrate gains that your client has achieved (Gateley & Borcherding, 2017). Here are some additional examples:

- *… with SBA using a grab bar*
- *… with hand-over-hand assist while standing at blackboard*
- *… Ⓘ while seated in wheelchair*
- *… with two verbal cues using a daily planner*
- *… with modified Ⓘ referring to a list of instructions*
- *… independently with arm supported on lap tray*
- *… with visual demonstration in crafts group*
- *… with modified independence using a timer*
- *… mod Ⓐ without shortness of breath*
- *… after set-up with one verbal cue for initiation*
- *… min Ⓐ while seated upright in bed*

In some instances, it is acceptable to use only the "A" or the "S," but you must use at least one of them (Gateley & Borcherding, 2017). For example, a client may have independence in a particular task but difficulty performing it due to a specific client factor such as low endurance or pain. In that case, you could eliminate stating an implied independent assist level but still state the conditions (Gateley & Borcherding, 2017). In the following examples, the measurable criteria are factors such as pain level, activity tolerance, quality of the task, and amount of time needed.

- *Client will carry laundry basket 20 feet with a* ***reported pain level of less than 5/10*** *by 6/13/22.*
- *Client will stand at stove 10 minutes to cook a meal* ***without shortness of breath*** *by expected discharge date 8/21/22.*
- *Student will demonstrate ability to carry lunch tray from cafeteria line to table* ***without spilling any items*** *by the end of the school year.*
- *Client will demonstrate improved decision-making skills by choosing one out of four possible projects* ***within 60 seconds*** *in OT craft group by the end of the week.*

Children sometimes exhibit a new behavior inconsistently before it is really established. Therefore, measurement used for children is more likely to reflect whether the behavior is established. For example:

- *Brady will use a Ⓡ pincer grasp to pick up and feed self 10 raisins* ***3/3 opportunities*** *by 4/28/22.*
- *Parker will demonstrate improved tolerance to tactile media as evidenced by self-initiation during art activities in* ***5/5 teacher reports*** *by the end of the month.*
- *Student will demonstrate ability to open combination lock on locker within 60 seconds* ***4/5 opportunities*** *by the end of the school year.*
- *Student will maintain upright sitting posture during classroom writing time without verbal reminders in* ***3/3 observations*** *by 6/24/22.*

You may find that some school settings use percentages in goals such as, *"Child will demonstrate ability to bring food to mouth with spoon without spilling 75% of the time by the end of school year."* However, it is more clear to say, *"Child will demonstrate ability to bring food to mouth with spoon without spilling 15/20 opportunities by the end of school year."* This way, anyone can observe the exact behavior and number of repetitions and determine if the criteria are met. Goals for children in public schools must be set in terms of a behavior that is needed in the classroom or school context. While you may be working with a student on sensory integration tasks (e.g., having the child maintain prone extension posture or cross-leg sitting on a scooter board or platform swing), as an intervention to improve client factors and skills (balance, motor planning, sensory processing, or strength), it must be written in language that is educationally based, relating to performance in the classroom setting.

T (Timeline)

This is the time frame within which the goal is expected to be accomplished. In a practice setting where notes are written monthly, the goal would be what you hope to accomplish in the next month. In an acute care setting, it might be your goal for tomorrow. In a school setting, goals in the Individualized Education Program (IEP) are considered annual goals with a time frame for the end of the school year. Benchmarks are then established to measure progress toward the annual goals. In a rehabilitation hospital or subacute unit, LTGs typically have time frames that coincide with the expected discharge date from the facility, which might only be 1 or 2 weeks. For example:

- While seated on tub bench, client will demonstrate ability to bathe upper body with SBA …
    - … by the end of the next intervention session.
    - … within 2 weeks.
    - … within 1 month.
    - … within three intervention sessions.
    - … by expected discharge on 08/16/22.

COAST Examples

C—Client will complete
O—setting the table
A—with SBA
S—using rolling walker and walker tray
T—within 1 week

C—Student will demonstrate ability to
O—open combination lock on locker
A—independently
S—and get to next class on time 5/5 opportunities
T—by the end of the school year

C—Child will
O—use left hand to stabilize paper when drawing
A—with min verbal cues
S—4/5 opportunities
T—within 1 month

C—Client will perform
O—toilet transfers
A—with min assist
S—using walker and adhering to total hip precautions
T—within 3 days

- *Client will perform all laundry tasks Ⓘ at laundromat by anticipated discharge on 06/13/22.*
- *Student will be able to change into his gym clothes within 5 minutes 3/3 opportunities by the end of the school year.*
- *Infant will be able to reach for a toy while supine by bringing Ⓡ UE to midline with min assist by 08/31/2022.*

Other Considerations for Goals

Demonstrating Progress for Specific Performance Components and Client Factors

Sometimes, a performance skill or client factor needs to be emphasized in a goal to show that the client is making progress with specific deficits, particularly for clients with cognitive or behavioral problems. As noted with the COAST method, an occupation-based task should be clearly identified in a goal along with the assist level, specific condition, and timeline. The following template is useful when particular performance skills or client factors must be addressed to prepare the client for function and demonstrate progress. However, the order of these components may sometimes need to be changed for the goal to make sense:

Client will demonstrate _____ _____ _____
  (use words such as improved   *(performance skill*   *(in order to do what occupation)*
      or an increase of)   *or client factor)*

_____ _____ .
(assist level and/or specific condition)   *(time frame—by when)*

- *Client will demonstrate improved time management skills for ADLs by completing a shower Ⓘ in 15 minutes or less within 1 week.*
- *Client will demonstrate improved attention to Ⓛ side when eating by locating all utensils and food items on Ⓛ side of meal tray with three verbal cues or less within 3 days.*
- *To reach clothes hanging in closet, client will demonstrate an increase of 20° shoulder flexion within 2 weeks.*
- *Infant will demonstrate improved proximal stability for play by maintaining prone extension while supported on elbows for 5 minutes within 1 month.*
- *Student will be able to place school work in folder Ⓘ by using both hands together spontaneously 5/5 opportunities by the end of the school year.*
- *Within 3 days, client will demonstrate increased assertiveness by asking a peer to share condiments during 3/3 meals without verbal prompting.*
- *In order to manage laundry, client will demonstrate improved dexterity to manipulate coins and insert (without dropping any) in coin-operated washing machine Ⓘ by anticipated discharge on 9/13/22.*

Skilled Occupational Therapy

It is important to remember that your documentation must demonstrate a clear need for skilled occupational therapy. Once a client reaches the level of minimal assistance, the changes become more subtle and may lead to denial of payment unless you specify the necessity of skilled occupational therapy. For example, dressing with minimal assistance does not necessarily indicate a need for skilled occupational therapy. However, documenting interventions such as *"Client needed minimal assistance and verbal instruction for over-the-head compensatory method of donning shirt"* could help to justify skilled occupational therapy. Client goals must also reflect the scope of reasonable, necessary, and skilled services that occupational therapy practitioners provide. In addition, the client's priorities must be addressed within the short time frames allowed for therapy. For example, a client residing in a nursing home may benefit more from goals that address independent wheelchair mobility, feeding, or ability to manage eyeglasses, rather than a goal that might only improve lower body dressing from moderate to minimum assistance (which still requires that another person help). Choosing what kind of goal to use and the specific criteria depend upon the individual's unique needs in addition to the type of setting and the funding source. As previously noted, goals in a school setting must be educationally related. Physical rehabilitation goals for adult and elderly clients generally focus on self-care, health management, work, or IADLs, as leisure activities are not generally considered a priority by Medicare and other payers. Goals in early intervention normally work toward achieving age-appropriate developmental milestones and safety in the home environment. Mental health goals aim for outcomes such as health, well-being, ability to participate in meaningful occupations, and role competence. Regardless of the setting, goals should be client-centered, occupation-based, written in measurable, objective terms, and include a timeline (Gateley & Borcherding, 2017).

The Client Is Not an Assist Level

Consider the following goal, which needs some improvement:

Liam will be min Ⓐ in dressing LEs in 10 days.

This goal needs to be written in terms of what the client **needs** rather than stating that he **will be** a particular assist level. It is a small distinction that shows more respect by wording the goal statement to acknowledge that the client is more than his ability to dress himself.

Specify the conditions under which this client will dress himself (including what parts of the task need assistance). Also indicate that he will dress the upper and lower *body* rather than that he will dress only his upper and lower *extremities*. For example:

Liam will be able to don lower body garments sitting EOB with min Ⓐ to pull pants and underwear over hips within 10 days.

Numbering the Short-Term Goals

Some occupational therapy practitioners number each STG. For example, if a client is working toward an outcome such as being able to complete laundry independently, the STGs might include specific activity demands that are problematic such as:

STG #1: *Consumer will demonstrate independence in laundry skills by selecting and inserting correct amount of money in coin-operated washing machine by 4/25/22.*

STG #2: *Consumer will demonstrate ↑ laundry skills by selecting proper cycles on washing machine by 4/25/22.*

In subsequent SOAP notes, the OT or OTA can refer to those numbered goals, providing a clear indication of the progress achieved. For example:

A: *STG #1: met. STG #2: consumer requires min verbal cues 50% of the time to select proper wash cycles for white and dark clothes.*

P: *Consumer will continue skilled instruction in IADLs until anticipated discharge in 4 weeks. At the time of discharge, consumer will be able to manage all laundry tasks Ⓘ at laundromat.*

HELPFUL HINT

DO NOT use participation in treatment as a goal. For example, it would not be very useful to say:

Client will do 20 reps of shoulder ladder with 1# wt. in order to ↑ endurance to become more Ⓘ in ADLs.

Instead, in a goal such as this, specify the amount of ↑ endurance you hope or expect to see for specific activities/occupations. For example:

Client will be able to participate in assembly line task > 10 minutes without rest breaks.

Client will be able to hang 10 clothing items in closet without shortness of breath.

Rather than saying:

Client will use therapy putty to ↑ left hand strength by 5 lbs.

It is better to say:

Client will ↑ left hand strength by 5 lbs in order to be able to open jars Ⓘ.

Rather than saying:

Client will play a board game with other clients.

It is better to say:

Client will demonstrate improved self-confidence by Ⓘ initiating a leisure activity with peers

Examples of Appropriate Goal Statements for Different Situations

Dressing

- *To prepare for recess, child will be able to manage zipper on coat with use of zipper pull within 1 month.*
- *In order to tie shoelaces Ⓘ, patient will demonstrate Ⓡ thumb MP flexion of at least 50° within 2 weeks.*

Hygiene

- *Client will complete grooming and hygiene activities with a reported pain level of < 3/10 within three intervention sessions.*
- *Student will be able to perform feminine hygiene Ⓘ to use bathroom at school by end of school year.*
- *Client will demonstrate 10-minute activity tolerance for standing at sink to brush teeth, comb hair, and shave within four OT sessions.*

Eating/Feeding

- *After set-up, resident will feed self a meal with correct use of adaptive equipment (nonslip placemat, lipped plate, rocker knife, and built-up angled utensils) with no more than one 5-minute rest break within 30 days.*
- *Zoey will be able to feed herself independently in preschool by maintaining upright posture and midline orientation in wheelchair throughout 15-minute snack time, within 1 month.*

Health Management

- *Consumer will choose at least two food items other than pizza that he is willing to include in his diet within 1 week.*
- *Client will remember to test blood glucose levels as directed by health providers and demonstrate ability to recognize symptoms of hypoglycemia, within 3 treatment sessions.*

Functional Mobility

- *Veteran will be able to propel w/c up ramp and through all doors with min Ⓐ in order to return to living at home within 2 weeks.*
- *Using walker, client will be able to perform transfers to tub bench with SBA within 2 weeks.*

Instrumental Activities of Daily Living

- *Client will demonstrate an ability to prepare a three-step stovetop meal Ⓘ after the fourth intervention session.*
- *Child will feed pet independently by accurately measuring and placing proper amount of dog food in bowl without verbal reminders within 1 month.*
- *Client will be able to unload clean dishes/utensils from dishwasher and place correctly in labeled cabinets/drawers with SBA within 2 weeks.*
- *In order to manage laundry Ⓘ, client will correctly sort white and dark clothes by the end of next session.*

Education

- *In order to complete writing activities, Jayden will be able to maintain upright posture at desk for > 5 minutes without verbal cues within 6 weeks.*
- *Student will be able to set up items on lunch tray Ⓘ by opening milk carton and unwrapping and placing straw 4/5 opportunities by the end of school year.*

Work

- *Client will ① request a job application from a restaurant within 1 week.*
- *In order to return to carpentry work, patient will demonstrate ® UE grip strength >70# within 4 weeks.*

Play

- *In order to engage in developmental play activities, toddler will sit unsupported for 3 minutes within 2 months.*
- *Keisha will use ⓛ UE as a functional assist 5/5 opportunities during spontaneous play within 2 months.*

Leisure

- *Client will identify at least three leisure activities that are not associated with drinking by 05/8/22.*
- *Within 1 month, client will demonstrate sufficient coordination to manipulate toothpaste caps, clothing fastenings, and knitting needles without dropping.*

Social Participation

- *Client will choose and participate in at least one social activity per week 3/3 weeks within 1 month.*
- *To demonstrate increased assertiveness skills, consumer will ask roommate to smoke outside the building within 2 days.*

Rest and Sleep

- *Client will remember to set alarm clock in order to wake up in time for work 5/5 days within 2 weeks.*
- *Client will turn off computer, cell phone, and TV in his bedroom by 11 PM without verbal reminders in order to get at least 7 hours of sleep nightly within 1 week.*

Learning Activity 15-1: Creating Occupation-Based Goals

The first column presents goals that need improvement because they lack occupation or are not specific enough. Column two includes examples showing how these goals can be revised to reflect specific occupations. In column three, it is your turn to practice completing goals to make them specific and occupation-based. Revise each of the first-column goals but choose a different occupation than the second-column example. Realize that for a "real" client the actual occupations, time frames, and specific criteria will, of course, differ according to what is appropriate for the individual's circumstances and practice setting.

Goal Lacking Occupation or Specificity	Goal that Reflects Specific Occupation	Your Turn to Complete Goal
Pt. will decrease left hand pain to a 4/10 reported pain level within 2 weeks	Pt. will be able to use computer keyboard at work with a reported pain level of 4/10 or less in left hand within 2 weeks	Pt. will be able to _____ with a reported pain level of 4/10 or less in left hand within 2 weeks
Resident will increase right shoulder flexion to 160 degrees within four treatment sessions	Resident will be able to reach overhead with RUE to place/retrieve clothing items on upper shelf in closet, within four treatment sessions	Resident will be able to _____ within four treatment sessions
Student will exhibit improved time management in school by the end of the school year	Student will exhibit improved time management by getting to all classes on time 5/5 days by the end of the school year	Student will exhibit improved time management by _____ by the end of the school year
Child will demonstrate good bilateral integration without verbal prompting within 3 months	Child will demonstrate improved bilateral integration by using both hands spontaneously to manage clothing fastenings ① within 3 months	Child will demonstrate improved bilateral integration by _____ within 3 months
Client will have decreased left neglect by expected discharge 4/10/2022	Client will shave both sides of face without need for verbal cues to attend to left side, by expected discharge 4/10/2022	Client will _____ by expected discharge 4/10/2022
Veteran will be able to sit unsupported on mat for 10 minutes with SBA while performing dynamic balloon toss activity within 2 weeks	Veteran will be able to maintain dynamic sitting balance EOB for 10 minutes at mealtimes, with SBA within 2 weeks	Veteran will be able to _____ within 2 weeks

Learning Activity 15-1: Creating Occupation-Based Goals (continued)

The first column presents goals that need improvement because they lack occupation or are not specific enough. Column two includes examples showing how these goals can be revised to reflect specific occupations. In column three, it is your turn to practice completing goals to make them specific and occupation-based. Revise each of the first-column goals but choose a different occupation than the second-column example. Realize that for a "real" client the actual occupations, time frames, and specific criteria will, of course, differ according to what is appropriate for the individual's circumstances and practice setting.

Goal Lacking Occupation or Specificity	Goal that Reflects Specific Occupation	Your Turn to Complete Goal
Patient will increase endurance for IADLs within 4 weeks	Patient will be able to sweep and use disposable wet mop pad to clean kitchen floor without shortness of breath within 4 weeks	Patient will be able to _____ without shortness of breath within 4 weeks
Toddler will exhibit improved hand skill development by attaining an inferior pincer grasp within 6 weeks	Toddler will utilize an inferior pincer grasp to feed self small finger foods (such as Cheerios, cheese puffs) within 6 weeks	Toddler will utilize an inferior pincer grasp to _____ within 6 weeks
Resident will demonstrate improved safety for ADLs by 6/12/2022	Resident will demonstrate improved safety awareness by remembering to hold onto grab bar when transferring on/off toilet by 6/12/2022	Resident will demonstrate improved safety awareness _____ by 6/12/2022
Client will be taught energy conservation techniques for IADLs within two treatment sessions	Client will demonstrate understanding of energy conservation techniques for laundry by sitting while folding clothes/ironing and using a rolling hamper to bring clothes to/from laundry room within two treatment sessions	Client will demonstrate understanding of energy conservation techniques _____ within two treatment sessions
Consumer will demonstrate improved social skills by the end of the month	Consumer will refrain from taking/using his roommate's personal items (e.g., food, toiletries) without asking by the end of the month	Consumer will _____ by the end of the month

Worksheet 15-1
Evaluating Goal Statements

Determine which of the following goals have all of the necessary COAST components to be useful in occupational therapy documentation. For each goal that is incomplete or inaccurate in some way, indicate what it lacks.

1.   *By the time of expected discharge in 1 week, client will be able to dress himself with min Ⓐ for balance using a sock aid and reacher while seated in wheelchair.*
_____This goal has all the necessary COAST components to be useful.

_____This goal lacks _____.

2.   *Client will tolerate 15 minutes of treatment daily.*
_____This goal has all the necessary COAST components to be useful.

_____This goal lacks _____.

3.   *Client will demonstrate increased coping skills in order to live at home with her granddaughter within 2 weeks.*
_____This goal has all the necessary COAST components to be useful.

_____This goal lacks _____.

4.   *Resident will demonstrate 15 minutes of activity tolerance without rest breaks using Ⓑ UE in order to complete self-care tasks before breakfast each morning.*
_____This goal has all the necessary COAST components to be useful.

_____This goal lacks _____.

5.   *In order to be able to toilet self after discharge, client will demonstrate ability to perform a sliding board transfer w/c → mat within the next week.*
_____This goal has all the necessary COAST components to be useful.

_____This goal lacks _____.

6.   *OTA will teach lower body dressing using a reacher, dressing stick, and sock aid within 2 intervention sessions.*
_____This goal has all the necessary COAST components to be useful.

_____This goal lacks _____.

7.   *In order to return to living independently, client will demonstrate ability to balance his checkbook.*
_____This goal has all the necessary COAST components to be useful.

_____This goal lacks _____.

Morreale, M. J. (2023). *The OTA's guide to documentation: Writing SOAP notes* (5th ed.). SLACK Incorporated.

Worksheet 15-2
Writing Goals That Are Client-Centered, Occupation-Based, and Measurable

Review the scenarios below and write goals that are client-centered, occupation-based, measurable, time-limited, and realistic. Goals are established with the client (under the supervision of the OT), so assume for this practice sheet that you have already collaborated with the client and your supervisor.

1. Your client, Maria, has difficulty with IADL tasks because she is unable to attend to task for more than a few minutes. Because she enjoys cooking and plans to resume cooking after discharge, you have been working with her in the kitchen. You would like to see her able to attend to task for 10 minutes by the time she is discharged next week. Write a goal to increase Maria's attention span.

C _____
   (Client will perform)

O _____
   (Occupation)

A _____
   (Assist level)

S _____
   (Specific conditions)

T _____
   (Timeline—by when?)

2. Now write a goal for Maria to be able to follow directions so that she can read the back of a boxed meal, and eventually a recipe, when she is cooking.

C _____
   (Client will perform)

O _____
   (Occupation)

A _____
   (Assist level)

S _____
   (Specific conditions)

T _____
   (Timeline—by when?)

3. Bill is having trouble performing dressing tasks after his stroke. You have been teaching him an over-the-head method for putting on his shirt and have given him a buttonhook to use. Write a dressing goal for Bill.

C _____
   (Client will perform)

O _____
   (Occupation)

A _____
   (Assist level)

S _____
   (Specific conditions)

T _____
   (Timeline—by when?)

Morreale, M. J. (2023). *The OTA's guide to documentation: Writing SOAP notes* (5th ed.). SLACK Incorporated.

Worksheet 15-3
Writing Goals That Are Client-Centered, Occupation-Based, and Measurable—More Practice

Review the scenarios below and write goals that are client-centered, occupation-based, measurable, time-limited, and realistic. Goals are established with the client (under the supervision of the OT), so assume for this practice sheet that you have already collaborated with the client and your supervisor.

1. Emma is recovering from an exacerbation of multiple sclerosis and has significant weakness. She desires to be able to care for her 4-month-old child and also go back to work as a receptionist. Write a goal to increase her activity tolerance. Anticipated discharge is in 2 weeks.

   C _____
      (Client will perform)

   O _____
      (Occupation)

   A _____
      (Assist level)

   S _____
      (Specific conditions)

   T _____
      (Timeline—by when?)

2. Alberto wants to live independently in the community, but he lacks basic money management skills. Write a goal for Alberto to improve his money management skills.

   C _____
      (Client will perform)

   O _____
      (Occupation)

   A _____
      (Assist level)

   S _____
      (Specific conditions)

   T _____
      (Timeline—by when?)

3. Katelyn has become increasingly more depressed over the past several weeks and was admitted to an inpatient behavioral health unit after a suicide attempt. You estimate that you will have her in groups for 1 week. You would like to see her mood change in that week. Write a goal that is occupation-based and will indicate an improved mood.

   C _____
      (Client will perform)

   O _____
      (Occupation)

   A _____
      (Assist level)

   S _____
      (Specific conditions)

   T _____
      (Timeline—by when?)

Morreale, M. J. (2023). *The OTA's guide to documentation: Writing SOAP notes* (5th ed.). SLACK Incorporated.

Worksheet 15-4
Writing Goals—Developmental Disability

Jake is an 18-year-old man with a developmental disability. He has just moved into a group home with five other clients. Jake exhibits mild to moderate cognitive impairment but can perform self-care occupations with supervision and occasional assistance. Muscle tone is minimally hypotonic but there are no other physical limitations. He has a fair frustration tolerance and occasionally exhibits some aggressive behavior. The plan is to improve Jake's social skills and allow him to be more independent in the group home and community.

Using the information in the above scenario, write a short-term occupation-based goal for each of the categories listed below. Make sure your goals are appropriate and realistic for this particular practice setting, keeping in mind the client's abilities and expected functional gains.

1. Instrumental ADL—meal preparation: _____

   _____

2. Instrumental ADL—household chore: _____

   _____

3. Instrumental ADL—shopping: _____

   _____

4. Instrumental ADL—money management/functional math skill: _____

   _____

5. Communication/interaction skills: _____

   _____

6. Prevocational skills: _____

   _____

7. Temporal organization/time management: _____

   _____

Morreale, M. J. (2023). *The OTA's guide to documentation: Writing SOAP notes* (5th ed.). SLACK Incorporated.

Worksheet 15-5
Goal Writing—ADL Performance Skills and Factors

There are instances when specific performance skills or client factors must be emphasized in goals to prepare the client for function and demonstrate progress. Create a client in your mind and consider the ADL task of tooth brushing. Using the client factors and performance skills below, write goals for the occupation of tooth brushing that address each listed component. Remember to include the assist level, specific condition, and timeline.

ADL: Brushing Teeth

1. Fine-motor skills: _____

_____

2. Hand strength: _____

_____

3. Standing balance: _____

_____

4. Unilateral inattention: _____

_____

5. Elbow range of motion: _____

_____

6. Problem solving: _____

_____

7. Spatial relations: _____

_____

References

American Occupational Therapy Association. (2020). Occupational therapy practice framework: Domain and process (4th ed.). *American Journal of Occupational Therapy, 74*(Suppl. 2), 7412410010. https://doi.org: 10.5014/ajot.2020.74S2001

Gateley, C. A., & Borcherding, S. (2017). *Documentation manual for occupational therapy: Writing SOAP notes* (4th ed.). SLACK Incorporated.

Chapter 16

Documenting Different Stages of Intervention

Information on evaluation reports was presented in Chapter 14. This chapter will focus on other types of notes written during the occupational therapy process. These include contact notes, progress reports/notes, reevaluation reports, transition plans, and discharge/discontinuation reports. Because the OTA's primary role is to implement planned interventions, OTAs are more likely to write contact notes and progress notes (but may also contribute to other types of notes), all under the OT's supervision (American Occupational Therapy Association [AOTA], 2018, 2020, 2021). Review the suggestions in Chapter 2 regarding the basics of documentation, including AOTA's list of fundamental elements that should be present in all occupational therapy documentation (AOTA, 2018). The client's identifying information should be on each page of the health record, although electronic records normally eliminate the need to manually reenter this every time an established client's file is opened and notes are added. If traditional paper records are what a setting uses, the client's identifying or demographic information is written onto each page of the health record or, possibly, stamped using an addressograph card.

Contact Note

Contact, visit, or treatment notes are used to document each encounter or occupational therapy session. Besides face-to-face contact with the client, these notes can also include information that was exchanged in pertinent telephone conversations or meetings with others such as the family/caregiver. As explained previously in Chapter 11, notes are also written stating why a scheduled session did not take place, ended prematurely, or involved unusual circumstances. In settings such as home health or acute care, formal contact notes are typically written in the health record each time a client is seen. In situations such as school settings or some skilled nursing facilities, occupational therapy practitioners might keep attendance records, logs, billing sheets, or informal contact notes, which are used for the purpose of writing a summary of progress later on at specified intervals. Practice settings vary regarding exact frequency, format, and content for treatment notes and this is also guided by payer requirements and applicable laws. Your facility or agency will normally supply you with designated printed forms or computerized formats to use. The *Guidelines for Documentation of Occupational Therapy* (AOTA, 2018) suggests the following criteria for contact notes:

Morreale, M. J. *The OTA's Guide to Documentation: Writing SOAP Notes, Fifth Edition* (pp. 237-246). © 2023 Taylor & Francis Group.

Contact Report (Daily Treatment Notes): Documents the contacts between the client and the occupational therapy practitioner, the goals, and the intervention types and approaches used in the occupational therapy process, and the therapy outcomes.

   a. *Client information*—Diagnosis, precautions, contraindications, and variables that influence the client's condition.

   b. *Therapy log*—Documentation of services provided that reflects the complexity of the client and the professional clinical reasoning and expertise of an occupational therapy practitioner required to provide safe and effective outcomes in occupational engagement and performance. Content includes date, length of service contact, type of contact, names and positions of persons involved, summary of significant information communicated during contact, client attendance and participation in intervention or reason service was missed, types and approaches of interventions used, client's self-report and response to intervention, adverse reaction or response to treatment, environmental or task modification, assistive or adaptive devices used or fabricated, statement of any training, education or consultation provided, and client's present level of performance. Significant, unusual, or unexpected changes in clinical or functional status are reported. Objective measures used to assess outcomes should be repeated in accordance with payer and facility requirements and clearly documented to demonstrate measurable functional progress toward the goals of the client.

Reproduced with permission from American Occupational Therapy Association. (2018). Guidelines for documentation of occupational therapy. *American Journal of Occupational Therapy, 72*(Suppl. 2),7212410010. https://doi.org/10.5014/ajot.2018.72S203

The following is an example of an acute care contact note that incorporates the AOTA guidelines:

Healthy Hospital
Acute Care Unit
Occupational Therapy Contact Note

Client: Klyent, Karl   **DOB:** 11/10/1940   **Health record #:** 34-6529
Dx: COPD   **Gender:** Male   **Physician:** Dr. Will Heelue
Precautions/Contraindications: Maintain O_2 levels at 95% to 100%
Date: 4/14/22   **Time:** 8:30 AM

S: Client reported, "I feel fair today. I had a long night."

O: In ICU, client participated in bedside session 18 minutes for instruction in ADL tasks and to increase activity tolerance. Client was also instructed in diaphragmatic and pursed lip breathing. Client required mod Ⓐ supine → sit. Upon sitting EOB, O_2 saturation dropped to ~85%. Client required min Ⓐ to return to supine. After ~2 minutes, O_2 levels returned to ~95%. With head of bed raised and ADL set-up, client washed face, combed hair, and brushed teeth with O_2 levels ~95% without rest breaks while incorporating proper breathing techniques c̄ min. verbal cues.

A: Client appears more willing and able to participate in therapy session as compared to his refusal of therapy yesterday. Activity tolerance still limited due to O_2 saturation levels upon exertion, which limits ability to participate in self-care tasks. Client would benefit from instruction in energy conservation as well as correct breathing techniques and positioning to ↓ exertion and ↑ activity tolerance for ADL tasks.

P: Continue skilled OT daily for 5 days or until discharge from acute care to ↑ activity tolerance and Ⓘ in ADL tasks. Client will complete grooming modified Ⓘ sitting EOB with rest breaks as needed within three intervention sessions.

Vera Veracity, COTA/L—Kimberly Kindness, OTR/L

Worksheet 16-1
Contact Notes

Use this worksheet as you are learning to write treatment notes. You may also use this worksheet to compare a "real" treatment note to AOTA's recommended criteria.

Criteria	How Does Your Note Comply With the Criteria?
Does the note state the client's full name and identifying number?	
Is information relating to the client's diagnosis and precautions/contraindications specified?	
Are the date (and time, if needed) of the contact indicated?	
Is the note identified as occupational therapy?	
Is the type of note indicated?	
Does the note state the type of contact and purpose of the encounter?	
Is there a summary of the interventions implemented or information communicated during the contact (e.g., modification of the task or environment, assistive/adaptive devices fabricated or used, education, training, or consultation provided, outcome measures used), and indication of client's present performance level?	
Is the client's attendance and participation in the contact (or the reason service was missed) indicated?	
Does the note indicate names/positions of persons involved?	
Are all abbreviations and terminology standard and acceptable for the setting?	
Are all errors noted and corrected properly?	
Is the note signed (and cosigned if needed)?	
Are professional credentials indicated next to the signature?	
Are intervention/procedure codes indicated if needed?	
Does the note reflect skilled occupational therapy happening?	

Morreale, M. J. (2023). *The OTA's guide to documentation: Writing SOAP notes* (5th ed.). SLACK Incorporated.

Progress Report/Note

Progress reports/notes are written on a regularly scheduled basis, which might be weekly, every 2 weeks, or monthly. The facility determines the specific time frame and format by considering the guidelines set forth by accrediting agencies and primary payers. Progress reports/notes provide a summary of the intervention process and include updated information about the client's condition (e.g., precautions/contraindications, new problems and so forth) along with a description of the client's progress toward established goals such as the client's present ability to engage in occupations, indication of relevant factors supporting or impeding progress and whether established goals have been met yet. Progress notes also specify frequency and duration of services provided, the types of assessments and measures implemented, the interventions furnished (i.e., occupational adaptations, assistive technology/adaptive equipment, orthotic devices, specific exercise programs, client/family education, and so forth), along with recommendations to continue or revise the plan (AOTA, 2018).

The following is an example of a progress note written in a SOAP format, although a narrative or other format could be used instead:

XYZ Behavioral Health Center
Occupational Therapy Progress Note

Client: Payshent, Patricia   **DOB:** 1/10/1979   **Health record #:** 54321
Dx: Depression   **Gender:** Female   **Physician:** Bea Well, MD
SOC: 10/01/21
Date: 10/12/2021

S: In assertion group on Tuesday, 10/10/21, client talked about how her life had taken a "downward spiral" since early September, and she had become more passive and less proactive in getting her needs met, although she had not been aware of it at the time.

O: Client attended assertion group 2/2, communication group 1/1, and IADL group 3/5 this week. She was on time to 4/6 groups without reminders, wearing neatly pressed clothing, makeup, and an ornament in her hair. In assertion group on Wednesday, 10/11/21, she shared (without prompting) two stories about her usual way of dealing with retail situations. In communication group, she spontaneously answered one question addressed to the group as a whole, and in IADL group, she offered to assist another client with his checkbook.

A: Client's spontaneous actions in groups and willingness to share verbally indicate an improved mood this week. Her unprompted attendance is up this week from 2/8 to 6/8 groups. Her improved dress, hygiene, and makeup also indicate an improvement in mood from last week. Client would benefit from planning a structure for her days to prevent another "downward spiral" after discharge, and she has expressed willingness to work on this.

Goals #1: (assertion) and #2: (communication) are met as of this date.

Goal #3: (leisure skills) is continued through expected discharge on 10/14/21 pending formulation of a plan.

Goal #4: (parenting skills) was discontinued on 10/10/21.

P: Client to participate in groups for 2 more days, with discharge anticipated on 10/14/21. IADL group and individual session, if needed, will be used for preparing the structured plan for using her time. Client will prepare a plan including at least one planned leisure activity per day for at least 5 days out of 7 after discharge and will discuss it with her husband and social worker by expected discharge on 10/14/21.

Evan Empathy, COTA/L—Sharon Sympathetic, OTR/L

Worksheet 16-2
Progress Note

Use this worksheet as you are learning to write progress notes. Review AOTA's *Guidelines for Documentation of Occupational Therapy* (2018) and use this worksheet to compare a "real" progress note to the recommended criteria.

Criteria	How Does Your Note Comply With the Criteria?
Does the note state the client's full name and identifying number?	
Is the date of the progress note specified?	
Is the note identified as occupational therapy?	
Is the type of note indicated?	
Has new data been obtained and presented?	
Is information relating to the client's condition and precautions/contraindications specified?	
Does the note state pertinent client updates, problems, or changes to the intervention plan?	
Does the note indicate the frequency of services and how long services have been provided?	
Does the note indicate what areas of occupation are being addressed?	
Is there a summary of techniques and strategies used? Does the note specify occupational adaptations, assistive technology/adaptive devices, orthotics, or other skilled services provided?	
Does the note indicate the type of education, training, or consultation that has been provided and to whom?	
Does the note indicate what progress (or lack thereof) the client is making toward established goals?	
Does the note indicate the client's response to occupational therapy services?	
Does the note reflect the client's occupational performance?	
Are any outcomes measures identified? Are they appropriate to the client's condition/situation and relate to function?	
Are recommendations indicated along with rationale? Will therapy be continued, discontinued, or is there need for referral?	
Does the note reflect the client's input to changes or continuation of the intervention plan?	
Are all abbreviations and terminology standard and acceptable for the setting?	
Are errors noted and corrected properly?	
Is the note signed (and cosigned if needed)?	
Are professional credentials indicated next to the signature?	

Morreale, M. J. (2023). *The OTA's guide to documentation: Writing SOAP notes* (5th ed.). SLACK Incorporated.

Data will need to be organized into whatever format is used for the electronic documentation system in place at your setting. However, as you can see by the examples, contact notes and progress notes fit neatly into the SOAP format. Reevaluation reports, transition plans, and discharge summaries may also use a SOAP format but generally require more organization, analysis, intervention planning, and a broader base of knowledge. The OT is responsible for developing and documenting these notes. However, OTAs can participate in all aspects of the intervention process and can contribute to documentation at all stages under the OT's supervision (AOTA, 2021). Therefore, we will take a brief look at reevaluations, transition plans, and discharge reports.

Reevaluation Reports

Practice settings vary regarding time frames for reevaluation. Clients might be reevaluated monthly, quarterly, or on an as-needed basis. The reevaluation is the responsibility of the OT, but certain functions might be delegated to the OTA (AOTA, 2020, 2021). According to the *Guidelines for Documentation of Occupational Therapy* (AOTA, 2018), a reevaluation report is warranted when there are new clinical findings, significant changes in the client's situation, further testing is indicated, or the client is not making progress as expected (AOTA, 2018). The reevaluation report should include any new information about the client's condition or situation along with a summary or update of challenges, changes, abilities, or specific concerns that relate to the occupational profile. In addition, the standardized and/or nonstandardized outcomes measures that were given initially are re-administered (along with new tests if indicated), and the results are compared with the results of prior outcome measures to determine the effectiveness of the intervention being provided. The OT identifies the factors that support or hinder occupational performance and participation and determines if revisions need to be made to the goals and plans (AOTA, 2018). New timelines are projected, and the OT also determines if any other recommendations or referrals are warranted.

XYZ Hand Clinic
Occupational Therapy Department
Reevaluation Report

Name: Doe, Jane   **DOB:** 4/01/81   **Gender:** Female   **Record #:** 123456

Primary diagnosis: Osteoarthritis in Ⓑ CMC joints

Secondary diagnosis: None

Precautions/contraindications: None

Referring physician: B. Paynefree, MD   **Date of referral:** June 27, 2022

Reason for referral: Client is 1 month post surgery (LRTI) to the Ⓛ CMC joint and Ⓛ CTR

Date of initial evaluation: 7/5/2022

Date of reevaluation: 8/31/2022

Funding source: University insurance

Occupational profile: Jane is a 41-year-old Caucasian female who works as an administrative assistant in the English Department at the University. She lives alone in a small two-story farmhouse 7 miles outside of town. The house is heated with wood that Jane cuts and stacks in the summer. Jane raises a large vegetable garden every year in addition to holding both a full-time job at the University and a part-time job in a department store. She began experiencing pain in the CMC joints of both hands approximately 3 years ago. She states she intends to continue her present living arrangement and both of her jobs. She was originally admitted to the outpatient hand clinic on July 5, 2022 at 1 month post-surgery for hand rehabilitation following a successful Ⓛ LRTI and a carpal tunnel release. She is being reevaluated this date (8/31/22) to determine whether further OT services are needed.

S: Client initially reported continuous pain at a level of 3/10 and pain on overexertion of the Ⓛ hand at a level of 5/10, resulting in difficulty performing bilateral work and daily living tasks, as well as some tasks requiring left hand use. On this date, she reports no continuous pain and pain at a level of 1/10 when typing for more than 45 minutes without rest breaks.

Initial ability to engage in work/ADL/IADL tasks (by client report):
- Unable to use keyboard with all fingers of Ⓛ hand. Types with one finger on standard keyboard.
- Unable to grasp cylindrical objects smaller than 1 ½ inches (broom handle, toothpaste tube) due to ↓ AROM
- Unable to wear watch or rings on Ⓛ hand due to edema
- Unable to turn door knob with Ⓛ hand to enter house when right hand is full

- Unable to lift laundry basket and other items requiring Ⓑ UE use. Unable to lift purse or other items needed for IADL tasks with left hand.

Current ability to engage in work/ADL/IADL tasks this date (by client report):

- Able to use new ergonomic keyboard for primary work task using all fingers
- Able to sweep the floors with a regular broom
- Able to fold laundry using Ⓑ hands
- Able to grasp small items needed for ADL and IADL tasks (toothpaste tube, key, lids), but not at prior level of function
- Able to turn doorknob if door is unlocked
- Able to hang out clothes on clothesline, including carrying basket and holding garments with left hand

O:

Initial evaluation of client factors 7/05/22	Reassessment of client factors 8/31/22
Total active motion of the left wrist: 125°	Total active motion of the left wrist: 160°
Total active motion of the left thumb: 110°	Total active motion of the left thumb: 130°
Grip strength Ⓡ 41#	Grip strength Ⓡ 43#
Grip strength Ⓛ 15# (37% of Ⓡ)	Grip strength Ⓛ 29#
Pinch not tested	Pinch not tested
Min edema Ⓑ thumbs	No edema

Client has participated in eight 45-minute sessions in outpatient hand clinic since admission on 7/05/22. AROM and PROM have been performed and taught to client, and home program has been modified as she progressed. Hot packs and paraffin were administered, and the client has purchased a home paraffin unit. Electrical stimulation has been used to elicit specific motion and facilitate strengthening of the flexor pollicis longus. A strengthening program has been added to the HEP, and client is able to demonstrate all exercises correctly. Client has received education on the structure and use of the hand, common features of CMC arthritis, ergonomics of the workstation, energy conservation, use of heat for pain relief, and adapted techniques for ADLs. Client reports understanding the education and has been given written material covering the same content.

A: Increase in grip strength of 14# left hand shows good progress in strength needed to perform functional tasks. Thumb AROM is now WFL, and total wrist AROM has increased 35°, allowing client to perform most work and ADL tasks Ⓘ in ways that do not damage the joint. Change to an ergonomic keyboard and understanding and correct self-administration of HEP indicate good potential to continue improvement without further OT services.

P: Results of reevaluation indicate no further need for OT services at this time. Client to follow the home program of heat, exercise, and adapted techniques. Client was advised to call hand clinic if questions arise.

Hans Handfixer, OTR/L, CHT

Transition Plans

A transition plan is developed and written whenever a client transfers within a service delivery system from one setting to another (AOTA, 2018). This is the responsibility of the OT, but, as with other stages of intervention, the OTA can contribute to this process (AOTA, 2021). The purpose of the transition plan is to provide client information to the new service providers to prevent any interruption in care. According to the *Guidelines for Documentation of Occupational Therapy* (AOTA, 2018), a transition plan summarizes the client's current occupational status, specifies what service setting the client is leaving and what setting the client is entering, and states how and when the transition will occur. It also lists what follow-up or recommended services would benefit the client, such as continued therapy, specific equipment, necessary modifications, and accommodations.

ABC Early Intervention Program
Occupational Therapy Department
Transition Plan

Name: Kidd, Kari   **Date of birth:** 4/29/19   **Gender:** Female   **Record #:** 87654

Date of plan: 4/11/2022   **Expected transition date:** May, 2022

Precautions/contraindications: Seizure disorder   **Funding source:** Medicaid

Occupational history: Kari experienced head and orthopedic injuries following an MVA at 9 days of age. Since that time, she has had multiple cranial, hip, and leg surgeries. She is currently under the management of a neurologist as well as an orthopedist. The mother carries out a home program daily, which is designed to stimulate development.

S: The mother reports that although Kari's seizures, multiple surgeries, and illnesses have slowed her development, the family is hopeful that Kari will progress more rapidly through her developmental milestones now that the surgeries are finished and the seizures are under control.

O: Child received her first occupational therapy screening in the hospital 1 week post injury. She received formal developmental assessments at 2, 4, 6, 12, and 24 months of age. Parents were instructed in a home program following the initial formal assessment. Regular OT intervention sessions were started at 12 months of age and have continued to this date. Child has been seen twice weekly in her home and monthly in the Birth-to-Three clinic. She is now eligible for preschool services as she is turning 3 years old.

Current occupational performance: Current problems being treated in occupational therapy include visual regard and visually directed reach, midline orientation, postural symmetry, and motor overflow. Current goals for Kari include functional reach, grasp and release, rolling, and ability to sustain anti-gravity positions for ADLs and developmental play activities.

A: At close to 3 years of age, Kari is at about a 4-month level of development. Although the mother provides a stimulating environment, Kari would benefit from continuation of regular occupational therapy, physical therapy, and speech therapy services to facilitate her continued progress through the developmental sequence.

P: Kari will receive her first preschool service evaluation next month in May of 2022. Parents have been instructed in a home program, which has been updated as child has progressed in treatment. Home program will continue through the transition to Preschool Services.

Alice Altruism, OTR/L

Discharge Report

When therapy is no longer necessary in a particular setting, a discharge report (also called a *discontinuation report*) is written. It provides a synopsis of the occupational therapy intervention provided and the client's changes or progress from start of care to the present time regarding ability to engage in occupation (AOTA, 2018). Discharge reports are the responsibility of the OT, but the therapist can delegate parts of this process to the OTA as appropriate (AOTA, 2021). Discharge notes often follow a specific format. Content should include the date and purpose of the referral; a summary of the client's condition; a comparison of initial evaluation findings to status at time of discharge; and a summary of course of treatment, such as frequency and number of sessions, types of interventions/programs implemented (i.e., ADL retraining, occupational adaptations, physical agent modalities, orthotic devices, assistive devices, client/caregiver education). Discharge reports also summarize progress and outcomes relating to occupational performance and specify any recommendations for follow-up care (AOTA, 2018). Recommendations might include continued therapy in a different setting; home exercise programs; adaptive equipment, assistive technology, or durable medical equipment; home, school, or workplace modifications; support groups or community services; etc. Client data will need to be organized into whatever format is used for the electronic documentation system in place at your setting. Discharge reports may also be written in a SOAP or narrative format, or the facility may have a special form that is used. Some facilities use the same (or similar) format for evaluation, reevaluation, and discharge, making it easier to prepare the discontinuation report. There are many reasons that an occupational therapy client is discharged or treatment is discontinued. It is important for the discharge report to indicate the circumstances or reasons for discharge. Table 16-1 indicates various reasons that can warrant occupational therapy discharge or discontinuation of treatment.

Table 16-1

Reasons for Discontinuing Occupational Therapy

- Occupational therapy outcomes were met.
- Client discharged from facility or agency.
- No further occupational therapy is medically or educationally necessary.
- Duplication of services
- Client not making progress.
- Client became ill/was hospitalized.
- Physician (or allowable nonphysician practitioner) discontinued therapy.
- Reimbursement issues/managed care (i.e., therapy not approved or used up allotted number of visits)
- Client requires more specialized services than can be provided at this facility/agency.
- Client noncompliant or refusing therapy.
- Poor attendance
- Client discharged self/did not return to therapy.
- Client expired.
- Client moved.
- Client decided to receive services elsewhere.

The following is an example of a discharge report using the SOAP format:

Reallygood Rehabilitation Center
Occupational Therapy Department
Discharge Report

Name: Rezzydent, Rosa   **Record #:** 246810   **DOB:** 11/10/48
Dx: Ⓡ THR   **Date of surgery:** 6/21/22 **Admission date:** 6/25/22
Date of Report: 7/19/22   **Time:** 3:00 PM   **Gender:** F

S: Client reports that she is "very pleased" with the outcome of her occupational therapy intervention, and with her ability to take care of herself at home. She reports no steps to the front entrance of a one-story home, and no architectural barriers inside the house. She reports owning the following adaptive equipment/DME: wheeled walker, reacher, dressing stick, sock aid, long shoehorn, tub bench, raised toilet seat, and grab bars around the toilet and tub area.

O: Client participated in OT bedside and in clinic area 20/20 sessions from SOC on 6/25/22.

ADL status on 6/25/22	ADL status on 7/19/22
Mod Ⓐ in transfers	SBA in transfers
Mod Ⓐ in toileting	SBA in toileting
Mod Ⓐ in feeding	Ⓘ in feeding after set-up
Mod Ⓐ in dressing	Dressing from arm chair requires set-up only, but SBA for standing and pulling pants up over hips
Max Ⓐ for safety in bathing	SBA in bathing with min Ⓐ w/c ↔ shower using tub bench

Client education in adaptive techniques and HEP were discussed with client, and client demonstrated ability to perform correctly and adhere to all total hip precautions. Written instructions provided. Home modifications discussed with client and caregiver.

A: Client has made good progress in self-care activities as shown by differences in admitting and discharge abilities. Because caregiver is available to provide SBA needed for safety in ADL tasks, all treatment goals have been met, and client is ready for discontinuation of occupational therapy services.

P: Client to continue home exercise program. Adaptive equipment recommended: walker basket and reacher holder for walker. Client to continue outpatient PT. No direct OT services recommended at this time.

Patty Patience, OTR/L

Now here is the same information using a narrative format:

Reallygood Rehabilitation Center
Occupational Therapy Department
Discharge Note

Name: Rezzydent, Rosa   **Record #:** 246810   **DOB:** 11/10/48
Dx: Ⓡ THR   **Date of surgery:** 6/21/22
Gender: F   **Admission date:** 6/25/22
Date of report: 7/19/22   **Time:** 3:00 PM

Course of Rehabilitation: Client participated in 20/20 sessions from SOC on 6/25/22. Skilled instruction in adaptive techniques for ADLs provided. Client's progress was good, and she demonstrated ability to adhere to total hip precautions. All treatment goals met. Client now requires SBA in all transfers, lower body ADLs, upper body ADLs, grooming/hygiene. Following set-up, client is able to perform dressing seated in armchair and using wheeled walker, but she needs SBA for standing and to pull pants up over hips. Client needs min Ⓐ w/c ↔ shower using tub bench but is able to complete bathing with SBA. She is able to complete toileting with SBA and feeding Ⓘ after set-up.

Client Education: Recommendations for additional adaptive equipment and modifications to home discussed with client and caregiver. Client and caregiver were instructed in home exercise program of exercise bands, free weights, wands, and other activities to choose from for Ⓑ UE strengthening. HEP discussed with client and client demonstrated ability to perform exercises correctly. Written instructions provided.

Discharge Recommendations/Referrals: Discharge with home caregiver. Continue home exercise program. Adaptive equipment recommended: walker basket and reacher holder for walker. Client already has wheeled walker, reacher, dressing stick, sock aid, long shoehorn, and functional bathroom equipment and she has demonstrated ability to use these correctly and safely. Client will continue outpatient PT. No further direct OT services are recommended at this time.

Patty Patience, OTR/L

References

American Occupational Therapy Association. (2018). Guidelines for documentation of occupational therapy. *American Journal of Occupational Therapy, 72*(Suppl. 2),7212410010. https://doi.org/10.5014/ajot.2018.72S203

American Occupational Therapy Association. (2020). Guidelines for supervision, roles, and responsibilities during the delivery of occupational therapy services. *American Journal of Occupational Therapy,* 74(Suppl. 3), 7413410020. https://doi.org/10.5014/ajot.2020.74S3004

American Occupational Therapy Association. (2021). Standards of practice for occupational therapy. *American Journal of Occupational Therapy,* 75(Suppl. 3), 7513410030. https://doi.org/10.5014/ajot.2021.75S3004

Chapter 17

Documentation in Different Practice Settings

This chapter will look at documentation for different practice settings, each of which has some requirements specific to the setting or the primary source of payment. Documentation for these situations is different in some ways from the examples you have learned so far. Realize that the present requirements are always subject to change based on federal and state regulations, payer requirements, or changes in clinical practice guidelines. Review Chapters 14 and 16 for more detail regarding the specific content of evaluation reports, progress notes, contact notes, and discharge reports and the roles of the OT and OTA.

Documentation in School-Based Practice

Occupational therapy practitioners working in the public school system use concepts and language that are unique to the educational setting. Therefore, documentation in school settings is different from the notes occupational therapy practitioners might write in other practice areas. Under Individuals with Disabilities Education Act (IDEA) Part B, the children with disabilities or qualifying health conditions in your school caseload will each have an intervention plan called an **Individualized Education Program (IEP)**. This IEP consists of strengths, challenges, goals, and interventions that are **educationally based**; that is, focused on behaviors and skills the student needs to participate and be successful in school. The IEP is a formal, multidisciplinary, written plan. It is established at an annual meeting for each child classified as needing special services. The plan is compiled together by therapists, teachers, and parents, plus any other appropriate professionals involved with the child (such as a psychologist, blind mobility specialist, sign language interpreter, social worker, or special educator). As each child's needs are different, not all students with an IEP require occupational therapy services.

There are two general purposes of an IEP (Center for Parent Information and Resources, 2017a):

1. To establish annual goals for the child that are measurable
2. To delineate the special education, related services and supplementary aids and services that will be provided to, or on behalf of, the child

The IEP team broadly considers the following three primary areas of school life for a child with a disability when creating an appropriate educational program (Center for Parent Information and Resources, 2017a):

1. General educational curriculum (e.g., science, language arts, math, history)
2. Extracurricular activities (e.g., school sports and clubs, yearbook, school newspaper, band, after-school programs)
3. Nonacademic activities (e.g., lunch, assemblies, rallies, field trips)

Morreale, M. J. *The OTA's Guide to Documentation:*
Writing SOAP Notes, Fifth Edition (pp. 247-276).
© 2023 Taylor & Francis Group.

In the school setting, extracurricular activities and nonacademic activities are typically voluntary, more social than academic, can be organized/supervised by teachers or other school personnel, and usually involve same-age peer groups (Center for Parent Information and Resources, 2017a).

If certain criteria are met, a state's Medicaid program will reimburse schools for *medically necessary* direct services (including occupational therapy) provided under IDEA for those children who are Medicaid eligible in that state. The child must have a qualifying health condition and the IEP must delineate what medically necessary skilled services are needed and will be provided for that condition (American Occupational Therapy Association [AOTA], 2022; Frolek Clark & Holahan, 2015). Some states might not allow an OTA to provide school services that are reimbursed by Medicaid (Frolek Clark & Holahan, 2015). Practitioners must follow the laws and requirements for services in their specific state, such as if a prescription is required, who meets the definition of a qualified health provider, and the specific documentation requirements needed to substantiate the skilled care furnished.

In 2004, President George W. Bush reauthorized IDEA as the Individuals with Disabilities Improvement Act to provide services to students needing academic and behavioral support but who are not classified as requiring special education. Additional aims of the 2004 reauthorization included improved standards, better educational outcomes, greater accountability, plus alignment with requirements of the No Child Left Behind Act (U.S. Department of Education, 2020). The 2004 regulations revised and outlined various requirements for general content of an IEP, including those listed in Box 17-1. Model forms were established by the U.S. Department of Education to help schools meet the IDEA requirements (U.S. Dept. of Education, n.d.a, n.d.b.).

In a school setting, the OT is responsible for directing the occupational therapy evaluation, establishing the occupational therapy component of the IEP, and implementing or overseeing occupational therapy intervention. The OTA might provide feedback throughout this process by implementing delegated assessments and interventions. The IEP is truly a shared effort. Based on each discipline's role and assessment, the IEP for each child details current educational status, strengths, challenges, goals, and interventions for the current school year. As the treatment principles, concepts, and outcomes for the entire team are collaborative, there may or may not be a distinct list of occupational therapy goals per se. However, the OT and OTA can play important roles in helping the child succeed in meeting curriculum standards and outcomes established by the district or team. Even though the child might have a particular medical condition or deficits in other areas of life, the IEP and interventions focus on the child's skills that need to be mastered in the educational setting. A student's challenges in school could involve a variety of areas, such as the following examples:

- Classroom behaviors and skills (attention to task, handwriting, scissors use, copying from blackboard, organizational skills, sitting at desk, handling art and science materials)
- Academic achievement
- Personal and toilet hygiene (washing hands, feminine hygiene, managing clothing for toileting)
- Dressing (putting on coat or boots for recess, changing for physical education class)
- Feeding (opening food containers/wrappers, managing finger foods or utensils, carrying meal tray)
- Ability to participate in extracurricular activities (school play, chorus, school sports and clubs)
- Ability to manage the activity demands for various school contexts (cafeteria, gym, recess, locker room, library, school bus)
- Ability to navigate around the school building/property (functional mobility, managing backpack, locker use, temporal considerations)
- Ability to communicate and relate successfully with school personnel and peers

It is also important to realize that, although a child may struggle academically in areas such as spelling, math, general knowledge, etc. due to a learning disability or cognitive impairment, occupational therapy may not be indicated in every case. Occupational therapy supports academic goals by addressing related underlying skills needed in the educational setting. The team determines what services are appropriate to best meet the challenges and needs of a particular child and occupational therapy may or may not be part of the plan.

Goal statements in the IEP are normally called *annual goals*, which are written for the duration of the school year, rather than using a timeline for each goal. **Benchmarks** or **objectives** are established to determine or grade the child's progress toward meeting his or her goals. A student's progress might be assessed quarterly along with the academic report cards or per other established intervals. In a school setting, it is important to set goals for specific educational components rather than underlying factors. Goals should be clear, objective, specific, measurable, and realistically attainable. Criteria for IEP goals could include district, state, or grade level standards, observable behaviors and skills, developmental milestones and so forth. School districts may vary in how the frequency and duration of occupational therapy sessions are delineated in the IEP. The IEP might specify a particular number of sessions

---

Box 17-1
IDEA GENERAL REQUIRED CONTENTS OF AN IEP

- A statement of the child's present levels of academic achievement and functional performance, including how the child's disability affects his or her involvement and progress in the general education curriculum;

- A statement of measurable annual goals, including academic and functional goals;

- A description of how the child's progress toward meeting the annual goals will be measured, and when periodic progress reports will be provided;

- A statement of the special education and related services and supplementary aids and services to be provided to the child, or on behalf of the child;

- A statement of the program modifications or supports for school personnel that will be provided to enable the child to advance appropriately toward attaining the annual goals; to be involved in and make progress in the general education curriculum and to participate in extracurricular and other nonacademic activities; and to be educated and participate with other children with disabilities and nondisabled children;

- An explanation of the extent, if any, to which the child will not participate with nondisabled children in the regular class and in extracurricular and nonacademic activities;

- A statement of any individual accommodations that are necessary to measure the academic achievement and functional performance of the child on State and districtwide assessments;

- Note: If the IEP team determines that the child must take an alternate assessment instead of a particular regular State or districtwide assessment of student achievement, the IEP must include a statement of why the child cannot participate in the regular assessment and why the particular alternate assessment selected is appropriate for the child; and

- The projected date for the beginning of the services and modifications, and the anticipated frequency, location, and duration of those services and modifications.

EXTRA IEP CONTENT FOR YOUTH WITH DISABILITIES

For students approaching the end of their secondary school education, the IEP must also include statements about what are called transition services, which are designed to help youth with disabilities prepare for life after high school.

IDEA requires that, beginning not later than the first IEP to be in effect when the child turns 16 years old, or younger if determined appropriate by the IEP team, the IEP must include:

- Measurable postsecondary goals based upon age-appropriate transition assessments related to training, education, employment, and, where appropriate, independent living skills; and

- The transition services (including courses of study) needed to assist the child in reaching those goals.

Also, beginning no later than one year before the child reaches the age of majority under State law, the IEP must include:

- A statement that the child has been informed of the child's rights under Part B of IDEA (if any) that will transfer to the child on reaching the age of majority.

Reproduced from Center for Parent Information and Resources. (2017a). Contents of the IEP. Retrieved October 4, 2021 from https://www.parent-centerhub.org/iepcontents/

---

weekly or monthly (e.g., two times a week for 30 minutes each, one session monthly for 45 minutes) or, instead, might specify only the total number of minutes that will be provided cumulatively by the end of the school year. Delineating a totality of minutes in the IEP allows for flexibility week to week according to the child's needs and the occupational therapy practitioner's discretion. How occupational therapy services will be provided is also outlined in the IEP, such as a direct service model (direct service to student in the classroom or pullout sessions), consultative model (providing recommendations to the teacher), or a combination of both (Steva, 2017). If Medicaid is the payer, it usually only pays for direct services provided to student present, not IEP meetings or consultation (Frolek Clark & Holahan, 2015). IEPs can be quite lengthy. The one provided in this chapter (Figure 17-1) has been condensed to show aspects that are representative or most pertinent to occupational therapy.

Individualized Education Program

Name: Truman T.   **Age:** 5 yr., 11 mo   **Grade Level:** Kindergarten

Present Level of Academic Achievement and Functional Performance: Truman will be 6 years old in just a few days. He was diagnosed with pervasive developmental disorder (PDD) at age 2 years. He attended the Early Childhood Special Education program for 2 years and is currently enrolled in a full-day kindergarten. The decision has been made by the IEP team to retain Truman in kindergarten for the upcoming school year. Truman's parents are in agreement with this decision and hope that another year in kindergarten will allow him to improve his academic performance and social skills prior to advancing to first grade. Truman does not qualify for Extended School Year services at this time.

Truman spends the majority of his day in the general education classroom with a paraprofessional present for support with classroom participation. He spends 60 minutes daily in the special education classroom for additional 1:1 and small group instruction in reading and writing skills. He also participates in adaptive physical education twice weekly for 45 minutes.

Truman's verbal skills are delayed in comparison to same-age peers, although he has demonstrated considerable improvement over the past year. He is now able to communicate in three- to five-word sentences consistently. He also uses a Picture Exchange Communication System (PECS) to supplement his verbal communication.

Truman is easily distracted by auditory and visual stimuli in and near the classroom and has difficulty remaining in his seat for more than 5 minutes at a time. He has difficulty with transitions between activities and locations, but this has improved following implementation of a visual schedule. Truman sometimes responds with negative behaviors (yelling, hitting, pinching) when classmates inadvertently touch or bump into him during classroom activities.

Truman is hesitant to engage in play activities with his peers. He prefers to play alone and does not initiate interactions with peers. Toward the end of last school year, he was beginning to participate in some simple ball activities with others during recess with significant support from his paraprofessional. He will continue participation in a weekly after-school peer communication group led by the elementary school counselor.

Truman is able to recognize all letters of the alphabet, but he does not yet read any words. He can copy the letters of his name when provided with a visual model, but legibility is inconsistent. His ability to copy other letters of the alphabet remains very inconsistent. Truman has difficulty achieving a tripod grasp on writing utensils and staying on the lines of standard writing paper. He also has difficulty with consistent letter size and spacing. His writing performance improves with the use of adaptive writing paper and rubber pencil grip. He does consistently copy basic shapes including circle, square, triangle, and cross.

Truman requires assistance to obtain and carry his tray in the lunchroom. He is easily upset by the noise in the lunchroom and often needs to be taken to a quieter room to finish lunch. Truman consistently indicates when he needs to use the restroom, but continues to have difficulty managing the button and zipper on his jeans. He needs hand-over-hand assistance to complete hand washing because he prefers to play in the water. Truman is now able to take his coat on and off independently. He can also manage Velcro tennis shoes independently.

Figure 17-1. Individualized education program. *(continued)*

Early Intervention

In early childhood settings, OTs and OTAs work toward helping children acquire those age-appropriate developmental skills needed to engage in childhood occupations (AOTA, 2017a). The five areas of child development addressed specifically in IDEA include physical, cognitive, communication, adaptive (i.e., daily living skills), and social/emotional (Center for Parent Information and Resources, 2017b; U.S. Department of Education, n.d.a). Children less than 3 years of age who are experiencing a developmental delay (or are at risk for developmental delay due to a diagnosed condition) in one or more of these areas are eligible for **Early Intervention** services under Part C of IDEA (U.S. Department of Education, n.d.a). States have discretion to expand the definition of "at risk" factors to include environmental or biological factors (U.S. Department of Education, n.d.a). Funding for early intervention programs is through private insurance or public programs such as Medicaid. The law mandates that early intervention services must be provided in the child's "natural environment," which can include the home or a community setting with nondisabled children such as a daycare center or preschool (Center for Parent Information and Resources, 2017b).

Type of Service	Anticipated Frequency	Amount of Time	Location of Service
Special Education: Special education teacher will provide intensive reading and writing instruction in both 1:1 and small group formats.	Daily	60 minutes	Special Education Classroom
Supplementary Aids & Services: Truman will have a paraprofessional present throughout the school day except when with the special education teacher.	Daily	340 minutes	General Education Classroom & Across Settings
Program Modifications: Adaptive P.E.	Weekly	90 minutes	Indoor/Outdoor P.E. Settings
Accommodations for Assessments: Truman will be allowed additional time for completion of classroom and state assessments.	Weekly	60 minutes	General and Special Education Classrooms
Related Services: Occupational Therapy	Weekly	30 minutes	General and Special Education Classrooms & Across Settings
Related Services: Speech Language Pathology	Weekly	90 minutes	General and Special Education Classrooms & Across Settings

Annual Goal #1: Using compensatory strategies, Truman will demonstrate legible handwriting in the classroom with appropriate baseline orientation, letter size, and spacing with 80% accuracy.

Evaluation Methods:
☐ Curriculum-Based Assessment
☐ State Assessments
☑ Data Collection Chart
☑ Work Samples
☐ Other:

Primary Implementers:
☑ General Education Teacher
☑ Special Education Teacher
☐ Physical Therapy
☑ Occupational Therapy
☐ Speech Language Pathology
☐ Other:

Measurable Benchmarks/Objectives:

1. Truman will demonstrate tripod grasp on writing utensils using adaptive pencil grip with 80% accuracy.
2. Truman will write his first name on adaptive paper without a visual model, demonstrating appropriate letter formation, size, and line orientation on 4 of 5 consecutive days.
3. Truman will copy 22/26 lowercase letters onto adaptive paper using a visual model, demonstrating appropriate letter formation, size, and line orientation on 4 of 5 consecutive days.

Date of Mastery:
1.
2.
3.

Figure 17-1 (continued). Individualized education program. *(continued)*

Annual Goal #2: Truman will demonstrate improved attention and work behaviors during classroom activities with no more than three sensory breaks per hour throughout the day on 4 of 5 consecutive days.

Evaluation Methods:	Primary Implementers:
☐ Curriculum-Based Assessment	☑ General Education Teacher
☐ State Assessments	☑ Special Education Teacher
☑ Data Collection Chart	☐ Physical Therapy
☐ Work Samples	☑ Occupational Therapy
☐ Other:	☐ Speech Language Pathology
	☐ Other:

Measurable Benchmarks/Objectives:	Date of Mastery:
1. Truman will remain seated at his desk or during circle time for 15 minutes with minimal verbal cues and no more than one sensory break.	1.
2. Truman will transition between classroom activities with minimal verbal cues using a visual schedule and without demonstrating negative behaviors (yelling, hitting, etc.) toward peers and staff on 4 of 5 consecutive days.	2.
3. Truman will tolerate unexpected touch from classmates without demonstrating negative behaviors (yelling, hitting, etc.) on 4 of 5 consecutive days.	3.

Annual Goal #3: Truman will demonstrate school-related self-care skills using adaptive strategies with no more than minimal assistance on 4 of 5 consecutive days.

Evaluation Methods:	Primary Implementers:
☐ Curriculum-Based Assessment	☐ General Education Teacher
☐ State Assessments	☐ Special Education Teacher
☑ Data Collection Chart	☐ Physical Therapy
☐ Work Samples	☑ Occupational Therapy
☐ Other:	☐ Speech Language Pathology
	☑ Other: Paraprofessional

Measurable Benchmarks/Objectives:	Date of Mastery:
1. Truman will complete toileting without assistance to manage clothing fasteners on 4 of 5 consecutive days.	1.
2. Truman will wash hands following a visual schedule with minimal verbal cues on 4 of 5 consecutive days.	2.
3. Truman will obtain/transport his lunch tray and remain seated in the cafeteria for the duration of the lunch period with minimal verbal cues on 4 of 5 consecutive days.	3.

Figure 17-1 (continued). Individualized education program. (Reproduced with permission from Gateley, C. A., & Borcherding, S. (2017). *Documentation manual for occupational therapy: Writing SOAP notes* [4th ed.]. SLACK Incorporated.)

In early intervention, a team of appropriate health disciplines (e.g., therapist, social worker, psychologist, nurse) evaluate the child and family and then meet with the parent(s)/guardian(s) to compile an **Individualized Family Service Plan (IFSP;** Box 17-2). The child's caregivers can also request that additional family members or an advocate be present at this meeting. The IFSP is a multidisciplinary plan that is family-centered and must be completed within 45 days of referral (Center for Parent Information and Resources, 2021). The plan must contain specific information about the child's developmental status, family situation, and assessment results. It also delineates the type, duration, and dates of services that will be provided to the child and family and the transition from Part C services (Center for Parent Information and Resources, 2021). The parents must give written consent for each service that will be provided, and the plan is reviewed every six months and updated at least yearly (Center for Parent Information and Resources, 2021). In addition, the IFSP specifies the individual who will be the service coordinator for that child's care, which can be an OT (AOTA, 2017a). A Model Form for an IFSP was developed by the U.S. Department of Education and can be viewed at www.parentcenterhub.org (Center for Parent Information and Resources, 2014).

Box 17-2
REQUIRED GENERAL CONTENTS OF AN IFSP

- The child's present developmental levels and needs in the areas of communication, cognitive, physical, social/emotional, and adaptive
- Family information which includes the resources, concerns, and priorities of the parents and other family members who are closely involved with the child
- The expected major results or outcomes for the child and family
- The specific services that will be provided to the child
- What is the natural environment (e.g., home, community) in which services will be provided (if the services will not be furnished in the child's natural environment, the IFSP must justify and state the reason why)
- When and where the child will receive services
- The number of sessions or days the child will receive each service and length of each session
- Who is responsible for paying for the services
- Identification of the service coordinator overseeing IFSP implementation
- The steps to be taken supporting the child's transition from early intervention into another program at the appropriate time
- Identification of other services the family might be interested in, such as information about raising a child with a disability or financial information

Adapted from Center for Parent Information and Resources. (2021). Overview of early intervention. Retrieved October 5, 2021 from https://www.parentcenterhub.org/ei-overview/

Occupational therapy practitioners collaborate with early childhood team members to assist and partner with the family in overcoming the identified challenges and support occupational participation. Documentation for early intervention services must follow the requirements of the specific payer to substantiate the need for services and the skilled care provided.

Acute Care

Occupational therapy practitioners working in acute care settings play a vital role, but they also face clinical challenges such as medically fragile clients and short lengths of stay. Inpatient clients with Medicare are reimbursed through Part A benefits based on the mandated Centers for Medicare & Medicaid Services (CMS) prospective payment system. Facilities are paid according to **Medicare Severity Diagnostic Related Groups (MS-DRGs)** which classify diagnoses and types of procedures needed through the reporting of ICD and CPT codes (CMS, 2022b). These groupings delineate the preset rate for totality of care on a discharge basis regardless of number of days but varies according to the specific DRG assigned to that beneficiary (CMS, 2022b).

Discharge planning often begins the day the client is admitted to the hospital and the health care team provides intervention directed toward the client's needs for the expected discharge environment. The therapist must be aware if the Medicare client was actually *admitted* to the hospital rather than just being *held for observation* (which could possibly involve an overnight stay). If therapy is provided during observation status, the rules for Medicare B would then apply as the client is technically still an outpatient.

When an order for occupational therapy is received, the OT begins the evaluation process and establishes the intervention plan. Some facilities utilize clinical pathways for standard diagnoses such as total hip replacement or total knee replacement. Clinical pathways provide a daily blueprint for the designated care that should be provided by each discipline, including occupational therapy. In this case, there are preplanned interventions and goals for each day of the client's hospital stay, although these interventions can be modified according to the individual's needs. Occupational therapy priorities in acute care reflect the client's occupational profile and the current medical concerns and challenges impacting safety, occupational participation, and expected roles/responsibilities upon discharge. As lengths of stay in acute care are usually brief, intervention will often focus on self-care, functional mobility, activity tolerance, safety, improving client factors for occupational performance, and client/family education. OTs and OTAs may also issue orthotic devices, adaptive equipment, and recommend durable medical equipment, occupational adaptations, or other services needed by the client at home.

Due to the client's rapidly changing status in the acute care environment, contact notes are normally written by the OT or OTA after each session to communicate the interventions being implemented, any progress or changes in the client's condition, and current functional abilities/limitations. Formal reevaluation reports are often not necessary due to the short time frames for care. If the client is transferred to another service delivery setting within the organization, a transition plan is developed; otherwise, a discharge or discontinuation note is written when the client is discharged from the facility or occupational therapy is no longer needed.

Inpatient Rehabilitation Facilities

An inpatient rehabilitation hospital (or the inpatient rehabilitation unit of a hospital) must meet certain criteria to be classified as an inpatient rehabilitation facility (IRF) for reimbursement purposes. Payment for Medicare clients is based on the inpatient rehabilitation system prospective payment system (CMS, 2013a). One major aspect that sets IRFs apart from other rehabilitation settings is the high physician supervision level needed for an intensive rehabilitation program (CMS, 2021e). CMS also mandates that at least 60% of inpatients served have one or more of the following medical conditions listed in Box 17-3 (CMS, 2013b).

All IRF patients are prescreened prior to admission then, once admitted, are evaluated by a physician to substantiate that IRF care is reasonable and necessary, in addition to directing the care provided (CMS, 2021c).

Box 17-3
MEDICAL CONDITIONS THAT MUST COMPRISE AT LEAST 60% IRF PATIENTS SERVED

• Stroke	• Burns
• Brain injury	• Active, polyarticular rheumatoid arthritis, psoriatic arthritis, seronegative arthropathies (under certain conditions)
• Amputation	
• Major multiple trauma	
• Fracture of femur (hip fracture)	• Systemic vasculidites with joint inflammation (under certain conditions)
• Spinal cord injury	
• Congenital deformity	• Severe or advanced osteoarthritis (under certain conditions)
• Neurological disorders (e.g., muscular dystrophy, polyneuropathy, multiple sclerosis, Parkinson's and motor neuron diseases)	• Knee or hip joint replacements (either bilateral replacement, obese with Body Mass Index > 50, or age 85 or older)

Adapted from Centers for Medicare & Medicaid Services. (2013b). *Medicare claims processing manual* (Pub. 100-04: Ch. 3, Section 140.1.1). Author. Retrieved from https://www.cms.gov/Regulations-and-Guidance/Guidance/Manuals/Downloads/clm104c03.pdf

---

Inpatient Rehabilitation Facility-Patient Assessment Instrument

CMS mandates that an **Inpatient Rehabilitation Facility-Patient Assessment Instrument (IRF-PAI)** be completed following admission and again upon discharge to classify a client's level of care needed, progress, and appropriateness of services (CMS, 2021a, 2021b). The current version being used is IRF-PAI Version 4.0 (effective as of October 1, 2020) and can be viewed on the CMS website (CMS, 2021a). The IRF-PAI is used for functional reporting of individual clients, usually submitted though the EHR system in place, and incorporates impairment codes that are the property of U B Foundation Activities, Inc. ©1993, 2001 (CMS, 2021a). In measuring level of impairment, the scoring scales indicate if a client is independent, needs set-up or clean-up assistance, or specific levels of assistance from another person to perform various functional tasks. A variety of areas are reported on, such as, cognition, mood, bowel and bladder, mobility, self-care, skin conditions, swallowing/nutrition, and others (CMS, 2021a).

Intervention and Team Meetings

IRF documentation in the medical record must clearly support CMS criteria, including *"a reasonable expectation that at the time of admission to the IRF the patient's condition is such that the patient can reasonably be expected to actively participate in, and significantly benefit from, the intensive rehabilitation therapy program"* (CMS, 2009b). The care plan must include "active and ongoing" multiple therapy disciplines, one of which must be occupational or physical therapy (CMS, 2009a). Intensive rehabilitation therapy is defined as a total of at least 3 hours of therapy daily for 5 days a week or, in some instance, 15 hours of therapy within 7 consecutive days (CMS, 2021d). If occupational therapy is one of the disciplines ordered by the physician, the OT will perform an evaluation, with contributions from the OTA as appropriate. Documentation must reflect the client's progress, functional improvement, and reflect intervention that focuses on enabling the client to return to a home or community-based environment safely upon discharge (CMS, 2014a). Documentation must also convey an interdisciplinary team approach with team conferences held at least once a week. Documentation of the team conference must delineate participation of each involved discipline and include decisions made, such as changes to the client's intervention, goals, and discharge planning (CMS, 2021f). If occupational therapy is involved in a client's care, an OT must attend these meetings and although OTAs can also participate in the meeting, they cannot take the place of an OT (CMS, 2021f). When occupational therapy is discontinued or the client is discharged from the facility, a discharge report is written.

Skilled Nursing Facilities

Resident Assessment Instrument

When any client is admitted to a Medicare- or Medicaid-certified skilled nursing facility (SNF), the federally mandated **Resident Assessment Instrument (RAI)** must be completed at specified intervals, usually integrated with the EHR system in place, and remains part of the client's health record (CMS, 2019a, 2021g). The RAI is a holistic, interdisciplinary approach to care that allows staff to initially determine and track each resident's strengths, challenges, and level/types of care needed. The aim of the RAI is to improve overall care, enhance quality of life for residents, and serve as a tool to provide consumers with quality-of-care comparisons regarding Medicare- and Medicaid-certified nursing homes in the United States (CMS, 2019a). It also is used to classify Medicare residents into Patient-Driven Payment-Model (PDPM) groupings (2019a).

The RAI consists of an interdisciplinary assessment tool used called the **Minimum Data Set (MDS)**. This can be viewed along with instructions at the CMS website (www.CMS.gov). The MDS is a quality measure that considers all aspects of the client, such as mood, cognition, mobility, ADL abilities, bowel and bladder function, nutrition, pain, skin condition, etc. Each item on the MDS is defined in specific terms and has a separate scoring system with detailed instructions. Various disciplines can contribute to the MDS to improve efficiency and team communication, and to facilitate a more holistic approach to care of the resident (CMS, 2019a). Facilities may vary in how ADL, cognitive, or other sections are divided between occupational therapy, nursing, or other disciplines. Each item pertaining to functional abilities is assessed separately to specify whether the resident is independent, requires supervision or cues from another person and level of physical assist needed (indicating one or two people; CMS, 2019a). Figure 17-2 shows a portion of the MDS relating to ADLs.

After completion, the MDS is interpreted through the *Care Area Assessment Process* to identify a client's problem areas (called *care area triggers*) for which the treatment team can determine need for further assessment of problem area and develop an individualized plan of care for desired outcomes (CMS, 2019a).

CMS requires that for residents to be covered for a Medicare Part A stay in a skilled nursing facility, the client must meet certain criteria including: a 3-day qualifying hospital stay prior to the SNF admission; be under the care of a physician; and require skilled nursing and/or rehabilitation services 7 days a week (minimum 5 days of therapy weekly if classified as a *rehabilitation stay*; CMS, 2018a, 2019b). All SNF Part A inpatient services are reimbursed according to the prospective payment system rates (CMS, 2018b). Medicare beneficiaries not meeting the criteria for a Part A stay may qualify for Part B benefits for skilled care furnished.

Resident _____   Identifier _____   Date _____

Section GG	Functional Abilities and Goals - Admission (Start of SNF PPS Stay)

GG0130. Self-Care (Assessment period is days 1 through 3 of the SNF PPS Stay starting with A2400B)
Complete only if A0310B = 01

Code the resident's usual performance at the start of the SNF PPS stay (admission) for each activity using the 6-point scale. If activity was not attempted at the start of the SNF PPS stay (admission), code the reason. Code the resident's end of SNF PPS stay (discharge) goal(s) using the 6-point scale. Use of codes 07, 09, 10, or 88 is permissible to code end of SNF PPS stay (discharge) goal(s).

Coding:

Safety and **Quality of Performance** - If helper assistance is required because resident's performance is unsafe or of poor quality, score according to amount of assistance provided.

Activities may be completed with or without assistive devices.

06. **Independent** - Resident completes the activity by him/herself with no assistance from a helper.

05. **Setup or clean-up assistance** - Helper sets up or cleans up; resident completes activity. Helper assists only prior to or following the activity.

04. **Supervision or touching assistance** - Helper provides verbal cues and/or touching/steadying and/or contact guard assistance as resident completes activity. Assistance may be provided throughout the activity or intermittently.

03. **Partial/moderate assistance** - Helper does LESS THAN HALF the effort. Helper lifts, holds, or supports trunk or limbs, but provides less than half the effort.

02. **Substantial/maximal assistance** - Helper does MORE THAN HALF the effort. Helper lifts or holds trunk or limbs and provides more than half the effort.

01. **Dependent** - Helper does ALL of the effort. Resident does none of the effort to complete the activity. Or, the assistance of 2 or more helpers is required for the resident to complete the activity.

If activity was not attempted, code reason:

07. **Resident refused**

09. **Not applicable** - Not attempted and the resident did not perform this activity prior to the current illness, exacerbation, or injury.

10. **Not attempted due to environmental limitations** (e.g., lack of equipment, weather constraints)

88. **Not attempted due to medical condition or safety concerns**

1. Admission Performance	2. Discharge Goal	
↓ Enter Codes in Boxes ↓		
☐☐	☐☐	**A. Eating:** The ability to use suitable utensils to bring food and/or liquid to the mouth and swallow food and/or liquid once the meal is placed before the resident.
☐☐	☐☐	**B. Oral hygiene:** The ability to use suitable items to clean teeth. Dentures (if applicable): The ability to insert and remove dentures into and from the mouth, and manage denture soaking and rinsing with use of equipment.
☐☐	☐☐	**C. Toileting hygiene:** The ability to maintain perineal hygiene, adjust clothes before and after voiding or having a bowel movement. If managing an ostomy, include wiping the opening but not managing equipment.
☐☐	☐☐	**E. Shower/bathe self:** The ability to bathe self, including washing, rinsing, and drying self (excludes washing of back and hair). Does not include transferring in/out of tub/shower.
☐☐	☐☐	**F. Upper body dressing:** The ability to dress and undress above the waist; including fasteners, if applicable.
☐☐	☐☐	**G. Lower body dressing:** The ability to dress and undress below the waist, including fasteners; does not include footwear.
☐☐	☐☐	**H. Putting on/taking off footwear:** The ability to put on and take off socks and shoes or other footwear that is appropriate for safe mobility; including fasteners, if applicable.

Figure 17-2. Component of MDS admission form for functional abilities and goals. (Reproduced from Centers for Medicare & Medicaid Services. (2019a). *Long-term care facility resident assessment instrument: Version 1.17.1* [Minimum Data Set (MDS)-Version 3.0 Resident Assessment and Care Screening: Nursing Home Comprehensive (NC) Item Set (p. 18 of 51). Retrieved October 21, 2021 from https://downloads.cms.gov/files/mds-3.0-rai-manual-v1.17.1_october_2019.pdf)

Patient Driven Payment Model

Under the prospective payment system, Medicare and Medicaid beneficiaries in SNFs were traditionally divided into **Resource Utilization Groupings (RUGs)**, most currently RUG-IV, according to the type and amount of reasonable and necessary skilled care an individual required (CMS, 2019a). **The Patient Driven Payment Model (PDPM)** replaced the RUG system for Medicare patients in SNFs as of October 1, 2019, but State Medicaid agencies have the option of using either PDPM or one of several versions of RUG classification systems (CMS, 2019a, 2019i). Payment under PDPM is based on a combination of six components. Five of these components involve a case-mix of OT, PT, speech-language pathology, nursing, non-therapy ancillary, plus the sixth non-case-mix component for other SNF resources utilized but unrelated to client characteristics (CMS, 2019k). OT and PT involve components that specify the clinical reason (primary diagnosis, including surgical intervention) for the SNF admission and resident's functional status so that the individual can be assigned to one of the delineated clinical groupings (CMS, 2019k). PT and OT clinical categories include: major joint replacement or spinal surgery; non-orthopedic surgery and acute neurologic; other orthopedic; medical management; plus therapists must also calculate a functional score for the client based on specific criteria (CMS, 2019k). Per-diem payment that the facility will receive is based on the PDPM categorized level of skilled care that is reasonable and medically necessary for the client according to the types of disciplines involved and amount of services needed (CMS, 2021h).

Minutes of Therapy for MDS

In order to substantiate a client's particular level of care, each rehabilitation professional involved in the client's care must keep track of (and document for the MDS) the exact, total number of therapy minutes provided weekly for each client with Medicare Part A or B, as explained in Box 17-4. For purposes of the MDS, a "day of therapy" for a discipline is counted if skilled intervention is furnished to the client for 15 minutes or more (CMS, 2019a). Each discipline tracks minutes separately for services furnished. A limit of 25% for group and concurrent therapy services for a client has been imposed by CMS (CMS, 2019j). As CMS directives often change, readers should consider this information only as general guidelines that could differ from the actual, current regulations that must be adhered to.

Box 17-4		
COUNTING MINUTES OF THERAPY FOR MINIMUM DATA SETS		
How to Count Weekly Minutes of Therapy for the MDS ***Provide Actual Number* *—Do Not Round Minutes*	*Resident With Medicare Part A*	*Resident With Medicare Part B* ****(Minutes for Billing Claims May Differ From These Minutes)*
Individual minutes	Count total minutes provided on an individual basis	Count total minutes provided on an individual basis (can be intermittent)
Concurrent minutes (treating two residents simultaneously)	Count minutes when the Part A resident and one other resident (with any payment source) received intervention at the same time while performing different types of activities. OT or OTA must be in line-of-sight.	Cannot be treated concurrently. Part B minutes are instead counted as group therapy whether similar or different activities performed.
Group minutes	Count minutes provided in a group of two to six residents performing same or similar activities supervised by OT or OTA. (The other individuals in group can have any payment source.) The practitioner cannot be supervising other individuals.	Count minutes provided for two or more residents at the same time whether performing same or similar activity or not (the second or additional residents can have any payment source). *(continued)*

Box 17-4 (continued)
COUNTING MINUTES OF THERAPY FOR MINIMUM DATA SETS

How to Count Weekly Minutes of Therapy for the MDS ***Provide Actual Number —Do Not Round Minutes	Resident With Medicare Part A	Resident With Medicare Part B ***(Minutes for Billing Claims May Differ From These Minutes)
Co-treatment minutes	Both disciplines practitioners count total number of minutes in full administered in co-treatment to the resident	Count total number of minutes administered in co-treatments to the resident for MDS but cannot each bill for same total service (either split time units with other discipline for billing claims or one discipline can bill all).
Set-up time	Count minutes for time to prepare areas or set up/adjust equipment preceding skilled therapy (set-up can be performed by OT, OTA, or even an aide). Add to the initial skilled treatment mode implemented by OT or OTA.	Count for MDS, not billing claims
Initial evaluation	Do not count toward MDS minutes.	Do not count toward MDS minutes but bill as 1 unit.
Therapy students	Document all time student spends with client(s). Must adhere to state and professional practice guidelines. For *individual* therapy, line-of-sight supervision not required but therapist must provide "skilled services and direction" to the student participating in therapy provision. Minutes are coded as individual therapy when only one resident is being treated by the therapy student and the supervising therapist/assistant is not supervising or treating other individuals and can immediately intervene/assist the student as needed. For *concurrent* therapy, student must be in line-of sight of the supervising therapist/assistant (who is not supervising others or treating individuals except those concurrently).	Qualified professional must be present in the room entire session. The qualified practitioner directs and is responsible for care, makes skilled judgment, and is not treating other clients or doing other tasks at the same time. Qualified professional must sign all documentation, but student may also sign.
Modalities	Count skilled time. Some modalities are not skilled or have both skilled and unskilled components of time.	Count skilled time for MDS. Some modalities are not skilled or have both skilled and unskilled time. Bill according to Part B/ Medicare Physician Fee Schedule guidelines
Family education	Minutes count if client present (must be documented in the record)	Minutes count if client present (must document in the record)
Non-therapeutic rest periods	Do not count	Do not count
Provision of unskilled or unnecessary services	Do not count	Do not count

Adapted from Centers for Medicare & Medicaid Services. (2019a). *Long-term care facility resident assessment instrument 3.0 user's manual: Version 1.17.1* (Chapter 3, MDS Items [O] Section O0400: Therapies). Retrieved October 21, 2021 from https://downloads.cms.gov/files/mds-3.0-rai-manual-v1.17.1_october_2019.pdf

CMS's RAI Version 3.0 Manual   **CH 3: MDS Items [O]**

O0400: Therapies (cont.)

O0400. Therapies

A. Speech-Language Pathology and Audiology Services

Enter Number of Minutes: `1 9 0`
1. **Individual minutes** - record the total number of minutes this therapy was administered to the resident **individually** in the last 7 days

Enter Number of Minutes: `7 0`
2. **Concurrent minutes** - record the total number of minutes this therapy was administered to the resident **concurrently with one other resident** in the last 7 days

Enter Number of Minutes: `7 5`
3. **Group minutes** - record the total number of minutes this therapy was administered to the resident as **part of a group of residents** in the last 7 days

If the sum of individual, concurrent, and group minutes is zero, → skip to O0400A5, Therapy start date

Enter Number of Minutes: `0`
3A. **Co-treatment minutes** - record the total number of minutes this therapy was administered to the resident in **co-treatment sessions** in the last 7 days

Enter Number of Days: `5`
4. **Days** - record the **number of days** this therapy was administered for **at least 15 minutes** a day in the last 7 days

5. **Therapy start date** - record the date the most recent therapy regimen (since the most recent entry) started

6. **Therapy end date** - record the date the most recent therapy regimen (since the most recent entry) ended - enter dashes if therapy is ongoing

`1 0 – 0 6 – 2 0 1 9`   Month Day Year   `- - – - - – - - - -`   Month Day Year

B. Occupational Therapy

Enter Number of Minutes: `1 1 3`
1. **Individual minutes** - record the total number of minutes this therapy was administered to the resident **individually** in the last 7 days

Enter Number of Minutes: `0`
2. **Concurrent minutes** - record the total number of minutes this therapy was administered to the resident **concurrently with one other resident** in the last 7 days

Enter Number of Minutes: `8 0`
3. **Group minutes** - record the total number of minutes this therapy was administered to the resident as **part of a group of residents** in the last 7 days

If the sum of individual, concurrent, and group minutes is zero, → skip to O0400B5, Therapy start date

Enter Number of Minutes: `6 0`
3A. **Co-treatment minutes** - record the total number of minutes this therapy was administered to the resident in **co-treatment sessions** in the last 7 days

Enter Number of Days: `5`
4. **Days** - record the **number of days** this therapy was administered for **at least 15 minutes** a day in the last 7 days

5. **Therapy start date** - record the date the most recent therapy regimen (since the most recent entry) started

6. **Therapy end date** - record the date the most recent therapy regimen (since the most recent entry) ended - enter dashes if therapy is ongoing

`1 0 – 0 9 – 2 0 1 9`   Month Day Year   `- - – - - – - - - -`   Month Day Year

O0400 continued on next page

Figure 17-3. Example of MDS form for documenting occupational therapy weekly minutes. (Reproduced from Centers for Medicare & Medicaid Services. (2019a). *Long-term care facility resident assessment instrument 3.0 user's manual: Version 1.17.1* (Chapter 3, MDS Items [O] Section O0400: Therapies, p. O-31). Retrieved October 21, 2021 from https://downloads.cms.gov/files/mds-3.0-rai-manual-v1.17.1_october_2019.pdf)

Realize that, due to how therapy minutes are calculated for the MDS, these numbers could differ from the number of allowable minutes that can be billed for Medicare Part B claims (CMS, 2019a). If the specified amount of therapy is not being implemented or is not documented properly on the MDS form, the client will be unable to get the level of care needed. Also, inaccurate assessments or unrealistic predictions about rehabilitation potential may result in reimbursement problems for care rendered. It is important to understand that rehabilitation professionals should never compromise ethics even if administrators are applying pressure to keep clients on program longer than necessary or to provide extra sessions of therapy that are not reasonable/necessary just so clients can remain in a higher payment category (AOTA, 2014, 2020a). CMS provides an example explaining how to document occupational therapy MDS weekly minutes which is shown in Figure 17-3 and Box 17-5.

Box 17-5
CMS Coding Example for Documenting Occupational Therapy Minutes on MDS Form

Occupational therapy services that were provided over the 7-day look-back period:

- Individual sitting balance activities; Monday and Wednesday for 30-minute co-treatment sessions with PT each day (OT and PT each code the session as 30 minutes for each discipline).
- Individual wheelchair seating and positioning; Monday, Wednesday, and Friday for the following times: 23 minutes, 18 minutes, and 12 minutes.
- Balance/coordination activities; Tuesday-Friday for 20 minutes each day in group sessions.

Coding:

- O0400B1 would be coded 113,
- O0400B2 would be coded 0,
- O0400B3 would be coded 80,
- O0400B3A would be coded 60,
- O0400B4 would be coded 5,
- O0400B5 would be coded 10092019, and
- O0400B6 would be coded with dashes.

Rationale:

- Individual minutes (including 60 co-treatment minutes) totaled 113 over the 7-day lookback period $[(30 \times 2) + 23 + 18 + 12 = 113]$; concurrent minutes totaled 0 over the 7-day look-back period $(0 \times 0 = 0)$; and group minutes totaled 80 over the 7-day look-back period $(20 \times 4 = 80)$.
- Therapy was provided 5 out of the 7 days of the look-back period.
- Date occupational therapy services began was 10-09-2019 and dashes were used as the therapy end date value because the therapy was ongoing.

Reproduced from Centers for Medicare & Medicaid Services. (2019a). *Long-term care facility resident assessment instrument 3.0 user's manual: Version 1.17.1* (Chapter 3, MDS Items [O] Section O0400: Therapies, pp. O-28 to O-29). Retrieved October 8, 2021 from https://downloads.cms.gov/files/mds-3.0-rai-manual-v1.17.1_october_2019.pdf

---

The MDS does not take the place of a "regular" occupational therapy evaluation. Occupational therapy documentation must justify that furnished services are skilled, reasonable, and necessary. This includes the CMS criteria for restorative care or skilled maintenance therapy that *requires* a qualified therapist for safe and effective care as described in Chapter 3. CMS clearly delineates the types of services that should *not* be considered as skilled therapy for the MDS or billing claims. These include moist heat only for comfort care, general supervision of routine exercises already taught, helping a client with self-care (e.g., rather than teaching or restoring skills), routine range of motion, or general care/use of an orthotic device that nursing staff can do and so forth (CMS, 2003). Documentation must substantiate medically necessary skilled services and include measurable, objective progress that the client is making (or justify client's need for a *skilled* maintenance program). OTs and OTAs must also keep track of day-to-day interventions implemented, the number of minutes and modes of therapy for each day. Documentation must clearly support the plan of care and meet MDS reporting requirements. Progress reports are written at specified intervals to note changes in the client's status and justify continued skilled care as appropriate. A discharge note is written when occupational therapy services are no longer necessary, or the client is discharged from the facility.

Outpatient Documentation

Private Insurance and Managed Care (Non-Medicare)

Documentation in outpatient settings depends on the requirements of the specific facility, accrediting agency, and payment source, such as if services are covered under early intervention, partial hospitalization programs, private insurance, Worker's Compensation, or Medicare Part B. Clients referred to outpatient occupational therapy will normally go through the evaluation process as described in Chapter 14. Documentation will be tailored to the particular practice area or specialization (such as adult physical rehabilitation, work hardening, cardiac rehabilitation, hand therapy, low vision, pediatrics, etc.) and the specifications of the EHR system in place. If managed care is involved, additional documentation or reports might be required to justify episodes of care. For example, a managed care company might only initially approve a set number of visits within a particular time frame (such as eight sessions within 30 days), depending on the plan's terms. If additional therapy is warranted after those approved visits are completed, the therapist might be required to contact the case manager and/or send additional reports, in accordance with HIPAA and facility guidelines.

Outpatient documentation usually includes progress notes at regular intervals, although attendance logs, checklists, or formal contact notes (e.g., SOAP notes) might also be required for each visit, depending on the setting and payer requirements. An OTA involved with the client's care will document skilled intervention and pertinent communication with the client/family/significant others, all under the OT's supervision. Any gains in specific functional abilities should be noted, as well as the limiting factors requiring continued occupational therapy. The supervising OT must co-sign an OTA's notes when required by the facility, state/federal or payer requirements (AOTA, 2018). Formal progress reports and reevaluation reports are written by the OT (with contributions from the OTA) according to facility guidelines and funding source requirements. An occupational therapy discharge or discontinuation note is also the responsibility of the OT when the client leaves the facility or therapy is no longer necessary.

Medicare B Documentation

Chapter 2 presents information regarding CMS quality initiatives and Chapter 3 explains the Medicare Part B criteria for reasonable and necessary client care, skilled occupational therapy services, and fundamentals of billing/coding. The current Medicare Part B requirements for occupational therapy documentation, including specific content of an occupational therapy evaluation, are delineated in Chapter 15 of the *Medicare Benefit Policy Manual*, which can be found at the CMS website (www.cms.gov). Using clinical knowledge and professional reasoning, the OT gathers pertinent client information and selects appropriate, objective measures to evaluate the client. The OT interprets the client data and establishes an intervention plan, which Medicare refers to as a *plan of care* (POC). The POC, at minimum, must include the client's diagnoses; the frequency, duration, type, and amount of occupational therapy services; occupational therapy measurable long-term goals; professional signature with credentials; and date (CMS, 2019e). Medicare also requires that the POC be **certified**, meaning the client must be under the care of a physician (or approved non-physician practitioner [NPP] such as a physician assistant or nurse practitioner) who approves of and signs (certifies) the occupational therapy plan (CMS, 2014b, 2019c). This certification is good for 90 calendar days (from the initial treatment date) or for the duration delineated in the POC, whichever is less. Once the certified POC is in place, any significant changes to that plan will require documented written or verbal approval from the physician/NPP (CMS, 2019c). OT services must be reasonable and necessary for the client's condition and situation and substantiated in the record (CMS, 2019d).

The purpose of **treatment notes**, according to CMS regulations, is to *"create a record of all treatments and skilled interventions that are provided and to record the time of the services in order to justify the use of billing codes on the claim. Documentation is required for every treatment day, and every therapy service"* (CMS, 2019e). Medicare does not specify the exact format of a treatment note but does require, at a minimum, the following content (CMS, 2019e):

- The date of treatment
- Each specific modality/intervention provided and billed for both timed and untimed codes (so that it can be verified with claims)
- Must record each service having timed code regardless of whether it is billable or not
- Total timed code treatment minutes
- Total treatment time in minutes (timed and untimed codes, not unbillable)

- May voluntarily include unbilled services information
- Qualified professional's signature and professional designation (who supervised or implemented the service) and individuals who participated in providing treatment (e.g., OTA)

If the occupational therapy supervisor did not actively communicate or participate in the session, it is not mandatory for the supervisor to cosign the OTA's note for clients with Medicare; although, state regulations, practice acts, or facility policies could require a co-signature (CMS, 2019e). OTs and OTAs use clinical judgment in determining additional kinds of information to include in the contact note, such as client self-report, changes in status, reaction to intervention, communication with other providers, etc., but must include these types of data in **progress reports** (CMS, 2019e). Periodic progress reports are required by Medicare at least every 10 treatment days and must be written by the OT (CMS, 2019e). The OT assesses the client's progress and modifies goals and interventions as needed. Progress reports may be written more frequently as needed to further justify therapy or note changes in the client's status. An OTA is allowed to write these additional progress notes in-between the required intervals so long as the OT participates in the client's care. An OTA documents objective information relating to the client but cannot make changes in the client's goals or intervention plan without the documented direction of the OT (CMS, 2019e). Formal reevaluations are implemented and documented by the OT at intervals determined by the OT's professional judgment or facility policy and a discharge report is completed when therapy is no longer indicated (CMS, 2019e).

Beginning in 2013, CMS required that therapists also report nonpayable, functional limitation G-codes and severity modifiers for each client with Medicare B (CMS, 2019f, 2019g). These G-codes were a means of identifying and classifying the client's functional impairment level for several broad categories (i.e., self-care, mobility) at specified points throughout the therapy process but were discontinued by CMS at the end of 2018 (CMS, 2019g).

Home Health

According to CMS, a client's residence can be a personal dwelling, relative's home, assisted living facility, or another place that the client considers to be their home, excluding institutions such as hospitals and skilled nursing facilities (CMS, 2020d). Clients with Medicare may receive benefits under Part A and/or B. Some benefits depend on whether the client had a qualifying prior 3-day hospital stay. The Medicare requirements for occupational therapy are outlined in Chapter 7 of the *Medicare Benefit Policy Manual*, which can be found on the CMS website (www.cms.gov).

A home health agency (HHA) must be Medicare-certified to provide Medicare Part A and B services. Funding is according to the prospective payment system bundled rates for 30-day payment periods. All services and routine/nonroutine supplies provided must be consolidated and billed through the HHA, except for DME (CMS, 2020a, 2020h). Medicare does not pay for 24-hour care and will not cover any personal care or homemaking services if other skilled care is not needed. To qualify for skilled services, the client must be under a physician's care, require skilled services, and be certified by physician (or allowed practitioner in that state such as PA or NP) that the patient is confined to home (homebound; CMS, 2020b, 2020c). CMS delineates that the following conditions in Box 17-6 must be met for a client to be considered as homebound (2020c):

Box 17-6
CMS HOMEBOUND CRITERIA

1. Criterion one: The patient must either: Because of illness or injury, need the aid of supportive devices such as crutches, canes, wheelchairs, and walkers; the use of special transportation; or the assistance of another person in order to leave their place of residence OR - Have a condition such that leaving his or her home is medically contraindicated. If the patient meets one of the criterion one conditions, then the patient must ALSO meet two additional requirements defined in criterion two below.

2. Criterion two: There must exist a normal inability to leave home; AND - Leaving home must require a considerable and taxing effort.

Reproduced from Centers for Medicare & Medicaid Services. (2020c). Medicare benefit policy manual (Pub. 100-02: Ch. 7, Section 30.1.1). Retrieved October 6, 2021 from https://www.cms.gov/Regulations-and-Guidance/Guidance/Manuals/Downloads/bp102c07.pdf

If your documentation states that your client is going to the neighborhood coffee shop every morning or routinely driving to the mall to shop, then payment for home health benefits will likely be denied as this indicates the client does not really meet the homebound criteria (CMS, 2020c). There are, however, some limited exceptions for leaving the home, such as going to medical appointments, religious services, or going out infrequently for nonmedical purposes (e.g., haircut, funeral, special family event; CMS, 2020c).

The skilled services requirement is delineated by CMS as the client needing either skilled nursing care intermittently *or* PT *or* speech-language pathology (SLP) services (CMS, 2020b). This means that any of those disciplines can be a stand-alone service to qualify for Medicare home health benefits. However, in order for a client to qualify for occupational therapy home health benefits under Medicare, CMS specifies that one of the other skilled services must have been needed in the current or prior certification period (CMS 2020f). Understand that Medicaid regulations differ from Medicare in that occupational therapy does not require another skilled service for eligibility (CMS, 2019h). Services provided must meet the standards for reasonable and medically necessary skilled care (CMS, 2020g). The client's physician or allowed practitioner in that state (e.g., PA, CNS, NP) must establish and approve a specific plan of care for all skilled home health services the client with Medicare will receive (CMS 2020e).

OASIS-D

Federal regulations mandate the gathering of specific outcomes data for non-maternity clients with Medicare or Medicaid who are 18 years of age or older and who receive skilled services at home (CMS, 2019h). The method used to collect the required data is called the **Outcome and Assessment Information Set (OASIS)** and the most current version is the **OASIS-D**, effective January 1, 2019 (CMS, 2019h, 2022c). A draft of OASIS-E has been developed but implementation of this new version has been delayed until January 1, 2023 (CMS, 2022c). All OASIS forms and instructions can be found at the CMS website.

The OASIS considers the holistic needs of the client, such as living situation and supports, falls and hospitalization risk, medication management, skin integrity, mood, self-care and IADL abilities, functional mobility, etc. and it remains part of the client's legal health record (CMS, 2019h). CMS mandates that the OASIS be completed at start of care (within 5 days), shortly before the end of each 60-day recertification period, upon client transfer to an inpatient facility (and resumption of care, if applicable), and within 48 hours following discharge or death at home, with some select assessment items only included at admission or discharge (CMS, 2019h).

If nursing is involved with the case, an RN must complete the OASIS at the start of the client's care, but subsequent assessments may be completed by an RN, OT, PT, or SLP if involved in that client's care (CMS, 2019h). If skilled nursing has not been ordered, a PT or SLP (not OT) can complete the initial OASIS for Medicare clients but any of the involved therapy disciplines can complete it for clients with Medicaid (CMS, 2019h). Completion of the OASIS at transfer or discharge/death is performed by only one clinician but reflects totality of care from all disciplines (CMS, 2019h). Figures 17-4 and 17-5 show a segment of the OASIS pertaining to self-care for different reporting periods.

For clients living at home or other noninstitutional settings (e.g., assisted living or congregate settings), Box 17-7 presents the CMS guidelines for reporting "availability of assistance" on the OASIS, meaning the frequency in which the individual has any other person available to assist in the home, not limited to ADLs/IADLs (CMS, 2019h). The caregiver does not have to live there but is willing and able to provide the assistance, which can include supervision and/or verbal cues (does not include telephone contact), not just physical help (CMS, 2019h).

Realize the OASIS does not take the place of a "regular" occupational therapy evaluation. If occupational therapy is indicated, the therapist assesses the client's situation and supports; functional status, capacities, limitations, safety, and so forth; creates an occupational profile; and establishes an intervention plan (AOTA, 2020b). Intervention in home care generally focuses on supporting safe occupational participation and performance for ADLs/IADLs in the home and community, and interventions to promote health and wellness, such as managing chronic conditions and minimizing risks of hospitalizations, falls, or pressure injuries. Provision of any therapy services must adhere to the CMS guidelines for skilled, reasonable, and necessary care (CMS, 2020g). CMS documentation requirements for Medicare beneficiaries in home health include reassessments completed by the OT (not OTA) at 30-day intervals, which begin the date of that discipline's first session (CMS, 2020g). Contact notes must be written for each visit to reflect the skilled services provided and communicate pertinent information to the health team (CMS, 2020g). CMS reminds practitioners to avoid subjective or vague descriptions and delineates the following elements for inclusion in therapy notes for each visit (CMS, 2020g):

ADL/IADLs, continued

(M1830)	**Bathing:** Current ability to wash entire body safely. **Excludes** grooming (washing face, washing hands, and shampooing hair).	
Enter Code	0	Able to bathe self in <u>shower or tub</u> independently, including getting in and out of tub/shower.
	1	With the use of devices, is able to bathe self in shower or tub independently, including getting in and out of the tub/shower.
	2	Able to bathe in shower or tub with the intermittent assistance of another person:
		(a) for intermittent supervision or encouragement or reminders, <u>OR</u>
		(b) to get in and out of the shower or tub, <u>OR</u>
		(c) for washing difficult to reach areas.
	3	Able to participate in bathing self in shower or tub, <u>but</u> requires presence of another person throughout the bath for assistance or supervision.
	4	Unable to use the shower or tub, but able to bathe self independently with or without the use of devices at the sink, in chair, or on commode.
	5	Unable to use the shower or tub, but able to participate in bathing self in bed, at the sink, in bedside chair, or on commode, with the assistance or supervision of another person.
	6	Unable to participate effectively in bathing and is bathed totally by another person.
(M1840)	**Toilet Transferring:** Current ability to get to and from the toilet or bedside commode safely <u>and</u> transfer on and off toilet/commode.	
Enter Code	0	Able to get to and from the toilet and transfer independently with or without a device.
	1	When reminded, assisted, or supervised by another person, able to get to and from the toilet and transfer.
	2	<u>Unable</u> to get to and from the toilet but is able to use a bedside commode (with or without assistance).
	3	<u>Unable</u> to get to and from the toilet or bedside commode but is able to use a bedpan/urinal independently.
	4	Is totally dependent in toileting.
(M1845)	**Toileting Hygiene:** Current ability to maintain perineal hygiene safely, adjust clothes and/or incontinence pads before and after using toilet, commode, bedpan, urinal. If managing ostomy, includes cleaning area around stoma, but not managing equipment.	
Enter Code	0	Able to manage toileting hygiene and clothing management without assistance.
	1	Able to manage toileting hygiene and clothing management without assistance if supplies/implements are laid out for the patient.
	2	Someone must help the patient to maintain toileting hygiene and/or adjust clothing.
	3	Patient depends entirely upon another person to maintain toileting hygiene.
(M1850)	**Transferring:** Current ability to move safely from bed to chair, or ability to turn and position self in bed if patient is bedfast.	
Enter Code	0	Able to independently transfer.
	1	Able to transfer with minimal human assistance or with use of an assistive device.
	2	Able to bear weight and pivot during the transfer process but unable to transfer self.
	3	Unable to transfer self and is unable to bear weight or pivot when transferred by another person.
	4	Bedfast, unable to transfer but is able to turn and position self in bed.
	5	Bedfast, unable to transfer and is unable to turn and position self.

Figure 17-4. Component of OASIS-D Start of Care Form. (Reproduced from Centers for Medicare & Medicaid Services. (2019i). Outcome and assessment information set OASIS-D guidance manual effective January 1, 2019 (Chapter 2, p.12 of 19). Retrieved October 10, 2021 from https://www.cms.gov/Medicare/Quality-Initiatives-Patient-Assessment-Instruments/HomeHealthQualityInits/Downloads/OASIS-D-Guidance-Manual-final.pdf)

Section GG	Functional Abilities and Goals

Section GG: Self-Care

GG0130. Self-Care

Code the patient's usual performance at Discharge for each activity using the 6-point scale. If activity was not attempted at Discharge, code the reason.

Coding:

Safety and **Quality of Performance** – If helper assistance is required because patient's performance is unsafe or of poor quality, score according to amount of assistance provided.

Activities may be completed with or without assistive devices.

06. **Independent** – Patient completes the activity by him/herself with no assistance from a helper.

05. **Setup or clean-up assistance** – Helper sets up or cleans up; patient completes activity. Helper assists only prior to or following the activity.

04. **Supervision or touching assistance** – Helper provides verbal cues and/or touching/steadying and/or contact guard assistance as patient completes activity. Assistance may be provided throughout the activity or intermittently.

03. **Partial/moderate assistance** – Helper does LESS THAN HALF the effort. Helper lifts, holds or supports trunk or limbs, but provides less than half the effort.

02. **Substantial/maximal assistance** – Helper does MORE THAN HALF the effort. Helper lifts or holds trunk or limbs and provides more than half the effort.

01. **Dependent** – Helper does ALL of the effort. Patient does none of the effort to complete the activity. Or, the assistance of 2 or more helpers is required for the patient to complete the activity.

If activity was not attempted, code reason:

07. **Patient refused**

09. **Not applicable** – Not attempted and the patient did not perform this activity prior to the current illness, exacerbation or injury.

10. **Not attempted due to environmental limitations** (e.g., lack of equipment, weather constraints)

88. **Not attempted due to medical conditions or safety concerns**

3. Discharge Performance ↓ Enter Codes ▼ in Boxes	
☐☐	**A. Eating:** The ability to use suitable utensils to bring food and/or liquid to the mouth and swallow food and/or liquid once the meal placed before the patient.
☐☐	**B. Oral Hygiene:** The ability to use suitable items to clean teeth. Dentures (if applicable): The ability to insert and remove dentures into and from the mouth, and manage denture soaking and rinsing with use of equipment.
☐☐	**C. Toileting Hygiene:** The ability to maintain perineal hygiene, adjust clothes before and after voiding or having a bowel movement. If managing an ostomy, include wiping the opening but not managing equipment.
☐☐	**E. Shower/bathe self:** The ability to bathe self, including washing, rinsing, and drying self (excludes washing of back and hair). Does not include transferring in/out of tub/shower.
☐☐	**F. Upper body dressing:** The ability to dress and undress above the waist; including fasteners, if applicable.
☐☐	**G. Lower body dressing:** The ability to dress and undress below the waist, including fasteners; does not include footwear.
☐☐	**H. Putting on/taking off footwear:** The ability to put on and take off socks and shoes or other footwear that is appropriate for safe mobility; including fasteners, if applicable.

Figure 17-5. Component of OASIS-D Discharge Form. (Reproduced from Centers for Medicare & Medicaid Services. (2019i). Outcome and assessment information set OASIS-D guidance manual effective January 1, 2019. (Chapter 2, p.11 of 13). Retrieved October 10, 2021 from https://www.cms.gov/Medicare/Quality-Initiatives-Patient-Assessment-Instruments/HomeHealthQualityInits/Downloads/OASIS-D-Guidance-Manual-final.pdf)

Box 17-7
CMS Availability of Assistance Definitions

- *Around the clock* means there is someone available in the home to provide assistance to the patient 24 hours a day.
- *Regular daytime* means someone is in the home and available to provide assistance during daytime hours every day with infrequent exceptions.
- *Regular nighttime* means someone is in the home and available to provide assistance during nighttime hours every night with infrequent exceptions.
- *Occasional/short-term assistance* means someone is available to provide in-person assistance only for a few hours a day or on an irregular basis, or may be only able to help occasionally.
- *No assistance* available means there is no one available to provide any in-person assistance.
- Clinical judgment must be used to determine which hours constitute "regular daytime" and "regular nighttime" based on the patient's specific activities and routines. No hours are specifically designated as daytime or nighttime ... If a person is in an assisted living or congregate setting with a call-bell that summons onsite, in-person help, this is considered in-person assistance. If its use is restricted to emergencies only, report the availability as occasional/short-term assistance unless other caregiver's availability meets a higher level.

Reproduced from Centers for Medicare & Medicaid Services. (2019h). Outcome and assessment information set OASIS-D guidance manual effective (Chapter 3, Section D, p. D-2) January 1, 2019. Retrieved October 10, 2021 from https://www.cms.gov/Medicare/Quality-Initiatives-Patient-Assessment-Instruments/HomeHealthQualityInits/Downloads/OASIS-D-Guidance-Manual-final.pdf

---

- Changes in client's status/response to prior treatment along with pertinent, measurable factors assessed on current visit
- Clear, objective description of the skilled services implemented
- Notation of changed behaviors due to client education provided
- Objective description of immediate response/reaction to the skilled intervention by client and/or caregiver
- Specific plan for "next steps" needed for immediate follow-up or next visit

Also, if skilled maintenance therapy is warranted, CMS regulations delineate that *"skills of a qualified therapist or by a qualified therapist assistant under the supervision of a qualified therapist are needed to perform maintenance therapy"* (CMS, 2020g). Therapists must follow specific criteria allowing for the necessity of *"safe and effective"* performance of the maintenance program, with documentation clearly indicating that skilled services are needed to either maintain the individual's condition or prevent/slow further deterioration, including *"a detailed rationale that explains the need for the skilled service in light of the patient's overall medical condition and experiences, the complexity of the service to be performed, and any other pertinent characteristics of the beneficiary or home"* (CMS, 2020g).

As a client is nearing discharge, a home maintenance program might be needed, which the client or family/caregiver is expected to follow through with. In this instance, CMS also requires that the qualified therapist designs, establishes, and performs the teaching (CMS, 2020g). CMS also clearly specifies that a home health visit solely to train HHA staff, such as a home health aide, is *not* a billable service because the HHA has responsibility for making sure its staff is trained to properly perform any service it furnishes (CMS, 2020g). Thus, the HHA must absorb the cost of a skilled therapist's visit for the purpose of training HHA staff as an administrative expense (CMS, 2020g).

Palliative Care

Occupational therapy practitioners who work in hospice or other practice settings where clients have terminal illnesses often provide palliative care rather than rehabilitation. Palliative care involves a philosophy of focusing on providing comfort, symptom relief, emotional support, and quality of life as clients prepare for death. Third-party payers look at therapy services slightly differently in these situations. As there is no expectation that the client will make progress in physical functioning, goals often center around quality of life, such as pain control and maintaining the client's ability to participate in meaningful occupations. Intervention might include traditional approaches such as energy conservation, adaptive equipment, positioning, and family/caregiver education. Sometimes nontraditional interventions are also used, including relaxation, active listening, and complementary and alternative therapies.

Documentation in Mental Health

If you go from a job in a rehabilitation center to one in a mental health (or behavioral health) setting, you might think that nothing you have learned about documentation applies. Some of the language used in mental health settings may appear more subjective and general than what you have learned already. Documentation and treatment will reflect different criteria and terminology regarding performance skills, client factors, goals, and interventions as compared to those typically assessed or addressed in physical rehabilitation settings, but will still relate to occupational participation and performance. Also, a multidisciplinary approach is often used in mental health settings to establish problems, goals, and interventions. Occupational therapy is often regarded as part of a broader treatment service designated as adjunctive therapy, expressive therapy, or activity therapy. Disciplines that fall under this umbrella can include therapeutic recreation specialists, music therapists, art therapists, and dance therapists. Intervention is often provided in groups or as part of a therapeutic environment or milieu. Reimbursement may not be discipline-specific and therapy services may be included in the comprehensive daily rate for the facility. For example, clients with Medicare who receive inpatient psychiatric hospital services come under the prospective payment system, which pays a predetermined, fixed per-diem rate based on the client's diagnosis and level of care needed (CMS, 2006). Thus, any occupational therapy services provided in those circumstances are not billed separately. However, outpatient occupational therapy is a separate covered service when provided through psychiatric hospital outpatient programs where the rules for Medicare Part B apply, such as requiring an individualized plan of care (CMS, 2022a).

Occupational therapy practitioners use a client-centered approach and consider the holistic needs of the people who receive their services. Using professional reasoning, OTs and OTAs consider pertinent inter-related areas such as a client's physical and mental factors (including cognitive and emotional components), specific performance skills, performance patterns, and internal/external contexts (such as psychosocial factors, family and community supports) that influence occupational role performance and quality of life (AOTA, 2017b, 2020b). OTs and OTAs in all practice areas advocate and intervene to promote desired outcomes such as health, well-being, occupational participation, and quality of life for individuals, groups, and populations (AOTA, 2017b, 2020b). Clients in behavioral/mental health settings often have significant psychosocial problems that create serious disruptions in their ability to take part in meaningful occupations. Occupational therapy practitioners in this practice area have a "toolbox" of psychosocial interventions that are a viable and fundamental component of occupational therapy practice.

Evaluation Reports and Intervention Plans

Initial evaluation reports may be performed by the OT (with contributions from the OTA). However, evaluation reports are often, instead, a collaborative effort involving all the disciplines included in activity therapy, thereby losing some of the individual professional identity of occupational therapy. Third-party payers often require that facilities bundle therapy into the daily or episode-based rate rather than billing individual therapies separately. Having an integrated activities or adjunctive therapy department is usually more cost effective than having a separate occupational therapy department. Even so, occupational therapy practitioners should consider an occupational profile essential so that appropriate and effective interventions can be planned (AOTA, 2020b). Depending on the specific condition and individual circumstances, clients with mental health conditions may exhibit a variety of symptoms and behaviors, for example, hallucinations, avoidant behaviors, poor coping strategies, misuse of alcohol or drugs, excessive eating or gambling, compulsive behavior, withdrawal from activities, poor interpersonal skills, and so forth. These can impact quality of life significantly and hinder ability to engage in meaningful occupations. The OT, with assistance from the OTA, analyzes the occupations that are disrupted by the client's condition, the client's capabilities and challenges, available supports, activity demands, and the client's goals (AOTA, 2017b, 2020b). The OT and OTA use this information to contribute to the health care team's multidisciplinary problem list and intervention plan.

The *therapeutic milieu*, or the setting's total environment, is often considered essential in caring for clients who have mental health conditions. Ideally, each discipline assesses the client's needs and strengths, and then the team meets to formulate and prioritize a list of the client's problems. Problems in a mental health (or behavioral health) practice setting are traditionally divided into two parts. First, the problem itself is stated in one or two words, such as *"substance use," "noncompliant behavior,"* or *"suicide risk."* Next, a description of the behavioral manifestations indicates the areas of occupation and underlying limiting factors involved. Here are several examples:

- **Problem**: Suicide risk
  - **Behavioral manifestations:** During the week prior to admission, the client verbalized suicidal ideation, stating that life was no longer worth living. On the day of admission, he had purchased a handgun.
- **Problem:** Substance use
  - **Behavioral manifestations:** Mark has been using alcohol since age 12 years with increasing frequency over the last year and admits to using cocaine, "crystal," opium, and marijuana, resulting in a failed marriage, loss of two jobs, and involvement with the criminal justice system.
- **Problem:** Noncompliant behavior
  - **Behavioral manifestations:** Blake disobeys foster parents by running away, refusing to follow rules or requests, and engaging in sexual activity, resulting in six foster home placements in the past 4 years.

From this problem list, each individual discipline might suggest goals, objectives, and interventions appropriate to that discipline. In community mental health settings, occupational therapy goals can be related more easily and clearly to specific areas of occupational engagement. An **individualized treatment plan (ITP)** is developed. This is a contract for change between the client and the health care team. Major concerns or problems identified in the evaluation are documented on the ITP, and each discipline's goals, objectives, and interventions are written into one comprehensive plan. The client collaborates in the intervention process and signs the treatment plan to demonstrate agreement with it. Similar types of plans are developed by teams in schools and rehabilitation settings, but mental health plans differ in that all team members generally work toward the same goals through different interventions. Because of short lengths of stay, a client may even be discharged before a comprehensive intervention plan can be formalized or all goals can be addressed. Some facilities utilize *critical care pathways* (also called *clinical pathways*) to save time. For multidisciplinary treatment plans to be successful, the client (and family or significant others, if they are a part of the client's present life) must be actively involved. Each member of the treatment team must be willing to cooperate in a coordinated effort to effect change. In addition, the plan must be periodically reviewed to assess its effectiveness and to change or modify any interventions that have not been effective.

Intervention Strategies

The *OTPF-4* identifies therapeutic use of self as a cornerstone of the occupational therapy process (AOTA, 2020b). OTs and OTAs use therapeutic communication qualities and techniques (such as empathy, active listening, genuineness, etc.) and implement a variety of individual and group interventions according to the type of setting and kinds of clients served. These interventions are directed toward enabling clients to be empowered, resilient, and hopeful in order to effect personal change and acquire/restore skills for occupational roles within the home, workplace, community, and other contexts (AOTA, 2016). OTs and OTAs can also help clients create an action plan for wellness recovery and provide instruction and practice to develop and support healthy habits and routines, life decision-making skills, coping strategies, organizational skills, communication/interaction skills, etc. (AOTA, 2016, 2017b).

Interventions may be specific to occupational therapy or may be broader and applicable to activity therapy. Often, the choice of interventions depends largely upon what treatment groups are being provided by the facility, such as expressive, ADL, leisure, or activity groups. Group members may consist of clients who have very different diagnoses from one another. The OT or OTA skillfully implements appropriate intervention strategies to the entire group while addressing each client's particular needs at the same time. When planning intervention strategies, the health care team considers the client's assets (e.g., intelligence, good verbal skills, self-awareness) as important tools that the client will use in overcoming problems. A *strength* in this context is an ability, skill, or interest that the client has used in the past or has the potential for using. Assets can include such things as the client's interests (e.g., enjoys playing music, gardening, going for walks); abilities (e.g., writes well, accepts personal responsibility, is well-organized); relationship skills (e.g., has a good relationship with spouse or adult children); and social support systems (e.g., Alcoholics Anonymous [AA group], clergy keeps in contact). Assets may also be past abilities that the health care team wants to encourage as treatment progresses (e.g., client was physically active before becoming ill). Some interests, of course, (e.g., enjoys going to bars or casinos on weekends) may not be assets.

Ideally, occupational therapy documentation in mental health programs should be objective, measurable, realistic, and reflective of the occupation base of the profession. This means that your documentation must center on the client's occupational profile and address the client's health, well-being, ability to participate in meaningful occupations, and role competence.

Contact and Progress Notes

The use of contact notes and progress notes vary by facility/agency and funding source. If a client with Medicare has a mental health diagnosis and is seen in home health, the Medicare standards for home health apply. In a situation where progress notes rather than contact notes are used, the occupational therapy practitioner keeps a log of attendance and might jot down informal notations about participation and behaviors that show progress each day. Although these may not be structured or formal entries into the record, they may be used later to compile a progress note in the health record at regular intervals.

When you begin thinking in the language of mental health, terms like *brightened affect, less delusional, improved mood, increased self-esteem,* or *better attention* begin to enter your vocabulary, and you may be tempted to write in less objective and measurable terms. However, there are definite *observable behaviors* that can help you determine and document how the client's affect is brighter, mood is improved, or attention and concentration are better. Perhaps you are seeing the client attend occupational therapy group with make-up applied or hair combed; initiate conversation three times in a group session; smile twice in 15 minutes; or respond to your "good morning" by making eye contact. You might also observe that the client now only needs 15 minutes to get out of bed and dress in the morning; is more easily persuaded to attend occupational therapy (perhaps needing only one verbal request); or is able to attend to and complete a particular craft project within 30 minutes without needing any redirection to task. All of these indicators are *measurable,* and it is very helpful to the health care team if you are able to report your skilled observations in measurable and behavioral terms.

Managed care, along with role diffusion, has made it more difficult to document occupational therapy as a service that offers good value for the dollars spent in mental health care. Individuals with serious mental illness or substance use disorder often have a myriad of factors that hinder their ability to engage in meaningful occupation. Occupational therapy practitioners need to focus on documenting functional changes that are cost effective and meaningful to both the payer and to the consumer.

Critical Care Pathways in Mental Health

As lengths of stay tend to be short for many psychiatric diagnoses, inpatient mental health/behavioral health settings might use critical care pathways (clinical pathways) for the most common problems seen in that setting. These methods save time and can be customized to the client by adding desired targeted outcomes and interventions tailored to the individual's needs. Critical care pathways in mental health are multidisciplinary and are conceptually the same as those in rehabilitation. The plan for the client's care is preplanned for each day and for each discipline. This makes the most efficient use of staff time during the client's short length of stay while still making sure the client's needs are met.

Computer-Generated Plans

An electronic documentation program might provide prompts from which the team or the individual clinician selects the problem statements, goals, objectives, and interventions or methods that will be used for the individual consumer. As previously noted, the problems might be expressed very briefly as *depressed mood, substance use,* or *suicide risk.* Then, the client's specific behavioral manifestations are written in. The treatment team chooses the client's goals from a menu of long-term goals, or outcomes, such as the following:

Client will report the absence of suicidal ideation.

—or—

Client will identify three new coping strategies to use when he feels the urge to use drugs.

During the client's hospitalization, all members of the multidisciplinary team work toward the selected client goals. The plan may contain a list of potential interventions that would also be selected and addressed by the team. Interventions on this menu might include such strategies as the following:

- Evaluate the client.
- Encourage the client to express emotions.
- Teach new coping skills.
- Encourage the client to verbalize alternatives to previous coping strategies.
- Assist the client to develop a discharge plan that will prevent recurrence.

Appropriate interventions are chosen for use with each client, and each discipline implements the interventions in its own way. Social work adapts interventions to individual and group therapy, nursing implements the interventions on the unit, but occupational therapy will implement the interventions in groups and individual activities relating to occupational performance. For example, an OTA might do the following to address the above identified intervention strategies:

- Assist the OT in data collection for the occupational profile.
- Assist the OT in determining specific problems in each area of occupation.
- Use occupational therapy media to encourage the client to express emotions.
- Use occupational therapy groups to teach new coping skills and help the client find alternatives to strategies that have not worked well in the past.
- Provide feedback to the OT and client regarding task behaviors and performance skills as they relate to occupational performance.
- Help the client develop a plan for any areas of occupation that were part of the previous problem.

The team can individualize the plan to the client by describing the client's behavioral manifestations of the problem and by adding and deleting outcomes and/or interventions. The plan also lists the staff members responsible for each intervention. Figure 17-6 shows an example of a computer-generated plan for alcohol use disorder. It is provided only as a representation of what might be seen in clinical practice. Each setting will have its own protocols, but this will give you an idea of how a problem might be handled.

Here is another example. Imagine a female client admitted to an acute psychiatric unit following a suicide attempt. In an electronic documentation program, appropriate choices for identifying this client's problems might include:

- Suicide attempt
- Anger
- Poor self-esteem

For each problem, there would be a place to identify the client's behavior in relation to the problem.

- **Problem:** Suicide attempt
  - **Behavioral manifestations:** During 2 days prior to admission, the client verbalized suicidal ideation, stating that her life was no longer worth living. On the day of admission, she took an overdose of sleeping pills and was brought to the ER by ambulance.
- **Problem:** Anger
  - **Behavioral manifestations:** For the past 6 months, client has been fighting with her husband, resulting in marital separation, physical destruction of household objects, and high levels of stress.
- **Problem:** Poor self-esteem
  - **Behavioral manifestations:** For the past month, client has shown diminished interest in her appearance, resulting in an unkempt look at home and work. She has been verbalizing self-deprecating statements regarding her looks, self-worth, and future plans.

Next follows a list of interventions commonly used for an identified problem, starting with evaluation and ending with discharge planning. Interventions on the list that do not apply to this client would be deleted, and any additional interventions unique to this client would be written in. The list of interventions would include some standard interventions such as, "*Encourage client to express emotions*" and "*Teach new coping skills.*" Other interventions would be added for this client as appropriate, such as, "*Encourage positive self-concept*," "*Facilitate attention to grooming and personal hygiene*," or "*Encourage interaction with peers.*" The groups provided by the facility would be listed as interventions, and the OT and OTA would plan for ways to make the daily occupational therapy groups meet the client's needs. There would be a list of desired outcomes for each client's identified problems, with a place to add outcomes specific to the client's situation.

Behavioral Health Multidisciplinary Treatment Plan

Client Name: **Record #:**
Problem #:   **Problem name:** Alcohol Use Disorder   **Date identified:**
Behavioral manifestations:

Desired Outcomes	Target Date	Date Achieved
1. Client will verbally acknowledge that alcohol use has been a problem and will state an intent to abstain from alcohol use.		
2. Client will have developed at least 3 new ways to manage stress and will have demonstrated use of these.		
3. Client will have an aftercare plan in place.		
4. Client will have established a 5-day period of sobriety and of attending AA meetings daily.		
5.		
6.		

Interventions	Staff Responsible
1. Evaluation of the client's alcohol intake and use patterns.	
2. Provide individual, group, and family therapy.	
3. Education re: the disease model of chemical dependency.	
4. Provide opportunities to express feelings.	
5. Teach coping skills.	
6. Assist client to restructure environmental situations.	
7. Evaluate and teach relationship skills.	
8. Facilitate peer confrontation and feedback.	
9. Introduce social/leisure activities that do not include alcohol.	
10.	
11.	

I agree with this plan.

_____
Client's signature

Figure 17-6. Computer-generated plan.

Different Formats for Notes

Facilities may use **checklists, flow sheets,** or other types of forms created by the facility instead of SOAP notes to save time. With these alternate formats, information might be categorized differently than if you are writing a SOAP note. Forms are a popular way to record an initial assessment because they allow quite a lot of information to be communicated with minimal time spent writing. **Narrative notes** are not formally organized into S, O, A, and P sections the way SOAP notes are and may present information in any order desired. However, good narrative notes will contain the same type of content as a SOAP note, usually in a paragraph format that flows easily. A narrative note can also be organized into specific categories (e.g., occupations, client factors, performance skills) to make it easier for the reader to locate specific information (e.g., ADLs, functional mobility, upper extremity function). Examples of the same note written in both SOAP and narrative formats are presented in Chapter 18.

Some facilities use **D.A.P.** notes (Data, Assessment, Plan), which are an adaptation of the SOAP format. In D.A.P. notes, the "D" (data) section contains both the "S" and the "O" information. Other formats of notes include **B.I.R.P., P.I.R.P.,** or **S.I.R.P.** notes. These types of notes are sometimes used in mental health practice settings with the information distributed as follows:

B: The **behavior** that is exhibited by the client
I: The treatment **intervention** provided by the OT or OTA
R: The client's **response** to the intervention provided
P: The therapist's **plan** for continued intervention, based on the client's response

P: The **problem/purpose** of the treatment
IRP   for intervention, response and plan, as above

S: The **situation**
IRP   for intervention, response, and plan, as above

Conclusion

In this chapter, you have learned that practice settings can vary greatly in their formats and requirements for documentation according to the client population/kinds of diagnoses seen, funding source, facility policy, state and federal guidelines. However, occupational therapy documentation in all practice areas should focus on the client's occupational participation and performance. The next chapter will present examples of occupational therapy notes for different stages of treatment and various practice settings.

Worksheet 17-1
Types of Documentation

Match each of the types of documentation below to the descriptions that follow. Use each item only once.

a. Contact note   h. Progress report
b. MDS   i. Reevaluation report
c. Initial evaluation   j. Intervention plan
d. Discontinuation report   k. Occupational profile
e. Transition plan   l. IFSP
f. IEP   m. Clinical pathway
g. OASIS   n. IRF-PAI
                                   o. POC

1. ____ Outcome measure required by Medicare and Medicaid for use in home care
2. ____ Yearly multidisciplinary plan established for a particular student requiring special services
3. ____ Contains goals and specific treatment approaches relating to desired client outcomes
4. ____ Written when occupational therapy services are no longer needed
5. ____ Interdisciplinary assessment used in a skilled nursing facility to determine a client's problem areas and care plan
6. ____ Summarizes course of treatment and progress toward achieving goals during specified intervals
7. ____ Written following a treatment session and includes intervention provided, information communicated, and client's response to furnished service
8. ____ Consists of an occupational profile and factors affecting engagement in occupation
9. ____ A determination of the client's present status as compared to start of care, including progress, problems, and revision of goals
10. ____ Includes the client's roles, responsibilities, and factors such as values, culture, physical and social environments, age, and educational level
11. ____ Written to provide consistency when a client switches from one setting to another during the treatment continuum
12. ____ A blueprint for a client's care preplanned for each day and for each discipline based on a specific diagnosis
13. ____ Part of the therapy report that must be certified by physician in home health
14. ____ Mandated assessment to determine care levels in an inpatient rehabilitation facility
15. ____ Established for children under age 3 years and identifies a service coordinator

Morreale, M. J. (2023). *The OTA's guide to documentation: Writing SOAP notes* (5th ed.). SLACK Incorporated.

References

American Occupational Therapy Association. (2014). Consensus statement on clinical judgment in health care settings AOTA, APTA, ASHA. Retrieved May 25, 2022 from http://www.aota.org/~/media/Corporate/Files/Practice/Ethics/APTA-AOTA-ASHA-Concensus-Statement.pdf?la=en

American Occupational Therapy Association. (2016). Fact sheet: Occupational therapy's role in mental health recovery. Retrieved October 6, 2021 from https://www.aota.org/About-Occupational-Therapy/Professionals/MH/mental-health-recovery.aspx

American Occupational Therapy Association. (2017a). Guidelines for occupational therapy services in early intervention and schools. *American Journal of Occupational Therapy, 71*(Suppl. 2), 7112410010. https://doi.org/10.5014/ajot.2017.716S01

American Occupational Therapy Association. (2017b). Mental health promotion, prevention, and intervention in occupational therapy practice. *American Journal of Occupational Therapy, 71*(Suppl. 2), 7112410035. https://doi.org/10.5014/ajot.2017.716S03

American Occupational Therapy Association. (2018). Guidelines for documentation of occupational therapy. *American Journal of Occupational Therapy, 72*(Suppl. 2), 7212410010. https://doi.org :10.5014/ajot.2018.72S203

American Occupational Therapy Association. (2020a). AOTA 2020 occupational therapy code of ethics. *American Journal of Occupational Therapy, 74*(Suppl. 3), 7413410005. https://doi.org: 10.5014/ajot.2020.74S3006

American Occupational Therapy Association. (2020b). Occupational therapy practice framework: Domain and process (4th ed.). *American Journal of Occupational Therapy, 74*(Suppl. 2), 7412410010. https://doi.org: 10.5014/ajot.2020.74S2001

American Occupational Therapy Association. (2022). Payment policy: Medicaid and occupational therapy. Retrieved May 25, 2022 from https://www.aota.org/practice/practice-essentials/payment-policy/pay-medicaid

Center for Parent Information and Resources. (2014). Module 6: Content of the IFSP. Retrieved October 5, 2021 from https://www.parentcenterhub.org/partc-module6/

Center for Parent Information and Resources. (2017a). Contents of the IEP. Retrieved October 4, 2021 from https://www.parentcenterhub.org/iepcontents/

Center for Parent Information and Resources. (2017b). Key terms to know in early intervention. Retrieved September 18, 2021 from https://www.parentcenterhub.org/keyterms-ei/

Center for Parent Information and Resources. (2021). Overview of early intervention. Retrieved October 5, 2021 from https://www.parentcenterhub.org/ei-overview/

Centers for Medicare & Medicaid Services. (2003). *Medicare benefit policy manual* (Pub. 100-02: Ch. 8, Section 30.5). Retrieved October 8, 2021 from https://www.cms.gov/Regulations-and-Guidance/Guidance/Manuals/Downloads/bp102c08.pdf

Centers for Medicare & Medicaid Services. (2006). *Medicare claims processing manual* (Pub. 100-04: Ch. 3, Section 190). Retrieved October 6, 2021 from https://www.cms.gov/Regulations-and-Guidance/Guidance/Manuals/Downloads/clm104c03.pdf

Centers for Medicare & Medicaid Services. (2009a). *Medicare benefit policy manual* (Pub. 100-02: Ch. 1, Section 110.2.1). Retrieved October 6, 2021 from https://www.cms.gov/Regulations-and-Guidance/Guidance/Manuals/Downloads/bp102c01.pdf

Centers for Medicare & Medicaid Services. (2009b). *Medicare benefit policy manual* (Pub. 100-02: Ch. 1, Section 110.2.3). Retrieved October 6, 2021 from https://www.cms.gov/Regulations-and-Guidance/Guidance/Manuals/Downloads/bp102c01.pdf

Centers for Medicare & Medicaid Services. (2013a). *Medicare claims processing manual* (Pub. 100-04: Ch. 3, Section 140). Retrieved October 6, 2021 from https://www.cms.gov/Regulations-and-Guidance/Guidance/Manuals/Downloads/clm104c03.pdf

Centers for Medicare & Medicaid Services. (2013b). *Medicare claims processing manual* (Pub. 100-04: Ch. 3, Section 140.1.1). Retrieved October 6, 2021 from https://www.cms.gov/Regulations-and-Guidance/Guidance/Manuals/Downloads/clm104c03.pdf

Centers for Medicare & Medicaid Services. (2014a). *Medicare benefit policy manual* (Pub. 100-02: Ch. 1, Section 110.3). Retrieved October 6, 2021 from https://www.cms.gov/Regulations-and-Guidance/Guidance/Manuals/Downloads/bp102c01.pdf

Centers for Medicare & Medicaid Services. (2014b). *Medicare benefit policy manual* (Pub. 100-02: Ch. 15, Section 220.1.1). Retrieved October 6, 2021 from https://www.cms.gov/Regulations-and-Guidance/Guidance/Manuals/Downloads/bp102c15.pdf

Centers for Medicare & Medicaid Services. (2018a). *Medicare benefit policy manual* (Pub. 100-02: Ch. 8, Section 30.6). Retrieved from https://www.cms.gov/Regulations-and-Guidance/Guidance/Manuals/Downloads/bp102c08.pdf

Centers for Medicare & Medicaid Services. (2018b). *Medicare claims processing manual* (Pub. 100-04: Ch. 6, Section 10). Retrieved October 6, 2021 from https://www.cms.gov/Regulations-and-Guidance/Guidance/Manuals/Downloads/clm104c06.pdf

Centers for Medicare & Medicaid Services. (2019a). *Long-term care Facility Resident Assessment Instrument 3.0 User's Manual Version 1.17.1* Retrieved October 13, 2021 from https://downloads.cms.gov/files/mds-3.0-rai-manual-v1.17.1_october_2019.pdf

Centers for Medicare & Medicaid Services. (2019b). *Medicare benefit policy manual* (Pub. 100-02: Ch. 8, Section 20.1). Retrieved July 10, 2021 from https://www.cms.gov/Regulations-and-Guidance/Guidance/Manuals/Downloads/bp102c08.pdf

Centers for Medicare & Medicaid Services. (2019c). *Medicare benefit policy manual* (Pub. 100-02: Ch. 15, Section 220.1.2). Retrieved October 6, 2021 from https://www.cms.gov/Regulations-and-Guidance/Guidance/Manuals/Downloads/bp102c15.pdf

Centers for Medicare & Medicaid Services. (2019d). *Medicare benefit policy manual* (Pub. 100-02: Ch. 15, Section 220.2). Retrieved October 6, 2021 from https://www.cms.gov/Regulations-and-Guidance/Guidance/Manuals/Downloads/bp102c15.pdf

Centers for Medicare & Medicaid Services. (2019e). *Medicare benefit policy manual* (Pub. 100-02: Ch. 15, Section 220.3). Retrieved October 6, 2021 from https://www.cms.gov/Regulations-and-Guidance/Guidance/Manuals/Downloads/bp102c15.pdf

Centers for Medicare & Medicaid Services. (2019f). *Medicare benefit policy manual* (Pub. 100-02: Ch. 15, Section 220.4). Retrieved October 6, 2021 from https://www.cms.gov/Regulations-and-Guidance/Guidance/Manuals/Downloads/bp102c15.pdf

Centers for Medicare & Medicaid Services. (2019g). *Medicare claims processing manual* (Pub. 100-04: Ch. 5, Section10.6). Retrieved October 6, 2021 from https://www.cms.gov/Regulations-and-Guidance/Guidance/Manuals/Downloads/clm104c05.pdf

Centers for Medicare & Medicaid Services. (2019h). *Outcome and Assessment Information Set OASIS-D Guidance Manual Effective January 1, 2019.* Retrieved October 13, 2021 from https://www.cms.gov/Medicare/Quality-Initiatives-Patient-Assessment-Instruments/HomeHealthQualityInits/Downloads/OASIS-D-Guidance-Manual-final.pdf

Centers for Medicare & Medicaid Services. (2019i). Patient Driven Payment Model Fact Sheet: Administrative level of care presumption under the PDPM. Retrieved October 8, 2021 from https://www.cms.gov/Medicare/Medicare-Fee-for-Service-Payment/SNFPPS/Downloads/PDPM_Fact_Sheet_AdminPresumption_v6_508.pdf

Centers for Medicare & Medicaid Services. (2019j). Patient Driven Payment Model Fact Sheet: Concurrent and group therapy limit. Retrieved October 8, 2021 from https://www.cms.gov/Medicare/Medicare-Fee-for-Service-Payment/SNFPPS/PDPM#fact

Centers for Medicare & Medicaid Services. (2019k). Patient Driven Payment Model Fact Sheet: PDPM Patient Classification. Retrieved October 8, 2021 from https://www.cms.gov/Medicare/Medicare-Fee-for-Service-Payment/SNFPPS/PDPM#fact

Centers for Medicare & Medicaid Services. (2020a). *Medicare benefit policy manual* (Pub. 100-02: Ch. 7, Section 10.1). Retrieved October 6, 2021 from https://www.cms.gov/Regulations-and-Guidance/Guidance/Manuals/Downloads/bp102c07.pdf

Centers for Medicare & Medicaid Services. (2020b). *Medicare benefit policy manual* (Pub. 100-02: Ch. 7, Section 30). Retrieved October 6, 20121 from https://www.cms.gov/Regulations-and-Guidance/Guidance/Manuals/Downloads/bp102c07.pdf

Centers for Medicare & Medicaid Services. (2020c). *Medicare benefit policy manual* (Pub. 100-02: Ch. 7, Section 30.1.1). Retrieved October 6, 2021 from https://www.cms.gov/Regulations-and-Guidance/Guidance/Manuals/Downloads/bp102c07.pdf

Centers for Medicare & Medicaid Services. (2020d). *Medicare benefit policy manual* (Pub. 100-02: Ch. 7, Section 30.1.2). Retrieved October 6, 2021 from https://www.cms.gov/Regulations-and-Guidance/Guidance/Manuals/Downloads/bp102c07.pdf

Centers for Medicare & Medicaid Services. (2020e). *Medicare benefit policy manual* (Pub. 100-02: Ch. 7, Section 30.2.1). Retrieved October 6, 2021 from https://www.cms.gov/Regulations-and-Guidance/Guidance/Manuals/Downloads/bp102c07.pdf

Centers for Medicare & Medicaid Services. (2020f). *Medicare benefit policy manual* (Pub. 100-02: Ch. 7, Section 30.4). Retrieved October 6, 2021 from https://www.cms.gov/Regulations-and-Guidance/Guidance/Manuals/Downloads/bp102c07.pdf

Centers for Medicare & Medicaid Services. (2020g). *Medicare benefit policy manual* (Pub. 100-02: Ch. 7, Section 40.2.1). Retrieved October 6, 2021 from https://www.cms.gov/Regulations-and-Guidance/Guidance/Manuals/Downloads/bp102c07.pdf

Centers for Medicare & Medicaid Services. (2020h). *Medicare benefit policy manual* (Pub. 100-02: Ch. 7, Section 50.4.1.1). Retrieved October 6, 2021 from https://www.cms.gov/Regulations-and-Guidance/Guidance/Manuals/Downloads/bp102c07.pdf

Centers for Medicare & Medicaid Services. (2020i). OASIS data sets. Retrieved October 5, 2021 from https://www.cms.gov/Medicare/Quality-Initiatives-Patient-Assessment-Instruments/HomeHealthQualityInits/OASIS-Data-Sets

Centers for Medicare & Medicaid Services. (2021a). *Inpatient Rehabilitation Facility Resident Assessment Instrument (IRF-PAI) and IRF-PAI Manual.* Retrieved October 8, 2021 from https://www.cms.gov/Medicare/Quality-Initiatives-Patient-Assessment-Instruments/IRF-Quality-Reporting/IRF-PAI-and-IRF-PAI-Manual

Centers for Medicare & Medicaid Services. (2021b). *Medicare benefit policy manual* (Pub. 100-02: Ch. 1, Section 110.1.5). Retrieved October 6, 2021 from https://www.cms.gov/Regulations-and-Guidance/Guidance/Manuals/Downloads/bp102c01.pdf

Centers for Medicare & Medicaid Services. (2021c). *Medicare benefit policy manual* (Pub. 100-02: Ch. 1, Section 110.2). Retrieved October 6, 2021 from https://www.cms.gov/Regulations-and-Guidance/Guidance/Manuals/Downloads/bp102c01.pdf

Centers for Medicare & Medicaid Services. (2021d). *Medicare benefit policy manual* (Pub. 100-02: Ch. 1, Section 110.2.2). Retrieved October 6, 2021 from https://www.cms.gov/Regulations-and-Guidance/Guidance/Manuals/Downloads/bp102c01.pdf

Centers for Medicare & Medicaid Services. (2021e). *Medicare benefit policy manual* (Pub. 100-02: Ch. 1, Section 110.2.4). Retrieved October 6, 2021 from https://www.cms.gov/Regulations-and-Guidance/Guidance/Manuals/Downloads/bp102c01.pdf

Centers for Medicare & Medicaid Services. (2021f). *Medicare benefit policy manual* (Pub. 100-02: Ch. 1, Section 110.2.5). Retrieved October 6, 2021 from https://www.cms.gov/Regulations-and-Guidance/Guidance/Manuals/Downloads/bp102c01.pdf

Centers for Medicare & Medicaid Service. (2021g). *Minimum Data Set (MDS) 3.0 Resident Assessment Instrument (RAI) Manual.* Retrieved October 7, 2021 from https://www.cms.gov/Medicare/Quality-Initiatives-Patient-Assessment-Instruments/NursingHomeQualityInits/MDS30RAIManual

Centers for Medicare & Medicaid Services. (2021h). Patient Driven Payment Model. Retrieved October 8, 2021 from https://www.cms.gov/Medicare/Medicare-Fee-for-Service-Payment/SNFPPS/PDPM

Centers for Medicare & Medicaid Services. (2022a). Medicare Learning Network: Medicare Mental Health. Retrieved May 26, 2022 from https://www.cms.gov/files/document/mln1986542-medicare-mental-health.pdf

Centers for Medicare & Medicaid Services. (2022b). MS-DRG classifications and software. Retrieved October 8, 2021 from https://www.cms.gov/Medicare/Medicare-Fee-for-Service-Payment/AcuteInpatientPPS/MS-DRG-Classifications-and-Software

Centers for Medicare & Medicaid Services. (2022c). *OASIS user manuals.* Retrieved May 26, 2022 https://www.cms.gov/Medicare/Quality-Initiatives-Patient-Assessment-Instruments/HomeHealthQualityInits/HHQIOASISUserManual

Frolek Clark, G., & Holahan, L. (2015). Medicaid FAQ for school occupational therapy practitioners. *OT Practice, 20*(20), 18-20.

Steva, B. J. (2017). Interventions to enhance occupational performance in education and work. In K. Jacobs, N. MacRae, & K. Sladyk (Eds.), *Occupational therapy essentials for clinical competence* (3rd ed., pp. 399-417). SLACK Incorporated.

U.S. Department of Education. (n.d.a). IDEA: Statute and regulations. Retrieved September 18, 2021 from https://sites.ed.gov/idea/statuteregulations/

U.S. Department of Education. (n.d.b). Model form: Individualized education program. Retrieved October 4, 2021 from www2.ed.gov/policy/speced/guid/idea/modelform-iep.doc

U.S. Department of Education. (2020). A history of the Individuals with Disabilities Education Act. Retrieved September 28, 2021 from https://sites.ed.gov/idea/IDEA-History

Chapter 18

Examples of Different Kinds of Notes

This final chapter provides examples of occupational therapy documentation for a variety of practice settings. The first group of notes illustrates different stages of the occupational therapy process, while the second set provides examples of single intervention sessions in different practice settings. Although formats in various electronic documentation systems will differ depending on the practice setting and specific software program involved, these examples illustrate the use of professional terminology and will give you an idea of the kind of information that is important to include. Many of the notes in this chapter were written by students, faculty, and practicing therapists. The signatures, names, and other details have been changed to make the notes anonymous. Other examples have been created to provide additional opportunities for learning. All names are fictitious and any specific resemblance to a real person is purely coincidental. Note that due to space limitations in this book, some required information may not be present on these examples but would be included in a "real" note. If you were writing an actual note in a client's health or education record, you would use the client's whole name and any other required identification and insurance information; demographic data; along with any pertinent background information, outcome measures, and other objective data needed. In addition, all notes must be signed with the occupational therapy practitioner's full name and credentials. An OTA's notes should also be cosigned by the OT when required by law, facility policy, or payer requirements (American Occupational Therapy Association [AOTA], 2018).

Examples of Notes for Different Stages of the Occupational Therapy Process

Examples of Notes for Different Kinds of Intervention Sessions

Morreale, M. J. *The OTA's Guide to Documentation: Writing SOAP Notes, Fifth Edition* (pp. 277-292). © 2023 Taylor & Francis Group.

Acute Care Hospital: OT Initial Evaluation Report

Name: Fraksure, Frieda   **Health Record #:** 34567   **Age:** 70
Primary Dx: Ⓛ THR   **Secondary Dx:** Hypertension
Precautions/contraindications: PWB Ⓛ LE
Primary payment source: Medicare   **Secondary payment source:** None
Admission date: 12/2/21   **Date of referral:** 12/3/21
DOB: 4/1/1951   **Gender:** Female
Estimated length of stay: 4 days   **Physician:** B. Paynefree, MD

History of present condition: Client reports that yesterday morning she went upstairs at home to use the bathroom because there was none on the first floor. She became lightheaded, fell down the stairs, and fractured her left hip. She was admitted for a total hip replacement yesterday.

Brief occupational profile: Client reports living alone and being Ⓘ in all ADLs prior to admission. Her husband died 3 years ago and her family lives out of town and cannot stay with her. She wants to return home. Client states she has supportive neighbors and lives in a small town where she is retired from her position as a second grade teacher. She lives in a two-story townhouse across the street from the elementary school. She is in the habit of visiting with the children and some of their families when school is out each day. She is also active in church activities and belongs to the choir.

Date: 12/3/21 **Time:** 9:30 AM

Occupational Therapy Evaluation Report

S: Client stated that she would like to "get this leg well" and go home to "live a regular life."

O: Client was seated in wheelchair and participated in 60-minute evaluation in hospital room to assess ADL capabilities and Ⓑ UE function after Ⓛ THR. Client educated on use of ADL equipment for self-care tasks and adherence to hip precautions. Client demonstrated ability to repeat 2/4 precautions. During ADL evaluation, client was observed flexing 8° to 10° beyond 90° and required four verbal cues to remain at or below 90° during the session. Other three hip precautions were followed Ⓘ. After set-up, client was able to complete sponge bath at sink for upper body and used dressing stick with washcloth and verbal cues for lower body. Client PWB Ⓛ LE and required min Ⓐ for balance with sit ↔ stand to bathe back and peri area. Client able to complete upper body dressing after set-up and able to don underwear and pants over hips using a dressing stick. She required min Ⓐ for balance with sit ↔ stand to pull up clothing. Client able to don socks using sock aid after set-up with min verbal cues. Client completed grooming tasks and oral care Ⓘ. Following min verbal cues, client demonstrated good problem solving by trying different body positions to perform ADLs while adhering to hip precautions and demonstrated understanding of adaptive aids by utilizing reacher and dressing stick correctly after instruction. Client demonstrated ↓ ADL activity tolerance as she required four 2-minute rest breaks during dressing tasks. Evaluation of client factors:

     Ⓡ hand dominant   Ⓑ UE strength: WFL
     Ⓑ UE AROM: WFL   Grip strength Ⓡ 47#, Ⓛ 43#
     Ⓑ UE sensation: intact   Lateral pinch Ⓡ 10#; Ⓛ 5#
          Tripod pinch Ⓡ 10#, Ⓛ 5#

A: Client demonstrated good motivation, problem-solving skills, and understanding of equipment use, all of which indicate excellent rehab potential. Upper body strength and AROM WFL are assets for learning adaptive self-care techniques and functional mobility. Although client is able to complete grooming tasks and oral care Ⓘ, decreased performance skills such as poor endurance, ↓ standing balance, and inconsistent compliance with hip precautions create safety concerns for lower body dressing and bathing. These problem areas negatively impact client's ability to be Ⓘ and safe in ADL tasks. Client would benefit from skilled instruction on hip precautions and use of adaptive equipment with ADL performance, and therapeutic activities that facilitate dynamic standing balance and ↑ ADL activity tolerance. Exploration of interim living arrangement or possible continued home visits and home equipment procurement will be needed if progress warrants discharge to home.

P: OT twice daily for 1 hour the next 3 days to ↑ Ⓘ in self-care tasks through instruction on hip precautions, use of adaptive equipment, and tasks to ↑ activity tolerance and dynamic standing balance.

LTG: By anticipated discharge on 12/7/21, client will:

1. Safely complete lower body dressing and bathing with modified Ⓘ utilizing adaptive equipment with 100% adherence to hip precautions.
2. Demonstrate safe toileting with modified Ⓘ using rolling walker and bedside commode.

STG:

1. By second intervention session, client will transfer SBA sit ↔ stand using bedside commode and rolling walker, and manage clothing with no more than 2 verbal cues.
2. By second session, client will don shoes & socks with modified Ⓘ, utilizing adaptive techniques & devices with 100% adherence to hip precautions.
3. By third session, client will ↑ activity tolerance for ADLs as demonstrated by no more than one 30-second rest break during lower body dressing task of donning underwear and slacks with SBA.
4. By third session, client will perform toileting with SBA using commode frame over toilet, grab bar, wheeled walker, and adhering to total hip precautions.
5. By fourth session, client will safely bathe her peri area with modified Ⓘ utilizing adaptive techniques and devices with 100% adherence to hip precautions.

Signature: Kim Kindness, OTR/L

OT Intervention Plan

Name: Fraksure, Frieda   **Health Record #:** 34567   **Age:** 70
Primary Dx: Ⓛ THR   **Secondary Dx:** HTN
Precautions/Contraindications: PWB Ⓛ LE
Strengths: UE strength & AROM WFL; intact cognition and motivation to return home
Date: 12/3/21
Functional Problem Statement #1: ↑ fatigue, decreased compliance with THR precautions, and low activity tolerance make client unsafe in ADL tasks.
LTG #1: By anticipated discharge on 12/7/21, client will safely complete lower body dressing and bathing with modified Ⓘ utilizing adaptive equipment with 100% adherence to hip precautions.

Short-Term Goals	Interventions
STG #1: By second session, client will don shoes & socks with modified Ⓘ utilizing adaptive techniques and devices with 100% adherence to hip precautions.	1. Instruct and have client verbalize 4/4 hip precautions. 2. Provide written handouts of hip precautions 3. Instruct in use of adaptive techniques and devices followed by demonstration of use in dressing activities.
STG #2: By third session, client will ↑ activity tolerance for ADLs as demonstrated by no more than one 30-second rest break during dressing task of donning underwear and slacks with SBA.	1. Educate client and provide written instructions on energy conservation techniques. Evaluate understanding by her application during ADL tasks; ask about how she performs ADL tasks at home. 2. Continue instruction in use of adaptive techniques/devices followed by demonstration of use in dressing activities. 3. Instruct in manipulation of clothing items while standing with rolling walker at sink while adhering to total hip precautions.
STG #3: By fourth session, client will safely bathe her peri area modified Ⓘ utilizing adaptive techniques and devices and 100% adherence to hip precautions.	1. Instruct in use of adaptive techniques/devices followed by demonstration of use in bathing activities. 2. Instruct in manipulation of clothing and bathing items while standing with rolling walker at sink while adhering to total hip precautions. 3. Assess for DME/home equipment needs and continued home care services if progress warrants discharge to home.

Functional Problem Statement #2: ↓ dynamic balance makes client unsafe during ADL tasks.
LTG #2: By anticipated discharge on 12/7/21, client will demonstrate safe toileting with modified Ⓘ using rolling walker and bedside commode.

Short-Term Goals	Interventions
STG #1: By second session, client will transfer SBA sit ↔ stand using bedside commode and rolling walker and will manage clothing with no more than two verbal cues.	1. Instruct client in safe transfer techniques; reinforce compliance with total hip precautions. 2. Provide dynamic balance activities through reaching and weight-bearing activities at sink and closet for grooming and dressing tasks and pushing up from chair and bedside commode.
STG #2: By third session, client will perform toileting with SBA using commode frame over toilet, grab bar, and wheeled walker, while adhering to total hip precautions.	1. Continue instruction in safe transfer techniques; reinforce compliance with total hip precautions. 2. Interview client regarding physical layout of home environment. Assess and discuss DME/adaptive equipment needs and placement in home. Explore possible interim living arrangements, family support, and educate client about community support services (e.g., Meals on Wheels, elderly transit) if discharge to home is warranted.

Outpatient Rehabilitation: Cancer OT Intervention Plan

Name: Klyent, Carol   **Record #:** 791115
Date of Birth: 2/2/87   **Age:** 35
Primary Dx: Ⓛ mastectomy 2° breast CA
Date: 3/10/22

Strengths: Prior to surgery, Carol was in good physical condition and employed full time as a library clerk. She has some social support from her sister who lives in another state.

Functional Problem Statement #1: Carol avoids social outings with friends due to ↓ self-esteem secondary to cosmetic alterations imposed by mastectomy procedure, which precludes her ability to return to work.

LTG #1: Carol will ↑ social interactions and activity to six outings/month within the next month, in preparation for return to work.

STGs (Objectives)	Interventions (Gateley & Borcherding, 2017)
STG #1: Carol will identify one support group of interest to her within 1 week in order to ↑ willingness to be out in public for work and social activities.	1. Educate Carol and provide written handouts re: available support groups and peer visitation groups, their contact persons and telephone numbers.
STG #2: Carol will attend one support group activity within 2 weeks in order to ↑ confidence in social and work situations.	1. Discuss with Carol her experiences with support groups. 2. Reminder phone call or e-mail to encourage attendance at support group.
STG #3: Carol will initiate conversation with at least one other support group member during her first visit to the group in order to ↓ negative impact of cosmetic alterations to body image.	1. Accompany Carol into the community the first time she goes out. 2. Encourage Carol to participate in group discussion.
STG #4: Carol will enroll in a women's exercise program in order to ↑ activity tolerance and positive body image within 10 days.	1. Educate Carol re: area exercise groups for clients who are post-mastectomy. 2. Follow-up phone call or e-mail to determine her exercise program enrollment.
STG #5: By next session, Carol will identify five assets she possesses other than physical in order to increase self-esteem and improve confidence in social and work situations.	1. Discuss Carol's assets with her, encouraging her to think of as many as she can. 2. Educate and provide written handouts of resources (websites, books, organizations) that address post-mastectomy concerns.

Functional Problem Statement #2: Carol is unable to return to work 2° Ⓛ UE 3/4 AROM, 4-/5 muscle strength, ↓ activity tolerance (fatigues after 1 hr.), and sensory changes.

LTG #2: Carol will return to work part time by 4/18/22.

STGs (Objectives)	Interventions (Gateley & Borcherding, 2017)
STG #1: Carol will demonstrate activity tolerance of 2 hours for work tasks within 3 weeks.	1. Scar massage and myofascial release to incision area along with client education on self-massage. 2. Instruction in self-ranging HEP. 3. Work reconditioning tasks/job simulation
STG #2: In order to perform work task of retrieving and placing books on overhead shelves, Carol will demonstrate ↑ of 20° in Ⓛ shoulder flexion within 2 wks.	1. PROM to Ⓛ shoulder 2. Instruction in self-ranging HEP. 3. Work reconditioning tasks. 4. Provide information and encourage participation in women's exercise group.
STG #3: In order to manage repetitive work tasks, Carol will transport fifteen 5-lb boxes 10 feet (from a table to shoulder level shelf) with reported pain level of less than 2/10 within 4 wks.	1. Active resistive ROM to Ⓛ UE. 2. Resistive strengthening with exercise bands, weights, and graded functional activities. 3. Work simulation with client education on energy conservation principles. 4. Provide home exercise program and modify as client progresses. 5. Encourage participation in women's exercise group.
STG #4: Carol will use correct body mechanics in seated and active work tasks in order to have pain level of <2/10 while working within 3 wks.	1. Educate in ergonomics and posture in order to prevent pain. 2. Provide written handouts. 3. Complete work simulation tasks.
STG #5: Carol will demonstrate sensory precautions in work and daily living tasks within 10 days.	1. Provide education on safety concerns with sensory loss. 2. IADL and work-simulation tasks to assess and facilitate application of adaptive techniques for sensory hazards.

OT Progress Note: Hand Therapy Clinic

Name: Lunate, Luna
Record #: 9876543
Date: 8/11/22   **Time:** 1:00 PM
Occupational Therapy Progress Note

S: Client reports pain 4/10 at the Ⓡ ulnar styloid with forearm supination. Client also reports she is still unable to start her car with her Ⓡ hand but can now use it to turn a doorknob.

O: Client participated in 45-minute therapy session to increase functional range of motion and strength in Ⓡ UE for IADLs. Moist heat applied to Ⓡ hand and forearm for 10 minutes at start of session. A/PROM Ⓡ hand and forearm were reassessed:

[KEY: ( ) PROM; - extension lag; + hyperextension]

Ⓡ Hand	MP	PIP	DIP
Index	0/90	0/105	0/75
Long	0/90	0/105	0/80
Ring	0/90	0/105	0/80
Small	0/85	-14/105 (0/105)	0/79

Ⓡ Wrist: ext/flex +45/40 (+60/50)
Ⓡ forearm: supination 62 (78)   Pronation 90

Client performed the following exercises with Ⓡ UE: Isometric forearm supination x10, AAROM supination x5, AROM forearm supination x5 followed by functional activities (carrying a tray and turning pages in a binder) which she completed successfully. Following exercises, client's supination ↑ to 77° AROM. HEP revised to include blue foam for finger flexion strengthening 2 to 3 x daily.

A: Client's 10° gains in DIP flexion AROM since last week is due to ↑ strength of flexors. Active wrist extension ↑ 9° and flexion ↑ 5° from last week. ↑ of 8° in active pronation is due to ↑ strength while client lost 14° of forearm supination since last week, which appears to be a result of muscle tightness. Client would benefit from continued skilled OT to regain functional AROM to complete IADLs and for general strengthening.

P: Client to continue OT 2 x wk for 45-minute sessions. Continue wrist exercises and modify intervention plan to include more supination stretching and strengthening. Client will demonstrate Ⓘ in HEP and sufficient ↑ in Ⓡ forearm supination to start her car with Ⓡ UE in 2 weeks.

Hans Handfixer, OTR/L, CHT

OT Progress Note: Inpatient Mental Health

Name: Ankshus, Annie
Record #: 76-5234
Date: 5/21/22   **Time:** 1600
Occupational Therapy Progress Note
S: During the first 2 days of admission, client elected not to attend OT group sessions, maintaining that she was too "anxious and overwhelmed."
O: Client stayed in her room most of the time for first 2 days despite consistent invitations to attend groups. On this date, the client attended a stress management group. Initially she was quiet, but she gradually began entering into the activity. She was able to identify specific physical, emotional, and behavioral symptoms that she experiences when feeling overwhelmed or anxious. Client stated that she had not been aware of these stress reactions.
A: The client is making progress as indicated by her initiating attendance to group, as well as relaxing and opening up socially during the group. Additional progress indicated by recognizing specific symptoms of stress as opposed to relating only general feelings.
P: Continue all goals as originally stated. Client to attend OT groups daily for 1 week to provide opportunities for client to learn basic stress management techniques so that she may recognize and control stress reactions when she begins feeling overwhelmed or anxious.
Bonnie Beneficence, COTA/L   Emmett Empathy, OTR/L

Acute Care Hospital: OT Discharge Note (SOAP Format)

Name: Payshent, Paul   **Admit Date:** 8/29/22   **Record #:** 246810
Dx: Multiple trauma 2° to MVA   **DOB:** 2/17/56
OT Order Received: 9/7/22   **OT Evaluation Completed:** 9/8/22
Number of Intervention Sessions: 5   **Discharge Date:** 9/14/22
S: Client reports "doing a lot better" and being "less confused" than he was on admission.
O: Client initially presented with multiple trauma 2° to MVA. OT evaluation on 9/8/22 indicated client had minimal deficits in short-term memory, safety awareness, attention to task, and ADL performance. Client participated in 30-minute sessions daily for 5 days for ADL retraining for dressing, grooming, and functional mobility. Client and family received skilled instruction on safety precautions in the home. Client's functional status upon admission and discharge are as follows:

Admit Status	Goal	Discharge Status
Min Ⓐ in grooming	Set-up/supervision	Set-up/supervision
CGA toilet transfers	SBA	SBA
Supine → sit c̄ min Ⓐ	SBA	SBA
Min Ⓐ upper body dressing	Set-up/supervision	Set-up/supervision

A: All goals achieved due to improved cognitive status, awareness of safety precautions, and skilled instruction in ADLs. Client will need supervision at home 2° remaining cognitive deficits (attention and short-term memory).
P: Client discharged to home. Recommend home health OT evaluation for safety in home environment and potential for necessary durable medical equipment. No home exercise program given. No other referrals at time of discharge. OT will follow up in 1 month by phone to check client's functional status in the home.
Laura Loyalty, OTR/L

Acute Care Hospital: OT Discharge Note (Facility Format)

Name: Klyent, Kayla   **Health Record #:** 97531
DOB: 11/10/1934   **Physician:** Harry Healer, MD
Room #: 537
Start of Care: 6/1/22   **Date of Discharge:** 6/10/22
Primary Dx: Ⓡ CVA   **Secondary Dx:** RA
    X Occupational Therapy   __ Physical Therapy   __ Communicative Disorders
Course of Treatment: Following admission for CVA, client participated in OT daily for 9 days, 30 minutes each session, to work on increasing independence in self-care skills, functional mobility, Ⓛ UE strengthening, energy conservation, & activity tolerance.
Status on Discharge: Client reports feeling "much better" and is ready to go home.

Discharge Status   **Admit Status**
Self-care modified Ⓘ and safe   Self-care mod Ⓐ
Ⓛ UE strength F+   Ⓛ UE strength F–
Functional mobility Ⓘ and safe   Functional mobility mod Ⓐ
Activity tolerance 10 minutes for ADL tasks   Activity tolerance 7 minutes for ADL tasks

Goals met: Client has met self-care and functional mobility goals using energy conservation techniques.
Goals not met: Activity tolerance goal of 15 minutes not met due to client declining last two intervention sessions when she learned she was being discharged.
Client/family education: Client instructed in HEP and demonstrates understanding. Handouts provided. Client reported having weights at home she can use for continued UE strengthening as instructed in her HEP. Client was instructed in use of a tub seat and grab bar for safe showering.
Recommendations: Discharge client to her sister's home due to functional goals being met. HEP for Ⓛ UE strengthening attached. No home health recommended at this time.
Bonnie Bestworker, OTR/L

OT Contact Note: Safety

Name: Empulziff, Earl   **Health Record #:** 192837
Dx: Right CVA
Date: 5/29/22   **Time:** 8:45 AM
Occupational Therapy Contact Note

S: Client stated he desires to return home and does not understand why he needs "so much therapy."

O: Client participated in therapy 45 minutes bedside for instruction in ADLs, use of adaptive equipment, and safety. As client was being instructed in method for safe transfer from bed to w/c, he did not follow verbal command to stay seated on EOB. He attempted to get out of bed before wheelchair was positioned in place and required mod Ⓐ to be seated safely in w/c 2° poor balance. Meal tray placed on w/c lapboard and client was instructed in use of non-skid matting and scoop dish for cereal. Client required mod verbal cues to locate items on Ⓛ side of food tray and to use Ⓛ UE as a functional assist when opening containers and holding breakfast sandwich. Mod verbal cues also were required for pacing of feeding as client pocketed food in Ⓛ cheek and drank liquids too quickly, causing him to cough.

A: Client's Ⓛ neglect and poor safety awareness create concerns for returning home. Poor safety awareness while eating poses risk for aspiration and necessitates constant supervision during meals. His improved motor return and ability to use Ⓛ UE as a functional assist with verbal cues will ↑ ability to manage bimanual tasks. Client would benefit from compensatory techniques and activities to ↓ Ⓛ neglect and ↑ safety awareness for ADLs.

P: Continue OT twice daily for 45-minute sessions to improve safety for transfers, feeding, and self-care. Post written safety reminders bedside, instruct in proper pacing and swallowing of food, and continue to work on sequencing and Ⓛ side awareness. By 6/5/22, client will locate items on food tray with min verbal cues and will verbalize safety reminders for feeding with two verbal cues to look at and read list of safety instructions.

Jane Justice, COTA/L   Sam Soopervizer, OTR/L

OT Contact Note: Acute Care (SOAP Format)

Name: Dystraktible, David   **Health Record #:** 45283
Dx: TBI
Date: 7/22/22   **Time:** 15:00
Occupational Therapy Contact Note
S: Client nonverbal. Client demonstrated startle response with position change.
O: Client participated in OT bedside 20 minutes to work on initiating and attending to self-care tasks. When asked to point finger, client required multiple verbal cues and demonstrations, and demonstrated poor response time. Client required max Ⓐ supine → sit but was able to maintain dynamic sitting balance EOB with CGA. Client also required multiple verbal cues and hand-over-hand Ⓐ 75% of the time to initiate holding on to washcloth. Client able to bring washcloth to water basin with one verbal cue but required hand-over-hand Ⓐ to bring washcloth to face. Client attended to looking at self in mirror for ~1 minute. Client required hand-over-hand Ⓐ to initiate brushing hair. AROM shoulder flexion and abduction lack 45° at end range due to ↑ tone.
A: Overall, client's motor planning, task initiation, and attention during intervention activities continues to be limited. Client would benefit from activities to increase shoulder AROM, as well as further interventions focusing on the skills of initiating and attending to task in order to complete ADL activities.
P: Client to continue OT daily for 20 to 30 minute sessions until discharge in ~2 weeks to work on self-care activities and the underlying performance skills and client factors necessary to complete tasks Ⓘ. Client will follow a one-step command in 1 week in order to attend to self-care routine.
Susan Smart, OTR/L

OT Contact Note: Acute Care (Narrative Format)

Name: Dystraktible, David   **Health Record #:** 45283
Dx: TBI
Date: 7/22/22   **Time:** 15:00
Occupational Therapy Contact Note
Client participated in OT bedside 20 minutes to work on initiating and attending to self-care tasks. Client is nonverbal and demonstrated startle response with position change. When asked to point finger, client required multiple verbal cues and demonstrations, and he demonstrated poor response time. Client required max Ⓐ supine → sit but was able to maintain dynamic sitting balance EOB with CGA. Client also required multiple verbal cues and hand-over-hand Ⓐ 75% of the time to initiate holding on to washcloth. Client able to bring washcloth to water basin with one verbal cue but required hand-over-hand Ⓐ to bring washcloth to face. Client attended to looking at self in mirror for ~1 minute. Client also required hand-over-hand Ⓐ to initiate brushing hair. AROM shoulder flexion and abduction lack 45° at end range due to ↑ tone. Overall, client's motor planning, task initiation, and attention during intervention activities continues to be limited. Client would benefit from activities to increase shoulder AROM, as well as further interventions focusing on the skills of initiating and attending to task in order to complete ADL activities. Client to continue OT daily for 20 to 30 minute sessions until discharge in ~2 weeks to work on self-care activities and the underlying performance skills and client factors necessary to complete tasks Ⓘ. Client will follow a one-step command in 1 week in order to attend to self-care routine.
Susan Smart, OTR/L

OT Contact Note: Cognition

Date: 4/5/22   **Time:** 10:00 AM
Name: Worheero, Warren   **Health Record #:** 89-1011
Dx: Left CVA

Occupational Therapy Contact Note

S: Veteran reported feeling "fine" but stated he does not remember the OTA's name that he has been working with.

O: In OT clinic, veteran participated in 30-minute session to improve cognition, Ⓡ UE AROM, strength, and fine motor coordination for ADLs. Veteran oriented to person, month, year, and place after two verbal cues. He followed two-step commands after max verbal cues and required mod physical assist to complete basic self-care tasks. Veteran was unable to grasp and release items with Ⓡ hand. He required mod physical Ⓐ and verbal cues to complete Ⓡ UE AROM used in tabletop activities.

A: Veteran is not oriented to surroundings at all times, which presents safety concerns. His ↓ cognitive functioning leads to ↓ attention to completion of tasks, specifically dressing, feeding, and bathing. Veteran would benefit from further cognitive skills training and safety instruction. Veteran also displays ↓ strength, coordination, and AROM in Ⓡ UE, which limits his ability to complete ADL activities. He would benefit from instruction in using Ⓡ UE as an assist as well as from activities to ↑ Ⓡ UE strength, AROM, and coordination to perform self-care activities.

P: Veteran to continue OT daily 1 hour for 4 weeks to improve cognitive skills, ↑ attention to task and safety awareness, and to ↑ Ⓡ UE strength, AROM, and coordination in order to complete self-care tasks. Next session, instruct client in use of calendar/daily schedule placed in room and work on improving task attention and integration of Ⓡ UE during breakfast and grooming tasks.

Patricia Patience, COTA/L   Duane Dogooder, OTR/L

OT Contact Note: Home Health Visit

Date: 8/14/22   **Time:** 9:30 AM
Name: Elderlee, Edward   **Health Record #:** 891011
Dx: Left TKR   **DOB:** 10/13/29
Physician: Bea Well, MD   **SOC:** 8/1/22

Occupational Therapy Contact Note

S: Client stated that he did not sleep well last night and is feeling tired this morning. Client's daughter reported that client is "transferring a little better."

O: Client participated in 45-minute session in his home for skilled instruction in ADLs, safety, transfers, and use of adaptive equipment. Client and daughter were instructed in use of transfer tub bench. Following skilled instruction, daughter demonstrated ability to transfer client safely w/c ↔ tub bench with client needing min assist for balance and to bring legs over edge of tub. Once set-up, client was able to sequence steps for bathing but required min assist to wash back and feet using long handle sponge. Recommended that client install grab bars in tub area for safety. Client stated he will ask his nephew, who is a carpenter, to do this ASAP.

A: Client demonstrates good progress in transfers from mod to min Ⓐ as compared to last week. Client's daughter demonstrates good carryover in safe transfer techniques. Client would benefit from further skilled OT instruction in transfers, self-care activities, and adaptive equipment to increase Ⓘ in home environment.

P: Client to continue OT 2 x wk for 45 minutes for transfer training, activities to promote self-care Ⓘ, and family education. Client will demonstrate transfers to tub bench modified Ⓘ with use of grab bar within three intervention sessions.

Jennie Joyful, COTA/L   Camilla Calmness, OTR/L

OT Contact Note: Inpatient Mental Health

Name: Sadnyss, Sadie   **DOB:** 9/23/71
Health Record #: 3572468   **Physician:** Helen Healer, MD
SOC: 4/15/22
Date: 4/16/22   **Time:** 4:00 PM

Occupational Therapy Contact Note

S: Client reported she is currently not volunteering and has not worked for the past 4 years due to her disability status. Regarding volunteering, she says, "I need the structure," and further stated that she wants to be productive. Currently, client reports she sleeps "too much" and is having relationship problems.

O: Client was admitted yesterday and attended 4/4 group sessions today. During activity group, client participated in baking with the rest of the group but did not eat anything. In expressive therapy group, when each group member identified current emotions, client identified hers as "miserable, angry, very anxious, overstimulated, frustrated, frightened, and alienated." During skills group, client identified a possible problem she may encounter upon discharge as "lack of organization," with her "red flags" being oversleeping and agitation. Client welcomed suggestions from others regarding restructuring her use of time.

A: Client is very perceptive of her emotions and limitations. Her refusal to eat with the group indicates continued appetite disturbance. Client would benefit from information about eating disorders. She would also benefit from continued group participation, with emphasis on increasing self-esteem and time management skills. Client's participation in all four group sessions today indicates good rehab potential.

P: Client will continue to attend all daily group sessions while on the acute unit to work on increasing self-esteem and ability to structure her time. Client will work on increased time management skills by developing five strategies she will use for gaining control of her daily time prior to discharge. Information will be provided to client regarding eating disorders and importance of a balanced diet.

Nancy Nice, OTR/L

OT Contact Note: Pediatric (Preschool Age)

Name: Tyke, Tess   **ID#:** ABC123
Dx: Cerebral palsy
Date: 3/7/22   **Time:** 3 PM

Occupational Therapy Contact Note

S: Tess said she wanted to play, but when the task was difficult for her, she said, "You do it. You fix it."

O: Tess participated in 30-minute OT session in her home to work on prerequisite skills for self-care and play including: bilateral use of UEs to ↑ spontaneous use of Ⓛ hand as a functional assist, sitting balance while tailor sitting unsupported, and functional mobility. Tess was engaged during ~90% of the session.
Bilateral UE Use: Tess required max Ⓐ to pull shirt over stuffed animal's arms with Ⓡ UE while holding it with Ⓛ UE. She spontaneously used Ⓛ hand to assist with stabilizing animal while pulling sleeve over its arm and shoulder with Ⓡ hand. Tess initiated snapping shirt, but needed max Ⓐ to use Ⓛ hand to stabilize shirt while fastening snaps. Both hands were used to hold animal steady during play.
Sitting Balance: Tess required five tactile cues from stand → sit using walker and mod physical Ⓐ from side sit → cross legged sit. She demonstrated adequate sitting balance to play for 5 minutes, requiring tactile cues twice to right herself from a lateral tilt.

A: Tess demonstrated bilateral integration and use of Ⓛ hand as a functional assist ~60% of the time, which is an increase from last week. When she is engrossed in activity, Tess is unable to concentrate on postural support and needs CGA assist to resume upright posture. She would benefit from continued skilled OT for activities that challenge postural support in order to gain protective responses, body righting, and vestibular integration in order to ↑ her Ⓘ during play.

P: Tess will continue OT weekly for 7 weeks to continue strengthening postural support in order to ↑ Ⓘ in play activities, promote bilateral hand use, and ↑ use of the Ⓛ hand as a functional assist during ADLs and play activities.

Patty Kake, OTR/L

OT Contact Note: Public School

Name: Stewdant, Stella   **ID #:** 653-4817
Date: 5/12/22   **Time:** 2:40 PM
Occupational Therapy Contact Note

S: Stella did not use verbal language to communicate, but did echo words spoken to her.

O: Stella participated in 25-minute OT session in classroom to improve fine motor skills needed for scissors use and writing. After 5 minutes of brushing to decrease tactile sensitivity, Stella worked on palmar pinch and tripod pinch using a "Fruit Loop" bracelet activity for 20 minutes. Stella used tripod pinch to manipulate tongs (in preparation for scissors use) to pull 15 Fruit Loops out of a bowl one at a time. Then, using a palmar pinch, she placed each Fruit Loop over a pipe cleaner. Five verbal cues were required for task completion.

A: Stella manipulates tongs well and exhibits a good awareness of positioning of tongs within her hands, which is an indicator that proper scissors use will be attained soon. Good attention to task for entire 25 minutes is an asset for completion of classroom craft projects.

P: Continue prehension activities 3 x wk using a variety of media in 20- to 30-minute intervals until proper scissors use goal is achieved. Stella will be able to cut a piece of 8-in. x 10-in. paper in 5 strips (each approximately 2 inches wide) using adaptive spring scissors Ⓘ 3/3 tries by the end of the school year.

Princy Pal, COTA/L   Dee Tention, OTR/L

OT Contact Note: Outpatient Clinic— Orthotic Device (SOAP Format)

Name: Carpus, Carl   **ID#:** 46103
Date: 9/21/22   **Time:** 1:15 PM
Occupational Therapy Contact Note

S: Client stated that the Ⓡ volar wrist orthosis he was issued last session "isn't causing any problems." Client also reported that he wore orthosis "all day at work" for the past 2 days and his pain level has decreased to 3/10.

O: Client participated in 45-minute session in OT clinic for assessment of orthosis use/tolerance and instruction in ergonomics for work. Client arrived at clinic wearing orthotic device. Skin checked following removal of orthosis and no pressure areas noted. Client demonstrated ability to don/doff orthosis Ⓘ. New stockinette liner issued per client request. Client was instructed in use of ergonomic equipment (split keyboard and wrist rest) for his software developer job. Following skilled instruction, client was able to demonstrate appropriate use of ergonomic devices while wearing orthosis. Client also provided with a catalog of ergonomic devices so that he can show them to his boss.

A: Client's ↓ pain from 6/10 last week to 3/10 since wearing orthosis shows good progress. Client would benefit from nerve gliding exercises, continued use of orthosis and further instruction in ergonomics for work.

P: Continue therapy 1x weekly for 4 weeks for instruction in ergonomics, median nerve gliding exercises, and continued assessment of orthosis use/tolerance to minimize pain when performing work tasks.

Dexter Dexterity, COTA/L   Patricia Putty, OTR/L

OT Contact Note: Outpatient Clinic—
Orthotic Device (Narrative Format)

Name: Carpus, Carl   **ID#:** 46103
Date: 9/21/22   **Time:** 1:15 PM
Occupational Therapy Contact Note
Client participated in 45-minute session at OT clinic for assessment of orthosis use/tolerance and instruction in ergonomics for work. He arrived wearing Ⓡ volar wrist orthosis he was issued last session. He stated orthosis "isn't causing any problems" and also reported that he wore orthosis "all day at work" for the past 2 days. Skin was checked following removal of orthosis and no pressure areas noted at this time. Client demonstrated ability to don/doff orthosis Ⓘ. New stockinette liner issued per client request. Client indicated improvement in Ⓡ hand symptoms with a reported pain level of 3/10 (was 6/10 last week). Client instructed in use of ergonomic equipment (split keyboard and wrist rest) for his software developer job. Following skilled instruction, client was able to demonstrate appropriate use of ergonomic devices while wearing orthosis. Client also provided with a catalog of ergonomic devices so that he can show them to his boss. Client's reduction in pain from 6/10 to 3/10 since wearing orthosis shows good progress. Client will benefit from continued OT 1x weekly for 4 weeks for further instruction in ergonomics, median nerve gliding exercises, continued assessment of orthosis use/tolerance to minimize pain when performing work tasks.
Dexter Dexterity, COTA/L   Patricia Putty, OTR/L

OT Contact Note: Wheelchair Mobility
Instruction (SOAP Format)

Name: Letzgo, Lester   **Record Number:** 42-6710
Date: 5/5/22   **Time:** 2:00 PM
Insurance: Medicaid
Occupational Therapy Contact Note
S: Client stated, "I can't wait to try out my new power wheelchair."
O: Client participated in 75-minute session in OT clinic for skilled instruction in power w/c mobility. Client was instructed in operating joystick control with Ⓡ hand using wrist stabilization orthosis. Following skilled instruction, client demonstrated ability to navigate w/c safely around obstacles, turn, and maneuver in tight spaces (e.g., bathroom). Client leaned to Ⓛ with posterior pelvic tilt when operating w/c. Preliminary instruction also provided for charging battery and care/maintenance of w/c.
A: Client demonstrates good potential for full Ⓘ in use and care of w/c. He would benefit from Ⓛ lateral support to maintain proper posture in w/c, continued instruction and practice regarding charging battery, and assessment of w/c mobility on uneven surfaces.
P: Continue OT daily until discharge in 3 days for further instruction in use of power w/c. By discharge, client will demonstrate Ⓘ in w/c mobility outdoors on uneven surfaces and will maintain upright posture in w/c with use of appropriate supports.
Roland Rollaway, COTA/L   Wilma Wheels OTR/L

OT Contact Note: Wheelchair Mobility Instruction (Narrative Format)

Name: Letzgo, Lester   **Record Number:** 42-6710
Date: 5/5/22   **Time:** 2:00 PM
Insurance: Medicaid
Occupational Therapy Contact Note
Client stated, "I can't wait to try out my new power wheelchair." He participated in 75-minute session in OT clinic for skilled instruction in power w/c mobility. Client was instructed in operating joystick control with Ⓡ hand using wrist stabilization orthosis. Following skilled instruction, client demonstrated ability to navigate w/c safely around obstacles, turn, and maneuver in tight spaces (e.g., bathroom). Preliminary instruction also provided for charging battery and care/maintenance of w/c. Client leaned to Ⓛ with posterior pelvic tilt when operating w/c and would benefit from a Ⓛ lateral w/c support. Client demonstrates good potential for full Ⓘ in use and care of w/c but requires further instruction and practice regarding w/c positioning and charging battery. Continue OT daily until discharge in 3 days for further instruction in use of power w/c and assessment of w/c mobility on uneven surfaces. By discharge, client will demonstrate Ⓘ in w/c mobility outdoors on uneven surfaces and will maintain upright posture in w/c with use of appropriate supports.
Roland Rollaway, COTA/L   Wilma Wheels, OTR/L

References

American Occupational Therapy Association. (2018). Guidelines for documentation of occupational therapy. *American Journal of Occupational Therapy*, 72(Suppl. 2), 7212410010. https://doi.org :10.5014/ajot.2018.72S203

Gateley, C. A., & Borcherding, S. (2017). *Documentation manual for occupational therapy: Writing SOAP notes* (4th ed.). SLACK Incorporated.

Appendix

Suggestions for Completing the Worksheets

If you are a student, new OTA, or instructor using this manual, you should be able to work your way through the exercises and check your work against those in this Appendix. Realize that the suggestions offered here for therapy notes and goals are examples of best practice and should be considered as only a few of the many possible "good" or "correct" answers. As you complete the documentation exercises, remember that your answer can be different and still be correct, as long as your therapy note or goal contains the essential elements. You should not sacrifice your own writing style to be more like someone else's, provided your information and protocol are essentially correct. SOAP notes are difficult to write without a real intervention session. Although there are many examples in this manual, there is no substitute for observing or working with actual clients. Only then will you be able to translate your intervention session onto paper or an electronic format in a meaningful way.

Chapter 1

Worksheet 1-1: Documentation Basics

1. __F__ OTs and OTAs can be referred to as occupational therapy practitioners or therapists. *Only the OT can be referred to as a therapist (AOTA, 2020a; Centers for Medicare & Medicaid Services [CMS], 2019).*

2. __F__ When skilled therapy is no longer needed, the OTA has responsibility for writing the discharge report if they treated the client for the final therapy session. *The OT is responsible for the discharge report although the OTA can contribute to this process (AOTA, 2018a)*

3. __T__ Most hospitals and physician offices in the U.S. utilize electronic health records (EHR).

4. __F__ The acronym SOAP stands for Subjective, Objective, Appraisal, and Plan. *The A represents Assessment.*

5. __F__ An occupational therapy note is only written when the OT or OTA has physical contact with the client. *Notes can include telehealth visits, phone calls, meetings with family/significant others.*

6. __T__ An alternate format to a SOAP note is a narrative note.

7. __T__ A transition note might be written when a client is transferring from special education to vocational services within the same system of service delivery.

8. __T__ It may be necessary for an OT or OTA to utilize various paper-based health forms in a setting that has an EHR system in place.

Morreale, M. J. *The OTA's Guide to Documentation: Writing SOAP Notes, Fifth Edition* (pp. 293-332). © 2023 Taylor & Francis Group.

9. __F__ The *OTPF-4* incorporates terminology and concepts compatible with the WHO health and disability framework *International Classification of Diseases (ICD)*. *This describes WHO's International Classification of Functioning, Disability and Health (ICF).*

10. __T__ In educational settings, benchmark reporting refers to documenting a student's progress for specific time periods during the school year.

11. __T__ To differentiate occupational therapy from other disciplines, OTs and OTAs should focus their documentation on the client's ability to engage in occupation.

12. __F__ An occupational profile is established once appropriate client goals are established. *The occupational profile is created at the beginning of the evaluation.*

13. __F__ ADL occupations include activities to improve or manage one's health, such as wearing an orthotic device, taking prescribed medication, or using a glucometer. *This describes the occupation of health management.*

14. __F__ An OTA should expect that a client's ability to perform an activity/occupation in the clinic will always be transferable to the client's home setting.

15. __F__ OTAs document performance skills such as reflexes and range of motion. *Reflexes and range of motion are client factors (body structures).*

16. __F__ Occupational therapy notes tend to be very consistent in content and style across different types of practice settings.

17. __F__ The OT cannot change an established occupational therapy intervention plan once treatment has been initiated. *The OT can modify goals/intervention plan during the intervention process. Some settings and/ or payers may require that the physician certify/approve changes in plan.*

18. __F__ Third-party payers always approve reimbursement for durable medical equipment or assistive technology if the client would benefit from it. *Payers have very strict requirements that must be met and substantiated in documentation for reimbursement of these types of items. Equipment must be deemed medically necessary (or educationally necessary in school settings) and are not just for comfort or convenience.*

19. __F__ Activity demand refers to a task the client insists on doing during an intervention session rather than what the OT or OTA is recommending. *Activity demands are the requirements of an activity such as the materials, space, methods, and skills needed for performance.*

20. __F__ Because leisure tends to improve one's quality of life, it is usually regarded by third-party payers as a reimbursable goal in physical rehabilitation settings. *However, in some practice settings, such as mental health, it might be appropriate to have leisure-related goals addressing problems in interpersonal skills, maladaptive behaviors, and so forth.*

Worksheet 1-2: The *Occupational Therapy Practice Framework: Domain and Process, Fourth Edition (OTPF–4)*

Correct answers are in bold and based on the *OTPF-4* (AOTA, 2020b).

1. Which of the following are examples of a performance pattern? *(Performance patterns include habits, routines, rituals, and roles.)*
   a. Tracing a client's hand during orthotic device fabrication
   b. **One's family or work role**
   c. Bilateral coordination
   d. **A religious ritual**
   e. **Bedtime routine**
   f. Two-point gait

2. Which of the following are examples of a performance skill? *(Answers b, e, and f are client factors.)*
   a. **Bending far enough to retrieve clothing from dryer**
   b. Muscle strength of Good (4/5) for shoulder flexion
   c. **Standing for 10 minutes**
   d. **Reciting a prayer from memory**
   e. Normal muscle tone
   f. Gag reflex

3. Which of the following are considered occupations?
   a. Spirituality *(a client factor)*
   b. **Social participation**
   c. Range of motion *(a client factor)*
   d. **Sleep**
   e. **Rest**
   f. **Play**

4. Which of the following are client factors?
   a. **Values**
   b. Sleep *(an occupation)*
   c. **Mental functions**
   d. Roles *(a performance pattern)*
   e. **Blood pressure**
   f. Age *(a context)*

5. Which of the following are examples of contextual factors?
   a. **Gender**
   b. **Completing high school or college**
   c. **Internet access**
   d. **Lack of public transportation for a client who is unable to drive**
   e. **Presence of lead or pesticides in client's home**
   f. **Income below poverty level**

6. A client is recovering from a stroke and has deficits in upper extremity function and difficulty performing ADLs/IADLs. Which of the following are examples of possible interventions to support occupations? *(Interventions to support occupations are methods/tasks that work toward developing/remediating/maintaining specific client factors/skills with goal of enabling occupational participation/improved quality of life (AOTA, 2020b). Answers c and d are activities.)*
   a. **Using pulleys to increase range of motion**
   b. **Squeezing therapy putty to improve grip strength**
   c. Practicing buttoning a shirt
   d. Measuring ingredients to make a cake
   e. **Passive range of motion to increase elbow flexion**
   f. **Fabricating and issuing an orthotic device**

7. Which of the following are activities?
   a. **Practicing writing one's name in cursive**
   b. Preparing a meal after shopping for ingredients *(an occupation)*
   c. **Peeling potatoes**
   d. A 50-year-old client stacking cones to improve upper limb function *(intervention to support occupations)*
   e. Maintaining balance while sitting on a therapy ball *(intervention to support occupations)*
   f. Completing morning grooming routine *(an occupation)*

8. Which of the following are examples of interventions to support occupations?
    a. Rolling out pie dough *(an activity)*
    b. **Performing wound care on a client**
    c. **Application of hot pack**
    d. **Using hand weights to increase upper extremity strength**
    e. Teaching client strategies to reduce stress *(education and training)*
    f. Washing lettuce for a salad *(an activity)*

9. Which of the following are delineated as the primary performance skills categories in the *OTPF-4*?
    a. **Motor skills**
    b. Emotional regulation skills
    c. **Social interaction skills**
    d. Sensory integration skills
    e. Preparatory skills
    f. **Process skills**

10. Which of the following are rituals?
    a. Biting one's fingernails when feeling anxious *(habit)*
    b. **Lighting candles on the Sabbath**
    c. Wearing a seatbelt when driving *(habit)*
    d. Showering, dressing, and buying coffee at Starbucks prior to work every day *(routine)*
    e. **Always making Irish soda bread for St. Patrick's Day**
    f. **Making the sign of the cross when entering a church**

Worksheet 1-3: Using the *Occupational Therapy Practice Framework*

Performance skills related to a clay or craft project might include observable behaviors such as the following: activity tolerance, sharing of materials, ability to organize time and materials, sequencing of steps, task initiation, decision making, asking for assistance, reaching for objects, sitting upright, speaking with others, gathering and searching for materials, attention to detail, coordination of both hands, crossing midline, frustration tolerance, pacing of activity, following directions or pattern, handling of tools, and many others.

Client factors related to a clay or craft project might include the following: UE AROM, strength, vision, hearing, touch, attention, eye-hand coordination, spatial awareness, concept formation, self-esteem, motor planning, gait patterns, muscle tone, stamina, temperament, attitude and values regarding crafts, standards for completion, and many others.

Worksheet 1-4: *Occupational Therapy Practice Framework*—More Practice

Performance skills related to a cooking task might include behaviors such as the following: knowledge of tools and equipment; carrying objects; adapting to environment; activity tolerance; ability to organize time, materials, and steps; task initiation; clean up; judgment, safety, and problem solving; reaching for objects; mobility; dynamic balance; lifting, stabilizing, pouring, and handling objects; gathering and searching for materials; coordination of both hands; pacing of activity; following directions; and many others.

Client factors related to a cooking task might include the following: appetite, attitude, and values regarding food, body image, UE AROM, strength, vision, hearing, smell, touch, eye-hand coordination, spatial awareness, depth and distance perception, concept formation, learned behaviors, motor planning, gait patterns, muscle tone, stamina, temperament, standards for completion, and many others.

Chapter 2

Worksheet 2-1: Internet and Chat Slang

Here are some suggestions for making the sentences more professional. Meanings of text and chat slang abbreviation (NetLingo, 2021) are indicated in brackets below and are generally not appropriate for use in professional communication. Various acceptable abbreviations are included in the abbreviations list in Chapter 4 and noted below.

1. TX, SLAP. Pt's DH and DD will be instructed in use of the equipment you suggested. [TX = thanks, SLAP = sounds like a plan, DH = dear/darling husband, DD = dear/darling daughter]
   Thank you. That seems like a good plan. Pt's husband and daughter will be instructed in the equipment you suggested.

2. Client AWOL today. Could not reach her by phone 2X. [AWOL = absent without leave]
   Client did not show up today. Two attempts to contact her by phone were unsuccessful.

3. K, I will call parents. FWIW the student did not hurt herself when she fell. TTYL. [K = ok, FWIW = for what it's worth, TTYL = talk to you later]
   Yes, I will call the parents. However, the student did not hurt herself when she fell. Let's discuss further this afternoon.

4. OMG, the client's wound stinks and has bad yellow drainage. Please TMB ASAP. [OMG = oh my goodness/God, TMB = text me back]
   The client's wound has purulent drainage. Please advise me ASAP.

5. IDK why the adaptive equipment was not ordered. Sorry, G2G [IDK = I don't know, G2G = got to go]
   Sorry, I do not know why the adaptive equipment was not ordered. I have to go to a meeting now.
   —or—
   I don't know why the adaptive equipment wasn't ordered. Sorry that I cannot continue this conversation right now but I have to see another client.

6. Resident negative for TB and AFAIK will be discharged in am. [AFAIK = as far as I know]
   The resident is negative for TB and I believe he will be discharged tomorrow morning.

7. Got ur message. IMHO client is unsafe transferring by herself and needs SBA. [ur = your, IMHO = in my humble opinion]
   I received your message. Client appears to be unsafe transferring by herself and needs SBA.

8. The MS pt. tires easily when AMB short distances and needs a w/c eval before discharge. TIA. [TIA = thanks in advance]
   The client with MS tires easily when AMB short distances. Please evaluate her for a w/c before discharge. Thanks in advance.

9. Transporting the CA victim to his room now. BRB. [BRB = be right back]
   I am presently transferring the client with CA to his room and will be right back.

10. Doc, WDYT about US and TENS to pt's wrist? [WDUT = what do you think]
    Dear Doctor Smart,
    Do you feel that US and TENS to pt's wrist would be beneficial at this time?
    —or—
    Doctor Smart,
    Please advise if you would like us to try US and TENS to help manage client's wrist pain.

Worksheet 2-2: People-First and Culturally Sensitive Language

Rewrite the following sentences using more appropriate people-first and culturally sensitive language (American Psychological Association [APA], 2020; Reed, et. al, 2019; U.S. Department of Education, 2017; Morreale & Amini, 2016, Harris, 2013).

1. The TBI was alert and oriented to person but not place or time.

    The client who sustained a traumatic brain injury was alert and oriented to person but not place or time.

2. The cerebral palsy child demonstrated difficulty fastening ½" buttons on her shirt because she is spastic.

    The child diagnosed with cerebral palsy demonstrated difficulty fastening ½" buttons on her shirt because she has spasticity in both upper extremities.

3. The first grader is fat and mentally retarded. She seems lazy.

    The first grader weighs 105 lb. and is diagnosed with an intellectual disability. She prefers sedentary activities and does not initiate performing chores/homework unless her parents offer reward incentives.

4. The resident diagnosed with polio is crippled and wheelchair bound.

    The resident diagnosed with polio is unable to ambulate and uses a wheelchair.
    —or—
    The resident diagnosed with polio is non-ambulatory and a wheelchair user.

5. The three Mexicans were teaching their classmates some Spanish phrases.

    The three students who emigrated to the U.S. from Mexico were teaching their classmates some Spanish phrases.

6. The client had a sex change.

    The client had gender affirmation surgery.

7. The OTA led an activity group consisting of two schizophrenics and two borderlines.

    The OTA led an activity group with two members diagnosed with schizophrenia and two members diagnosed with borderline personality disorder.
    —or—
    Diagnoses of the four group members in the OTA's activity group included schizophrenia and borderline personality disorder.

8. The Haitian stroke victim speaks only Creole.

    The client diagnosed with stroke is Haitian and speaks only Creole.
    —or—
    The client has a diagnosis of CVA. He is from Haiti and speaks only Creole.

9. The client suffers from amyotrophic lateral sclerosis and lives in an old folks home.

    The client diagnosed with amyotrophic lateral sclerosis resides in a skilled nursing facility.
    —or—
    The client diagnosed with amyotrophic lateral sclerosis lives in a boarding home for the elderly.
    —or—
    The client with a diagnosis of amyotrophic lateral sclerosis resides in an assisted living facility.

10. The quad has an upper respiratory infection. He is being very difficult and won't come to therapy.

    The individual with quadriplegia has an upper respiratory infection. He has refused therapy yesterday and today.

Worksheet 2-3: Written Communication

Resources: Morreale, 2022, Davis & Rosee, 2015

1. Proofread written communication and ensure that any auto-correct changes are accurate. This note contains a misspelled word (i.e., correct word is "horrible" rather than "horible") plus poor punctuation and grammar ("Lets" should be "let's").

2. Slang chat abbreviations such as, "Prof" "ur" "OMG" or "TTYL", are too casual to use in a professional note. It is best to avoid using slang terms.

3. Use a suitable greeting or salutation such as "Dear."

4. Use the person's full, appropriate title (i.e., Professor Smith, Mrs. Smith). **Ensure you have spelled the person's name correctly.** This author has often experienced students spelling the author's surname incorrectly on homework assignments and emails (i.e., Morreal or Morales rather than the proper spelling of Morreale).

5. Do not use all capitals in a word or sentence as this denotes shouting.

6. The use of emoticons, emojis, or creative signature designs does not give a professional appearance.

7. Consider the tone of what is written and how it may be perceived by the recipient. This note conveys an angry, accusatory, and demanding attitude.

8. In a professional note it is better to spell out certain standard abbreviations such as "as soon as possible."

9. Use a closing phrase before your name such as "Sincerely."

10. Use your full name to identify yourself, as the professor could have more than one student with the same first name.

Here is the same note written in a more useful format:

Dear Professor Smith,

Please let me know a convenient time that we can meet to discuss my activity analysis grade. Thank you.

Sincerely,

Stewart Stewdious

Chapter 3

Worksheet 3-1: Delegating Tasks to Aides

1. *Y* Help maintain inventory of adaptive equipment and supplies.

2. *Y* File OT department paperwork.

3. *N* Instruct the client in new therapy putty exercises.

4. *N* Perform retrograde massage to decrease hand edema.

5. *Y* Assist the OT practitioner with a client transfer by stabilizing chair or walker.

6. *N* Upgrade a client's exercise program.

7. *Y* Photocopy a home exercise program for client's chart.

8. *Y* Transport a stable client in a wheelchair from their hospital room to the OT room.

9. *Y* While the OTA is leading a sensory group, encourage a client in that group to handle and share the tactile objects.

10. *Y* Assist client in filling out routine client information forms.

11. *N* Teach a client how to use lower extremity adaptive equipment following a total hip replacement.

12. *N* Determine what adaptive feeding equipment is needed for a client who has a CVA with right hemiparesis.

13. *Y* Schedule OT appointments.

14. *N* Select activities for a client's fine motor exercises.

15. *Y* Assist the OTA with client wound care by opening packages of bandages and instruments without touching sterile materials inside.

16. *N* Adjust settings on a TENS unit when client reports not feeling the treatment modality work.

17. *Y* Sit and talk with a client while client is receiving a hot pack or other modality.

18. *Y* Assist a child with scissors skills when more practice is needed after child learns the task and condition is stable.

19. *Y* Obtain therapeutic equipment that the OTA will be using with client.

20. *Y* Cut out Velcro tabs and straps for an orthosis that the OTA is fabricating.

21. *N* Administer part of a standardized assessment.

22. *Y* Add more paraffin to unit when paraffin levels are low.

23. *Y* Maintain temperature log of hydrocollator.

24. *N* Determine if a client should have a paraffin treatment rather than a hot pack that day.

25. *Y* Set up client's meal tray in preparation for an occupational therapy feeding session.

26. *Y* Clean equipment and treatment tables/mats.

27. *Y* Place reality orientation calendar in client's room.

28. *N* Determine if a client is adhering to weight-bearing precautions during morning ADLs.

29. *Y* Call a client as a reminder to bring orthosis to tomorrow's therapy appointment.

30. *Y* To work on a client's dynamic balance, play catch with the client as the OTA is providing contact guard assist.

Worksheet 3-2: Billing and Reimbursement Terms

1.	*h. (Coinsurance)*	The 20% out-of-pocket expense that a Medicare Part B beneficiary pays for a covered service
2.	*f. (Medicaid)*	A combined federal-state health program with income eligibility guidelines
3.	*o. (IDEA Part B)*	Mandates an appropriate and free public education in the least restrictive environment for children with disabilities
4.	*n. (CMS-1500)*	A claim form
5.	*t. (Beneficiary)*	The person covered by an insurance plan
6.	*d. (Deductible)*	The initial out-of-pocket expenses an individual must pay to providers before the insurance company begins paying for those covered services
7.	*k. (Medicare Advantage Plan)*	Medicare Part C
8.	*j. (Fee schedule)*	Used by insurers to indicate set prices for covered services
9.	*q. (CPT codes)*	Used on claim forms to identify specific therapy services provided based on units of time
10.	*s. (CO modifier)*	Used to indicate services provided by an OTA under an OT plan of care
11.	*p. (Medicare Part D)*	A prescription drug program
12.	*a. (Third-party payer)*	An entity that pays for health services that is not the individual or provider
13.	*r. (ICD codes)*	Used to indicate a client's specific diagnosis or condition
14.	*l. (Workers' Compensation)*	A mandatory insurance that businesses pay to cover employees injured on the job
15.	*e. (IDEA Part C)*	Establishes early intervention services up to age 3 years
16.	*c. (Copayment)*	A set amount individuals pay to a health provider at each visit, in addition to what the insurer pays
17.	*i. (KX modifier)*	Used to indicate therapy services that exceed financial threshold limits
18.	*g. (Medigap insurance)*	A plan that helps pay for out-of-pocket Medicare expenses
19.	*m. (ABN)*	This must be provided prior to therapy exceeding Medicare Part B financial limits
20.	*b. (GO modifier)*	Used to indicate that occupational therapy services were provided

Worksheet 3-3: Billing and Coding

For each of the items below, indicate if it is true (T) or false (F).

1. *F* Tub seats and elevated toilet seats meet the CMS criteria for DME. *(Considered comfort/convenience items.)*

2. *F* A sock aid and long shoehorn for a client with total hip precautions are billed as DME. *(Does not meet criteria.)*

3. *T* Billing CMS for missed client appointments is fraud.

4. *F* For a client in occupational therapy, ADL practice supervised by an aide for 18 minutes should be billed as 1 unit. *(Services by an aide cannot be billed as skilled therapy.)*

5. *T* The modifier on claim forms that indicates an occupational therapy service is "GO."

6. *T* For Medicare Part B, a covered timed 25-minute occupational therapy skilled procedure is billed as 2 units.

7. *F* An OT who performs an occupational therapy evaluation (for a client with Medicare Part B) for 60 minutes should bill 4 units. *(An evaluation is untimed and billed as only 1 unit.)*

8. *F* The yearly financial limitation in 2021 for Medicare Part B therapy services is $2110 combined for physical, occupational, and speech therapy before any exceptions are applied. *($2110 for occupational therapy and an additional $2110 for physical and speech therapy combined)*

9. *T* CPT codes are maintained by the American Medical Association.

10. *F* HCPCS Level I codes are used to bill for items such as prosthetics and durable medical equipment (DME). *(Level II codes are used for these items.)*

11. *F* An OT and PT work together simultaneously with a client (skilled transfer training) for 15 minutes, which allows them to each bill Medicare Part B 1 unit of therapy. *(15 minutes equals one unit which can be billed by OT or PT but not both.)*

12. *F* ICD Codes are established by CMS. *(World Health Organization)*

13. *F* Total timed treatment time in minutes includes the time spent providing skilled interventions and documenting in the client's health record. *(Does not include non-billable time such as documentation.)*

14. *T* Twenty-one minutes of transfer training plus 8 minutes for client rest periods is billed as 1 unit. *(Time for rest periods is non-billable.)*

15. *T* The bundling of services reimbursed at a reduced rate is called the multiple procedure payment reduction.

Worksheet 3-4: Billing and Reimbursement Scenarios

For each scenario, fill in the blanks with the correct dollar amounts that the third-party payers and client would each have to pay for services furnished. Realize the numbers used are for illustrative purposes only.

1. *Client has Medicare Part A and B and has already met deductibles.*
    - Occupational therapy outpatient service—$90 charged by occupational therapy clinic
    - Medicare B allowable amount (MPFS)—$68
    - Medicare B pays **$54.40 (80% of $68)**
    - Medicare A pays **$0 (Part A does not cover outpatient therapy)**
    - Patient is responsible for paying **$13.60 (Coinsurance is 20% of $68)**
    - Total reimbursement to occupational therapy clinic for this service is **$68 ($54.40 + $13.60)**

2. *Client has private insurance that pays 90% of allowable amount. Client also has a remaining $150 deductible.*
    - Occupational therapy service—$60 charged by outpatient clinic
    - Insurance company allowable amount—$55
    - Physical therapy service—$60 charged by outpatient clinic
    - Insurance company allowable amount—$55
    - Insurance company pays **$0 (Insurance company does not pay anything until the client's deductible is met)**
    - Patient pays **$110 (Must pay out-of-pocket until $150 deductible is met)**
    - Total reimbursement to outpatient clinic for both services is **$110 ($55 + $55)**

3. *Client has Medicare Part B, Medigap insurance, and no deductible.*
    - Occupational therapy outpatient service —$110 charged by occupational therapy outpatient clinic
    - Medicare B allowable amount (MPFS)—$82
    - Medicare B pays **$65.60 (80% of $82)**
    - Medigap insurance pays **$16.40 ($20% of $82)**
    - Patient pays clinic **$0**
    - Total reimbursement to occupational therapy clinic for this service is **$82 ($65.60 + $16.40 is   the allowable amount paid fully by both insurances due to coordination of benefits)**

4. *Client has private insurance which pays 80% of covered services in-network and 75% out-of-network at allowable rates.*
   - Occupational therapy service—$120 charged by outpatient therapy clinic in-network provider
   - Insurance company allowable rate—$96
   - Insurance company pays **$76.80 (in-network pays 80% of $96)**
   - Client pays **$19.20 (remaining coinsurance amount is 20% of $96)**
   - Total reimbursement to occupational therapy clinic for this service is **$96 ($76.80 + $19.20)**
5. *Client has private insurance which requires a co-pay of $15 per outpatient therapy session.*
   - Occupational therapy service—$90 charged by occupational therapy outpatient clinic
   - Insurance company allowable amount—$72
   - Physical therapy service—$90 charged by outpatient clinic
   - Insurance company allowable amount—$72
   - Insurance company pays **$144 ($72 + $72)**
   - Patient pays **$30 (Has a co-pay for each service $15 + $15)**
   - Total reimbursement to outpatient clinic for both services is **$174 ($144 plus two $15 co-pays)**

Chapter 4

Worksheet 4-1: Using Abbreviations

1. Pt. Ⓘ ADLs.
   Patient is independent in activities of daily living.
2. Client reports ↓ pain Ⓡ shoulder p̄ HP.
   Client reports decreased pain in right shoulder following application of a hot pack.
3. Resident w/c ↔ EOB with SBA.
   Resident transferred from the wheelchair to edge of bed and transferred back to wheelchair with stand-by assist.
4. Client c/o pain in Ⓡ index MCP joint p̄ ~2 min PROM.
   Client complained of pain in the right index finger metacarpophalangeal joint after approximately 2 minutes of passive range of motion.
5. Client w/c → mat c̄ sliding board max Ⓐ x2.
   Client transferred from his wheelchair to the mat using a sliding board and maximum assistance of two people.
6. Pt. O x 4.
   Patient is oriented to person, place, time, and situation.
7. Client has SOB p̄ 30 reps of UE PRE.
   Client has shortness of breath after performing 30 repetitions of upper extremity progressive resistive exercises.
8. Pt. has ↓ STM and OCD which limit IADLs.
   Patient has decreased short-term memory and obsessive compulsive disorder, which limit instrumental activities of daily living performance.
9. Pt. min Ⓐ AMB bed → toilet 2° ↓ balance.
   Patient requires minimal assistance to ambulate from bed to toilet secondary to decreased balance.
10. Child's FM WFL to don AFO Ⓘ.
    The child's fine motor skills are within functional limits to put on ankle-foot orthosis independently.

Worksheet 4-2: Using Abbreviations—Additional Practice

1. Client requires minimal assistance to stand and pull up clothing with partial weight-bearing status of right lower extremity.
   Client min Ⓐ to stand and pull up clothing c̄ PWB Ⓡ LE.

2. Patient is able to feed herself independently with the use of built-up utensils.

   Pt. Ⓘ feeding c̄ built-up utensils.

3. Client has intact sensation in both upper extremities but reports minimal pain.

   Client has intact sensation Ⓑ UE but reports min pain.

4. Client has fifty-five degrees of passive range of motion in the left index distal interphalangeal joint, which is within functional limits.

   55° PROM in Ⓛ index DIP is WFL.

5. While sitting on edge of bed, client is able to put on her socks with standby assistance, but requires moderate assistance with putting on and taking off left shoe.

   Client dons socks c̄ SBA while sitting EOB but requires mod Ⓐ to don & doff Ⓛ shoe.

6. Student is independent in wheelchair mobility and activities of daily living.

   Student Ⓘ w/c mobility and ADLs.

7. Patient requires moderate assistance of two people to transfer from wheelchair to toilet and from toilet to wheelchair.

   Pt. mod Ⓐ x2 w/c ↔ toilet.

8. Patient's toe-touch weight-bearing status limits her performance of instrumental activities of daily living.

   Pt.'s TTWB limits IADLs.

9. Constraint induced movement therapy protocol was initiated to improve function of weak left upper extremity for activities of daily living.

   CIMT initiated to ↑ Ⓛ UE function for ADLs.

10. Client was lying on her back with head of bed raised. Client was able to correctly state her own name, the name of facility, and today's date. Neuromuscular electrical nerve stimulation was applied for ten minutes to right glenohumeral joint to help minimize subluxation.

    Client supine c̄ HOB raised. Client A&O X 3. NMES applied 10 min to Ⓡ glenohumeral joint to ↓ subluxation.

Worksheet 4-3: Deciphering Doctors' Orders and Abbreviations

1. Dx s/p Ⓡ TKR 2° OA, WBAT
   OT 2x/wk for BADLs, IADLs

   Diagnosis: status post right total knee replacement secondary to osteoarthritis, weightbearing as tolerated.
   Occupational therapy ordered two times weekly for basic and instrumental activities of daily living.

2. X-ray + Ⓛ index finger MCP Fx 2° GSW

   X-ray is positive for a left index finger metacarpophalangeal joint fracture, which is secondary to a gunshot wound.

3. 5 y.o. child has pain 2° bone CA Ⓛ LE

   Five-year-old child has pain secondary to bone cancer in left lower extremity.

4. Dx Ⓡ DRUJ Fx c̄ ORIF
   OT 3x/wk for PAMs PRN, P/AROM, ADLs, CPM

   Diagnosis is right distal radioulnar joint fracture with open reduction and internal fixation.
   Occupational therapy ordered three times weekly for physical agent modalities as needed, passive and active range of motion, activities of daily living, continuous passive motion.

5. 1° Dx PTSD, 2° Dx HTN

   Primary diagnosis is post-traumatic stress disorder; secondary diagnosis is hypertension.

6. 1° Dx DJD Ⓡ hip, 2° Dx COPD & CHF

   Primary diagnosis is degenerative joint disease right hip and secondary diagnoses are chronic obstructive pulmonary disease and congestive heart failure.

7. Dx CAD, TIA, PEG

   Diagnoses are coronary artery disease, transient ischemic attack, percutaneous endoscopic gastrostomy.

8. Dx Ⓡ BKA, CABG, HBV

   Diagnoses are right below-knee amputation, coronary artery bypass graft, and hepatitis B virus.

9. s/p Ⓛ TKR, PWB, OOB c̄ walker

   Client is status post left total-knee replacement. Client has partial weight-bearing status and is allowed to get out of bed using a walker.

10. Dx: C6 SCI, HTN, UTI

OT: eval for w/c and DME

Diagnoses: Spinal cord injury at 6th cervical level, hypertension, and urinary tract infection. Occupational therapy ordered to evaluate client for wheelchair and durable medical equipment needed.

Worksheet 4-4: Deciphering Abbreviations—More Practice

1. The infant remained in the NICU for 2 wks 2° to low birth wt of 2100 gm.

The infant remained in the neonatal intensive care unit for two weeks due to low birth weight of 2100 grams.

2. The resident reported LBP. He needed mod Ⓐ to don Ⓡ KAFO and CGA to transfer safely EOB → w/c using WBQC and FWB Ⓡ LE.

The resident reported low back pain. He needed moderate assistance to don right knee-ankle-foot orthosis. Contact guard assistance was needed to transfer safely from edge of bed to the wheelchair using a wide-base quad cane and full weightbearing of the right lower extremity.

3. To ↓ pain and edema Ⓛ elbow, client was instructed in RICE.

To reduce pain and edema in left elbow, client was instructed to rest the elbow, apply ice and a compression wrap, and elevate the extremity.

4. Client needs DME recommendations and ADL instruction following LVAD.

Client needs durable medical equipment recommendations and instruction in activities of daily living following left ventricular assist device surgery.

5. This yr the OT and PT were part of the school district committee that developed new policies and procedures regarding HIB and IEPs.

This year the occupational therapist and physical therapist were part of the school district committee that developed new policies and procedures regarding harassment, intimidation, bullying and Individualized Education Programs.

6. Dx: PDD-NOS, ADHD

OT: ADLs, SI, FM

2 x/wk X 12 wks

Diagnoses are pervasive developmental disorder not otherwise specified and attention deficit hyperactivity disorder. Occupational therapy ordered for activities of daily living, sensory integration, fine-motor skills.
Twice weekly for twelve weeks.

7. EMG pos. Ⓡ CTS and neg. TOS

Electromyogram is positive for right carpal tunnel syndrome and negative for thoracic outlet syndrome.

8. Dx: s/p Ⓛ THR, pt. NWB Ⓛ LE

OT eval. and tx; ADLs, Ⓑ UE PREs

3x/wk X 4 wks

Diagnosis is status post left total hip replacement. Patient has non-weight-bearing status for left lower extremity. Occupational therapy ordered for evaluation and treatment, activities of daily living, bilateral upper extremity progressive resistive exercises.
Three times weekly for 4 weeks.

9. MRI + TBI, VS stable, BRP c̄ assist

Magnetic resonance imaging is positive for traumatic brain injury. Vital signs are stable. Patient is allowed bathroom privileges (able to get out of bed and use the bathroom) with assistance.

10. CXR neg. TB but pos. URI. Pt. has DOE and FUO.

Chest x-ray is negative for tuberculosis but positive for an upper respiratory infection. Patient has dyspnea upon exertion and fever of unknown origin.

Worksheet 4-5: Additional Practice

1. *Pt. participated in OT session bedside for instruction in ADLs. Supine → sit at EOB c̄ min Ⓐ. Max Ⓐ to don lower body garments over feet and mod Ⓐ sit → stand to pull up clothing. Mod Ⓐ to don upper body garments.*

2. *Resident to OT via w/c escort. Resident leans ⓛ and needs verbal cues and min physical assist to maintain symmetrical posture in midline while seated. Standing pivot transfer w/c → toilet mod Ⓐ for balance. Verbal cues and feedback using a mirror needed to maintain upright posture.*
    —or—
    Resident to OT via w/c escort. Resident leans ⓛ and needs verbal cues and visual feedback from mirror to maintain upright symmetrical posture in midline. Standing pivot w/c → toilet mod Ⓐ for balance.

3. *Pt. 10 wks s/p ⓛ DRUJ Fx and presently has URI. Pt. participated in 40-minute session in OT clinic for assessment of selected, relevant client factors. Strength ⓛ shoulder and elbow flex. & ext. 4/5, wrist flex. & ext. 3-/5, grip strength 8#. Light touch intact. Ⓡ UE strength and sensation WFL.*

4. *Client is a 65 y.o. ♀ diagnosed with MS and low vision. OT eval included COPM, visual acuity, visual-perception, ROM, MMT. PMH: sleep apnea for ~ past 18 mos. and uses CPAP nightly. Hx of HTN 5 yrs.*

5. *10-y.o. male student in 4th grade dx c̄ ADHD. LTGs in IEP include: 30-min sustained sitting at desk during class s̄ verbal cues from teacher and ability to complete art class project during time allotted s̄ needing redirection to task.*

Worksheet 4-6: Generating Abbreviations

Here are some suggestions from the abbreviations list in this manual:
Lower extremity weight-bearing status:
  NWB, TTWB, PWB, WBAT, FWB
Different types of range of motion:
  ROM, PROM, AROM, AAROM, TAM, TPM
Physical agent modalities:
  US, W/cm², MHz, HP, CPM, TENS, NMES, °C, °F, HVPC

Chapter 5

Worksheet 5-1: Quoting and Paraphrasing

1. *C*   The child stated that she was extremely hungry.
2. *I*   The child stated that "she was starving."
3. *I*   The child "stated I am starving."
4. *C*   The child verbalized that she was "starving."
5. *I*   The child stated "I am starving".
6. *I*   The patient asked how to put her orthosis on?
7. *I*   The patient asked "How do I put my orthosis on"?
8. *C*   The patient asked about the proper way to put on her orthosis.
9. *C*   The patient asked, "How do I put my orthosis on?"
10. *I*   The patient asked "how to put her orthosis on."
11. *C*   The client requested a new buttonhook.
12. *I*   The client asked if "she could have a new buttonhook."
13. *I*   The client asked, "Can I have a new buttonhook"?
14. *C*   The client asked for a new buttonhook.
15. *C*   The client asked, "Can I have a new buttonhook?"
16. *I*   The client stated "he felt dizzy" as he stood at the kitchen counter.
17. *C*   The client reported feeling "dizzy" while standing at the kitchen counter.
18. *I*   While standing at the kitchen counter, the client stated "he felt dizzy."
19. *I*   The client, while standing at the kitchen counter, stated I feel "dizzy."
20. *C*   The client reported dizziness while standing at the kitchen counter.

Worksheet 5-2: Spelling

Place a check mark next to the word that is spelled correctly.

1. _____ defered   ___✓___ deferred
2. _____ definately   ___✓___ definitely
3. ___✓___ dining   _____ dinning
4. _____ excercise   ___✓___ exercise
5. _____ parraffin   ___✓___ paraffin
6. _____ transfering   ___✓___ transferring
7. _____ recieve   ___✓___ receive
8. _____ pnumonia   ___✓___ pneumonia
9. _____ rotator cup   ___✓___ rotator cuff
10. _____ tolorate   ___✓___ tolerate
11. _____ therapy puddy   ___✓___ therapy putty
12. ___✓___ independent   _____ independant
13. ___✓___ tremors   _____ tremers
14. ___✓___ phlegm   _____ phlem
15. _____ diaphram   ___✓___ diaphragm
16. _____ urinary track   ___✓___ urinary tract
17. _____ anasthesia   ___✓___ anesthesia
18. ___✓___ brachial plexus   _____ brachial plexis
19. ___✓___ incontinence   _____ incontinents
20. _____ illiac crest   ___✓___ iliac crest
21. ___✓___ oculomotor   _____ occulomotor
22. ___✓___ vitiligo   _____ vitilago
23. _____ diaphorretic   ___✓___ diaphoretic
24. ___✓___ boutonniere deformity   _____ boutinniere deformity
25. ___✓___ homonymous hemianopsia   _____ homonomous hemianopsia

Worksheet 5-3: Spelling—More Practice

Place a check mark next to the word that is spelled correctly.

1. ___✓___ counseling   _____ counselling
2. ___✓___ diarrhea   _____ diarrea
3. _____ hemhorrage   ___✓___ hemorrhage
4. ___✓___ benefit   _____ benifit
5. ___✓___ interfered   _____ interferred
6. _____ eyesite   ___✓___ eyesight
7. _____ pullies   ___✓___ pulleys
8. _____ extention   ___✓___ extension
9. _____ hygeine   ___✓___ hygiene
10. ___✓___ preparation   _____ preperation
11. ___✓___ therapeutic   _____ theraputic
12. _____ flexability   ___✓___ flexibility
13. ___✓___ strength   _____ strenth
14. _____ assymetrical   ___✓___ asymmetrical
15. ___✓___ toilet   _____ toliet

16. __✓__ leisure   _____ liesure
17. __✓__ nauseous   _____ nauseus
18. _____ eccymosis   __✓__ ecchymosis
19. __✓__ paresthesia   _____ parasthesia
20. __✓__ pulse oximeter   _____ pulse oxymeter
21. _____ glycometer   __✓__ glucometer
22. _____ bollis   __✓__ bolus
23. __✓__ jejunostomy   _____ jujenostomy
24. __✓__ sphygmomanometer _____ sphygnomanometer
25. _____ electromyelogram   __✓__ electromyogram

Worksheet 5-4: Using Words Correctly

1. The home health *aide* gave the patient a shower.
2. The client refused to *accept* the doctor's diagnosis.
3. The traumatic brain injury will have a tremendous *effect* on activities of daily living.
4. If the client falls, she probably will *break* her hip due to osteoporosis.
5. The patient became short of *breath* after ambulating to the bathroom.
6. The client stated she wanted to *lose* 10 pounds.
7. The patient injured her *dominant* right hand, which prevented her from writing.
8. The occupational therapy room is *farther* down the hallway than the physical therapy room.
9. The *current* caseload consists of 10 clients, as compared to 15 clients last week.
10. The OT asked the patient to *lay* the scissors down on the table.
11. The weight of the pan was more *than* the patient could manage.
12. The clients in the craft group put *their* projects away in the closet.
13. The child was able to remain quiet and *stationary* while standing in line.
14. The *principal* of the school attended the IEP meeting.
15. The resident regained *continence* of bowel and bladder.

Worksheet 5-5: Using Words Correctly—More Practice

1. The client has difficulty *gripping* the steering wheel.
2. The client was able to navigate his wheelchair throughout the store's *aisles* without knocking anything over.
3. The patient refused to take *personal* responsibility for his actions.
4. The patient reported pain when his biceps muscle was *palpated* by the OTA.
5. The client was able to *perform* all bathing tasks without assistance.
6. The child asked for a *piece* of candy.
7. The client had difficulty swallowing liquids due to *dysphagia*.
8. The student was denied *access* to the client's medical record.
9. The client followed the OTA's *advice* and purchased a shower chair.
10. A buttonhook can be a useful assistive *device* for clients with impaired dexterity.
11. The student was *adept* at playing the violin.
12. The client developed a lung infection due to *aspiration* of food.
13. The resident was very *impulsive* during transfers as she would not wait for the wheelchair to be properly positioned and locked before trying to stand up.
14. The occupational therapy assistant handed the client an *emesis* basin because the client was nauseous.
15. The child's *residence* was unsafe due to the presence of lead.

Worksheet 5-6: Capitals

Underline the words that do not correctly follow the rules for capitals.

1. The OTA put the chart on the <u>Occupational Therapist's</u> desk.
2. The <u>Patient</u> was going to see his <u>Doctor</u> this afternoon.
3. The OT <u>Aide</u> used <u>velcro</u> and Scotch <u>Tape</u> to fix Mrs. Smith's lapboard during the occupational therapy session.
4. The <u>Doctor</u> spoke to the child who has <u>Chicken Pox</u>.
5. The OTA <u>Student</u> performed a <u>Sensory Test</u> on the client.
6. The client took Tylenol and <u>Antacids</u> before his <u>Business Meeting</u>.
7. The <u>Nurse</u> told the new mother that the infant has <u>down</u> syndrome.
8. The <u>Physical Therapist</u> informed the OTA that their client was admitted to the <u>Hospital</u> due to <u>Pneumonia</u>.
9. The <u>Occupational</u> therapy assistant worked in the outpatient department.
10. The OT used the Miller <u>assessment</u> for <u>preschoolers</u> to assess the child with <u>Autism</u>.
11. The <u>Skilled Nursing Facility Resident</u> diagnosed with <u>guillain-barre</u> syndrome also has <u>Dementia</u>.
12. The OT <u>club</u> at the local <u>Community College</u> volunteered at a <u>Food</u> pantry last weekend and donated canned goods, <u>kleenex</u>, <u>band-aids</u>, and paper towels.
13. The OTA <u>Student</u> attended an <u>Inservice</u> to learn more about kinesiology.
14. The OTA students had opportunities to observe OTs working in <u>Hand Therapy Clinics</u>, <u>Long-Term Care</u> facilities, and <u>Elementary</u> schools.
15. The local newspaper wrote an article about We-Care Rehabilitation Hospital <u>occupational therapy department</u>.

Worksheet 5-7: Pronouns, Plurals, and Possessives

Look at the following sentences and determine the incorrect components in each sentence. The corrections are provided in bold.

1. The three *clients'* appointments were all rescheduled because their OTA was ill.
2. The *OTA's* lab coat was new.
3. The OTA *student's* résumé was reviewed by the OT.
4. The *child's parents* attended most therapy *sessions*.
5. The children almost hurt *themselves* when they collided with each other in the hallway.
6. The *nurses'* patient gave them all flowers.
7. The *PTs* and *OTs* had the day off.
8. The occupational *therapist's* paperwork was on the *administrative assistant's* desk.
9. One of the *clients* left an *orthotic* device on the food tray.
10. The OT took the *OTA's* lab coat home by mistake.
11. Sarah told her math and social studies *teachers* she did the homework by *herself*.
12. The broken wheelchairs were repaired by the two *PTAs*.
13. The student had difficulty opening the *combination* lock on the locker.
14. The client diagnosed with depression completed a three-*step* craft *project* independently.
15. The parents **were** given a variety of *equipment* to help improve the *triplets'* motor skills.

Chapter 6

Worksheet 6-1: Choosing a Subjective Statement

In this instance, a pending visit by the client's grandson is not really relevant to the intervention session or to how the client sees her progress. For a different situation, it might be important to note. For example, if the client were planning to go to live with her grandson after discharge, it might be very relevant and a topic the OT or OTA would explore further with the client.

Even though the client may have been cooperative, and even though this may have been important in this intervention session, it is an assessment of the situation and does not belong in the "S" category of the note. The client's social conversation might be important in some situations. However, there is a better choice for this particular note.

Feeling "pretty good" today might be important, because it might show progress or a change in her condition. In this case, however, it is not the best choice.

The client's observations and statements about her upper extremity seem most pertinent to this intervention session as use of the Ⓡ UE is relevant in all aspects of this session.

A report of safety concerns by nursing might be relevant to this client's treatment. However, it is not the best choice for the "S" category of this note for several reasons. A concern by nursing staff should be documented in the nursing notes. The OTA should report what they see rather than what some other staff member believes. Finally, the subjective section of the SOAP note is used to document the client's views about treatment rather than the staff's views, except in rare instances.

Worksheet 6-2: Writing Concise, Coherent Statements

Client reports using adaptive equipment to don pants and socks while maintaining hip precautions without difficulty. She reports no pain in Ⓛ hip when transferring to toilet using raised seat. Client states her daughter now has bathroom equipment in home that was ordered by OT last week.

Chapter 7

Worksheet 7-1: Organizing the "O" With Categories

Some or all of the following categories might be used to make this note easier to read:

- *Ⓛ UE use or reach/grasp/release*
- *Ⓡ UE use or stabilization for sitting balance*
- *Feeding*
- *Attention/attention to task/attention span*
- *Orthotic device*

Depending on the categories selected, the note might read:

Child engaged in 60-minute OT session in daycare setting to work on increasing functional use of Ⓛ UE and feeding skills. Child wore a Ⓛ soft thumb spica orthosis throughout the intervention session.

Reach/grasp/release: *With min Ⓐ for facilitation of elbow movement, child demonstrated ability to use Ⓛ UE to reach, grasp, and release 5 objects with 1 to 2 verbal cues per object.*

Stabilization/sitting balance: *Child used Ⓡ UE to stabilize self for unsupported sitting at table.*

Feeding: *Child was able to feed self Ⓘ with ~50% spillage, but demonstrated significant limitations in chewing action with ~3 rotary chews and swallowing ~90% of the food without chewing.*

Attention: *Child required verbal cues throughout the session to maintain attention to task.*

Worksheet 7-2: Using Professional Terminology

Here are some suggestions to make these sentences sound more professional. You may come up with other wording that may also be acceptable.

1. The client said she had pain just past the pinky knuckle in her bad hand.
   Client reported pain in her involved hand just proximal to small finger MP joint.
   -or-
   Client states pain present in affected hand just proximal to small finger MP joint.
2. Five minutes after the treatment session started, the patient said he had to go to the bathroom.
   5 min into session, client needed to use restroom.
   -or-
   Five minutes after session began, client asked to use the restroom.
3. The client afflicted with Alzheimer's occasionally has an accident in his diaper.
   The client, diagnosed with Alzheimer's disease, has occasional episodes of fecal incontinence.
   -or-
   The client is diagnosed with Alzheimer's disease and exhibits occasional incontinence of feces.
4. The OTA gave the client therapy putty for home use.
   Client was issued therapy putty for home use.
   -or-
   Client was issued therapy putty for use in home exercise program.
5. The teenager complained of cramps because it was that time of the month for her.
   Teen reported having cramps now due to menses.
   -or-
   Teen stated she is not feeling well due to menstrual cramps.
6. The client's left glenohumeral joint crackled when passive range of motion was done to it.
   Crepitation noted in left glenohumeral joint upon PROM.
7. The client suffers from multiple sclerosis and says she has difficulty putting on her lower extremity garments.
   The client has multiple sclerosis and reports difficulty donning lower body garments.
   -or-
   Client reports difficulty donning lower body garments due to her MS symptoms.
8. The OTA gave the senile client a mental status exam.
   Mental status exam administered to client diagnosed with Alzheimer's disease.
   -or-
   Client has Alzheimer's disease. Mental status exam was administered during today's OT session.
9. It was determined that the very obese client needed an oversized electric wheelchair and he was instructed in wheelchair ambulation.
   Client fitted for bariatric power wheelchair and instructed in wheelchair mobility.
10. The dyspraxic child said she tripped on her shoelaces and fell on her bottom, sustaining a large black and blue.
    Child has dyspraxia and reports falling recently due to tripping on her shoelaces. She sustained large ecchymosis on buttocks.

Worksheet 7-3: Using Professional Terminology—More Practice

Here are some suggestions to make these sentences sound more professional. You may come up with other wording that may also be acceptable.

1. On the way to school, the child threw up on the school bus and became sweaty and clammy.
   While riding bus going to school, child vomited and became diaphoretic.
2. The paraplegic client developed a bedsore on his sit bones.
   The client with paraplegia has a sacral pressure injury.
3. The preschool accepted normal and abnormal children.
   The preschool accepted children with typical and atypical development.

4. The client was unable to wash her right armpit because she could not actively lift her bad right shoulder.
   Client dependent in washing right axilla 2° inability to actively flex or abduct affected right shoulder.
   -or-
   Client unable to wash right axilla due to poor muscle strength (2/5) for right shoulder flex/abd.

5. The OTA showed the client a different way to put on upper extremity clothes so that the client could do this by herself.
   Client instructed in compensatory techniques for upper body dressing.

6. The child asked for a tissue because he had snot running down his face.
   Child had rhinorrhea and requested a tissue.

7. The client's hearing improved after the doctor removed excessive earwax.
   Client's hearing improved following removal of cerumen by physician.

8. After going to the bathroom the autistic child rubbed some poop on the bathroom wall.
   After defecating, the child diagnosed with autism rubbed feces on the wall.

9. The brain-damaged client said he has double vision.
   The client has a diagnosis of traumatic brain injury and reports diplopia.

10. The client takes nitroglycerin under his tongue and takes an insulin shot in his stomach.
    Client takes nitroglycerin sublingually and injects insulin into his abdomen.

Worksheet 7-4: Trademarked Versus Generic Therapy Terms

For each of the following brand names, indicate the generic equivalent term you might use in documentation.

1. Purell (*alcohol-based hand sanitizer*)
2. Velcro (*hook and loop fastener*)
3. Dycem (*non-slip matting*)
4. Polyform, Aquaplast, Ezeform (*thermoplastic material*)
5. Ace bandage (*elastic bandage*)
6. Kinesio Tape (*kinesiology tape*)
7. Pampers (*disposable diapers*)
8. Theraputty (*therapy putty*)
9. Theraband (*exercise band, resistance band*)
10. Neosporin (*anti-bacterial ointment*)
11. Advil (*ibuprofen*)
12. Tylenol (*acetaminophen*)
13. Q-tip (*cotton-tipped swab, cotton-tipped applicator*)
14. Chux (*disposable underpads*)
15. Nerf ball (*foam ball, sponge ball*)
16. Thick-It (*thickener*)
17. TED stockings (*anti-embolism stockings, anti-embolism hose*)
18. Hoyer lift (*mechanical lift, hydraulic lift*)
19. Jobst glove (*compression glove*)
20. Coban, CoFlex (*self-adherent bandage*)

Worksheet 7-5: Being More Concise

Client participated in 30-minute session in room for skilled instruction in ADLs. He ambulated ~3 ft to shower stall c̄ SBA for balance. Client showered (took ~20 minutes) and dressed with verbal cues to sit for both activities. SBA also needed to manage IV lines. Following shower, client required SBA for balance in order to stand and adjust clothing and to ambulate and transfer back to bed safely.

—or—

Client participated in 30-minute ADL session in room for skilled instruction in safe showering and dressing. Client ambulated ~3' SBA for balance. After verbal cues to sit, client showered in 20 min with SBA to manage IV lines. Dressed upper body ① while seated and lower body with verbal cues to remain seated. Following shower, client required SBA to ambulate and transfer to bed safely.

Worksheet 7-6: Using Professional Language

1. *Resident diagnosed with Parkinson disease. She is oriented to person and place but not always oriented to time. Uses wheeled walker and exhibits shuffling gait when ambulating. Client requires occasional verbal reminders to avoid pulling up from walker when rising (from bed, chair, and toilet), which is unsafe. When experiencing urinary urgency, resident tends to ambulate too quickly to the bathroom to avoid an episode of incontinence and is unsteady. These factors create risk for falling at home.*

2. *Client's dressing skills were assessed. Client donned bathrobe and slippers with three verbal cues needed to tie belt and two verbal cues to determine ® and ⓛ slippers. Client performed functional ambulation bed to chair with wheeled walker and required CGA for balance. While seated in chair, client was positioned with pillows to support and elevate affected upper extremity and promote upright trunk posture in midline orientation.*

3. *® volar wrist extension orthosis was fabricated and issued to minimize CTS symptoms which client reports as pain and numbness in hand. Following skilled instruction, client demonstrated ability to don/doff orthosis ⓛ.*

4. *Logan participated in 30-minute OT session in second-grade classroom for assessment of assistive technology needed to enable independent computer tablet use. Logan's cerebral palsy symptoms (spasticity, decreased voluntary control and unwanted movements of upper extremities) create difficulty with accurate touchscreen use. He exhibits fair/good midline orientation in wheelchair and good head control. Following skilled instruction in low-tech device use of a tablet stand and mouthstick, Logan was able to write his name 5 times without any errors.*

Worksheet 7-7: Understanding Health Care Terms

1. B
2. A
3. C
4. A *(The term indicates a client is "stuck" on certain words or behavior.)*
5. C
6. C
7. D
8. B
9. B *(This term relates to "crackling" of joints when moved.)*
10. C
11. A
12. D
13. D
14. C
15. B
16. A *(This term refers to moving objects from the fingertips into the palm.)*
17. D *(An oversize wheelchair is needed due to the client's excessive weight.)*

18. A
19. B (*A different term, dysphagia, relates to eating and swallowing.*)
20. C (*Presbycusis is age-related hearing loss. The only choice that helps compensate for hearing loss is C.*)

Chapter 8

Worksheet 8-1: De-Emphasizing the Treatment Media

1. Client played a game of catch using bilateral UEs to facilitate grasp and release patterns.
   Client worked on dynamic gross grasp/release patterns needed to manipulate household objects.
2. Resident put dirt into pot to halfway point, added seedling, and filled remainder of pot with dirt, which was transferred by cup. Resident completed three more pots while standing 8 minutes before requiring a 5-minute rest. Resident then resumed standing position for approximately 5 minutes to water completed pots.
   Resident demonstrated standing tolerance of 13 minutes with a 5-minute break after 8 minutes, in order increase endurance and standing balance needed for ADL tasks.
3. Client painted some picture frames in crafts group to be able to see that she could do something successfully.
   Client completed a series of quick-success projects to increase self-esteem.
4. Child traced around a can to make a circle and then cut out the circle to work on his visual-motor skills. He also drew a face in the circle and glued it onto a paper bag to make a puppet.
   Child worked on improving visual-motor skills for classroom activities by completing an activity involving tracing, cutting, drawing, and pasting.

Worksheet 8-2: Being Specific About Assist Levels

Without having seen the intervention session, it is impossible to know what part of the tasks required assistance. However, here are some suggestions for how the statement might have been worded:

1. Client supine → sit with min Ⓐ; bed → w/c with mod Ⓐ.
   - *Client supine → sit with min Ⓐ to initiate activity; bed → w/c with mod Ⓐ for balance.*
   - *Client supine → sit with min Ⓐ to pull up using trapeze; bed → w/c with mod Ⓐ to lift body weight.*
   - *Client supine → sit with min Ⓐ to sequence movement; bed → w/c with mod Ⓐ to bend forward to 45° when rising.*
   - *Client supine → sit with min Ⓐ swinging legs to EOB; bed → w/c with mod Ⓐ for postural control.*
2. Client required SBA in transferring w/c ↔ toilet.
   - *Client required SBA for proper hand placement in transferring w/c ↔ toilet.*
   - *Client required SBA to remind him of steps of the transfer when transferring w/c ↔ toilet.*
   - *Client required SBA to remind him to lock w/c brakes and lean forward in order to rise from chair when transferring w/c ↔ toilet.*
3. Client retrieved garments from low drawers with min Ⓐ.
   - *Client retrieved garments from low drawers with min Ⓐ to open drawers.*
   - *Client retrieved garments from low drawers with min Ⓐ to release trigger on reacher.*
   - *Client retrieved garments from low drawers with min Ⓐ to judge halo placement in space.*
   - *Client retrieved garments from low drawers with min Ⓐ to grasp handles of drawers.*
4. Brushing hair required max Ⓐ.
   - *Brushing hair required max Ⓐ to hold brush.*
   - *Brushing hair required max Ⓐ to reach back of head.*
   - *Brushing hair required max Ⓐ to flex shoulder past 35°.*

5.   Client completed dressing, toileting, and hygiene with min Ⓐ.
   • *Client completed dressing, toileting, and hygiene with min Ⓐ for sitting balance.*
   • *Client completed dressing, toileting, and hygiene with min Ⓐ for sequencing.*
   • *Client completed dressing, toileting, and hygiene with min Ⓐ for activities requiring fine motor dexterity.*
   • *Client completed dressing, toileting, and hygiene with min Ⓐ to adhere to hip precautions.*

Chapter 9

Worksheet 9-1: Organizing Your Thoughts for Assessment

Problems:
   • *Safety of transferring to and from the toilet*
   • *Client factors that were not WFL (AROM shoulder abduction).*
   • *Decreased performance skills (activity tolerance and dynamic balance)*

Progress/potential:
   • *Verbalized an understanding of safety instructions*
   • *PROM Ⓡ shoulder abduction WNL*

   A: *Safety concerns (impulsivity, ↓ dynamic standing balance) noted when client attempts to transfer sit → stand during toileting. Client verbalized an understanding of safety instructions and has potential to progress to independence. Client's ↓ AROM in right shoulder, ↓ activity tolerance, and ↓ dynamic standing balance all interfere with ability to complete ADL tasks safely and independently. Client would benefit from Ⓡ UE AROM and strengthening exercises along with continued skilled instruction on safety and energy conservation techniques.*

Worksheet 9-2: Justifying Continued Treatment

Which of the following require the skill of an OTA (AOTA 2018a, 2020a, 2020b, 2021a, 2021b)?
Note that OTA tasks are performed under the OT's supervision.

1. *No*   Administering paraffin irrelevant to occupational performance (*Stand-alone PAMS are not considered occupational therapy* [AOTA, 2018b].)
2. *Yes*   Instructing the client in leisure skills for stress management
3. *No*   Having a client watch a video on assertiveness training without further instruction or without role-playing the techniques (*Need instruction and practice*)
4. *Yes*   Analyzing and modifying functional tasks/activities through the provision of adaptive equipment or techniques
5. *Yes*   Determining that the modified task is safe and effective
6. *No*   Carrying out a routine maintenance program
7. *No*   Upgrading the intervention plan (*This is the role of the OT.*)
8. *Yes*   Teaching the client to use the breathing techniques he has learned while performing his ADL activities
9. *No*   Interpreting initial evaluation results and establishing the intervention plan (*This is the responsibility of the OT.*)
10. *Yes*   Providing individualized instruction to the client, family, or caregiver
11. *No*   Giving the client a replacement piece of hook and loop fastener (*Anyone can give the client a piece of hook and loop fastener. If the OTA was modifying a piece of equipment or an orthotic device, then that might be considered skilled occupational therapy.*)
12. *No*   Making the decision to discharge a client from occupational therapy (*This is the role of an OT; although, the OTA can provide recommendations to the OT.*)
13. *Yes*   Writing out a home exercise program and instructing the client
14. *Yes*   Teaching compensatory skills

15. *No*   Gait training with goal of increasing ambulation distance *(This is the role of PT. OT practitioners address functional ambulation for specific occupations and activities, such as being able to carry items from refrigerator to table or obtain clothing from closet.)*

16. *Yes*   Making recommendations to a parent for a child's positioning and feeding

17. *Yes*   Educating clients to eliminate safety hazards

18. *Yes*   Teaching adaptive techniques such as one-handed shoe tying

19. *No*   Helping a client in the bathroom *(An aide or family member can simply help a client; OTAs provide skilled instruction or modification of the task.)*

20. *No*   Telling a client about a new computer app *(Skilled occupational therapy is not just conversing with a client. However, if the OTA was providing instruction or making specific recommendations as part of the client's intervention plan, then that would be considered a skilled service.)*

Worksheet 9-3: Assessing Factors Not Within Functional Limits

1. Child wrote poorly due to immature pencil grasp and difficulty with spatial orientation of letters.
   Poor visual-spatial perception and immature pencil grasp interfere with writing skills.
2. Client demonstrated difficulty with balancing her checkbook due to memory and sequencing deficits.
   Memory and sequencing deficits cause difficulty with IADL tasks such as balancing checkbook.
3. Client problem solved poorly while performing lower body dressing as evidenced by multiple attempts to button shirt and don socks.
   Client's ↓ ability to problem solve limits her ability to dress herself without Ⓐ and raises safety concerns in all ADL areas.
4. Client was unable to hang clothes in closet or place dishes in upper kitchen cabinets due to P/AROM shoulder flexion/abduction limited to 105°.
   Client's shoulder contracture limits performance of home management tasks.

Worksheet 9-4: Social Skills Worksheet

1. What **problems** are evident in the above "S" and "O"?
   - *Unkempt appearance*
   - *Interrupts others when talking*
   - *Does not stay on topic of conversation*
2. What **areas of occupation** are affected by these problems?
   - *Social participation*
3. What evidence of **progress** and/or **potential** do you see?
   - *Engages in conversation*
   - *States that she understands the purpose of the group*
   - *Willingness to participate in the group*
   - *Spontaneously shared her ideas and experiences*

   A: *Client's unkempt appearance, interrupting behaviors, and need for redirection to topic of conversation interfere with her ability to engage in social participation with peers. Her expressed interest in groups and her willingness to engage in conversation and share her ideas show good potential to develop relationships and to express herself verbally in place of acting out. Client would benefit from participating in groups where conversational skills are stressed along with further facilitation of attention to social cues, and from assistance with ADL activities stressing hygiene and appearance.*

Chapter 10

Worksheet 10-1: Determining the Plan

P: *Continue OT 5 X wk for 1 week for skilled instruction in safe transfers and toileting. Home program for AROM and strengthening exercises for ® shoulder will be taught.*

—or—

P: *Continue OT for 1 hour 5 X wk for 1 week to work on safe transfers, toileting, and improving activity tolerance. Client will be instructed in HEP to improve ® shoulder AROM and strength.*

Worksheet 10-2: Completing the Social Skills Plan

P: *Client to continue daily OT for the next week to ↑ interpersonal skills and ADLs needed for social participation in a variety of contexts.*

—or—

P: *Client to continue social skills group 3 X wk and to be given individual feedback daily on her attention to appearance and social cues.*

Worksheet 10-3: Completing the Plan—Additional Practice

P: *Client to continue OT 2 X wk for 3 wks to ↑ ® hand strength, functional fine motor skills, and ADLs. Next session, client will be instructed in one-handed shoe tying technique and will be assessed for return demonstration of HEP.*

—or—

P: *Client to continue OT twice weekly for 3 weeks for instruction in compensatory techniques and remediation of ® fine motor skills and hand strength to enable ADL performance. Client will be instructed in adaptive equipment needed to manage all clothing fastenings Ⓘ. HEP to be upgraded by increasing resistance of therapy putty next week.*

Chapter 12

Worksheet 12-1: Mechanics of Documentation

1. Time of day not recorded
2. No health record number or identification number present
3. Last name is not listed first (may not be required by facility to list last name first)
4. Spaces present without line drawn (for a handwritten note)
5. Error not corrected properly—should have date and initials above or next to the error for a handwritten note or follow established procedures for EHR
6. No co-signature (will depend on facility and legal guidelines)
7. Type of note not indicated (contact note)
8. Occupational therapy department not indicated
9. Spelling errors (escorted, deferred)
10. OTA's first name only indicated by initial
11. License not designated in credentials—COTA/L (if required in that state)
12. Punctuation error (nurses should be nurse's)

Worksheet 12-2: Documentation Basics

For each of the following SOAP note sentences, correct any errors in spelling, grammar, abbreviations, and basic mechanics of documentation.

1. The client used **compensitory** techniques to **donn** his shoes and socks.

   The client used compensatory techniques to don his shoes and socks.

2. The client **preformed** bed mobility Ⓘ, then sat on **SOB** with SBA to doff his shirt.

   The client performed bed mobility Ⓘ, then sat on EOB with SBA to doff his shirt.

   (SOB is the abbreviation for shortness of breath.)

3. Child **was seen** for 20 minutes in classroom **to help** her put her coat on.

   Child participated in 20-minute session in classroom to improve skills needed for donning her coat.
   —or—
   Child participated in 20-minute session in classroom for skilled ADL instruction.

   (Remember to show active client participation in therapy. Also, as a teacher or aide could help the child put a coat on, be sure to indicate the skilled services that the occupational therapy practitioner is providing.)

4. Client stated he will "not wear **his orthosis** to work."

   Client stated he will not wear his orthosis to work.
   —or—
   Client stated, "I will not wear my orthosis to work."

5. The **CVA pt.** demonstrated ability to transfer bed ↔ commode with SBA and **VC**.

   The pt. diagnosed with CVA demonstrated ability to transfer bed ↔ commode with SBA and verbal cues.
   —or—
   The pt. who sustained a CVA demonstrated ability to transfer bed ↔ commode with SBA and verbal cues.

   (Always use people-first language. Also, VC is the abbreviation for vital capacity per Table 4-1.)

6. The child demonstrated progress by using her **bad** hand to stabilize the paper when writing.

   The child demonstrated progress by using her affected hand (or involved or weak hand) to stabilize the paper when writing.

   (Don't use "bad" or "good" to delineate limbs.)

7. During her **Occupational Therapy** session, the pt. worked on ↑ Ⓛ **neglect and** ↓ **safety** to perform ADLs.

   During her occupational therapy session, the pt. worked on activities to ↓ Ⓛ neglect and ↑ safety to perform ADLs.
   —or—
   During her occupational therapy session, the pt. worked on increasing awareness of Ⓛ side and improving safety during ADLs.

   (In the incorrect example, it seems to indicate that therapy is working to increase the client's neglect and decrease her safety rather than what is intended.)

8. **I** instructed the client in **arom** exercises to improve her ability to braid her two **daughter's** hair.

   Client was instructed in AROM exercises to improve her ability to braid her two daughters' hair.

   (Focus on the client and not the practitioner.)

9. While eating her pudding **desert**, the client performed self-feeding with **modified assistance**.

   While eating her pudding dessert, the client performed self-feeding with modified independence.
   —or—
   While eating her pudding dessert, the client performed self-feeding with moderate assistance.

   (Modified assistance is not a standard term.)

10. The **THR client's** Ⓛ hip is sore because **the PT made her walk too long**.

    The client with a Ⓛ THR reported Ⓛ hip soreness following PT session.
    —or—
    The client who had Ⓛ hip replacement surgery reported soreness in Ⓛ hip.

    (Use people-first language and do not make subjective or judgmental statements about another professional in your note.)

11. The student **was** mod assist to write his name.

    Due to hand spasticity, the student needed mod assist to hold the pencil when writing his name.
    —or—
    When writing his name, the student needed mod assist with spatial orientation of the letters.
    —or—
    The student required mod assist to attend to task when writing his name.
        (Indicate that the client needs assist rather than the client is an assist level. Also, describe what part of the task needed assistance.)

12. The child had a rash around her **naval** which she kept **itching.**

    The child had a rash around her navel which she kept scratching.

Chapter 13

Worksheet 13-1: SOAPing Your Note

1. O Client supine → sit in bed Ⓘ.
2. O Client moved kitchen items from counter to cabinet Ⓘ using Ⓛ hand.
3. S Parent reports child's handwriting has improved significantly within the past month.
4. A Problems include decreased coordination, strength, sensation, and proprioception in left hand, which create safety risks in home management tasks.
5. S Client reports that his fingers are stiff this morning and that he is having trouble handling small items like buttons.
6. P By the end of next intervention session, client will demonstrate ability to don/doff orthosis Ⓘ.
7. A Increase of 15 minutes in activity tolerance for UE activities permits her to prepare a light meal Ⓘ.
8. O Child participated in 30-minute OT session to promote development of FM skills for ADLs.
9. A Deficits in proprioception and motor planning limit client's ability to dress herself.
10. P Continue ROM and retrograde massage to Ⓡ hand for edema control and to enable grasp of objects needed for ADLs.
11. P Consumer will be seen 2X weekly to improve attention to task in order to obtain a job.
12. S Client reports that she cannot remember her hip precautions.
13. A Client would benefit from further instruction to incorporate total hip precautions into lower body dressing, bathing, and toilet hygiene.
14. A Learning was evident by client's ability to improve with repetition.
15. A Client's request to take rest breaks demonstrates knowledge of her limitations in endurance.
16. O Client required three verbal prompts to interact with peers in OT social group.
17. A Fair plus muscle grade in Ⓡ wrist extensors this week shows good progress toward goals.
18. A Poor temporal organization interferes with getting to work on time.
19. P Next session, instruct parent in proper positioning of infant for bottle feeding.
20. O Client demonstrated ability to perform sliding board transfer w/c ↔ mat with min assist to position board properly.

Worksheet 13-2: Writing the "S"—Subjective

S: *Client reported significant arthritis in ⓡ shoulder and ⓡ knee, and a preference to approach transfers from the affected side. Client stated it hurts to bear weight on her ⓡ leg and reported pain as 7/10. She also stated w/c → bed sliding board transfers are the most difficult, and reported feeling tired at start of session.*

—*or*—

S: *Client stated she felt tired. She reported "bad arthritis" in ⓡ shoulder and ⓡ knee and stated knee pain is 7/10 when bearing weight on ⓡ LE. Pt. able to verbalize needs regarding sliding board transfer (placement of board and approach from affected side).*

Worksheet 13-3: Making Opening Lines Better

1.   Client practiced laundry tasks for 45 minutes.

  Client participated in 45-minute session in her laundry room at home to increase ⓘ in IADLs, improve safety during functional mobility, and to provide instruction on proper use of adaptive equipment for home management tasks.

  —*or*—

  Client participated in OT 45 minutes in hospital room for skilled instruction on total hip precautions and use of adaptive equipment to safely perform home management tasks.

  —*or*—

  In hospital room, client participated in 45-minute session for education on safety concerns during IADLs and skilled instruction in use of adaptive equipment for laundry tasks.

  —*or*—

  In OT clinic, client participated in 45-minute session for education in use of adaptive equipment and hip precautions during performance of home management tasks.

2.   Consumer seen at workshop for 1 hour to improve job skills.

  At workshop, consumer participated in 1-hour session to address time management, cognitive, sensory, and bilateral integration barriers to performing work tasks effectively.

  —*or*—

  Consumer participated in OT for 1 hour at workshop to work on sequencing, bilateral coordination, concentration, and time management skills while completing work task of package handling.

  —*or*—

  In order to improve time management and sequencing skills, increase bilateral coordination, and decrease distractibility for package handling at work, consumer participated in 60-minute OT session at workshop.

  —*or*—

  Consumer participated in 1-hour session at workshop for skilled instruction in task sequencing, bilateral coordination, and techniques to improve time management and decrease distractibility for job skills.

3.   Client seen in his hospital room bedside for 30 minutes for feeding.

  Client participated in 30-minute session bedside for instruction in adaptive equipment for feeding and to minimize unilateral neglect.

  —*or*—

  Client participated in 30-minute session bedside to increase ⓘ self-feeding and to decrease ⓛ neglect.

  —*or*—

  Client participated in 30-minute session bedside for education in compensatory methods for feeding and to ↑ awareness of left side.

  —*or*—

  At bedside for 30 minutes, client participated in OT for skilled instruction in self-feeding methods and to improve perceptual skills for ADLs.

4. Worked with client in kitchen for 1 hour to ↑ Ⓘ in cooking.

Client participated in 1-hour session in OT kitchen to increase activity tolerance for standing and increase awareness of affected UE for safety in cooking.

—or—

In OT kitchen, client participated in 1-hour session to address safety concerns regarding standing tolerance and left unilateral neglect.

—or—

Client participated in 60-minute OT session in kitchen to work on cooking tasks with attention to standing tolerance, position of affected left upper limb, and safety.

—or—

In OT kitchen, client participated in 1-hour session for skilled IADL instruction to improve safety, standing tolerance, and attention to weak UE.

Worksheet 13-4: Writing the "O"—Objective

First an opening line is needed stating where, for how long, and for what purpose the client was seen. One possibility is:

Client participated in 45-minute OT session in room for skilled instruction in ADL tasks and assessment of orthotic device needs.

—or—

Client participated in 60-minute session bedside for skilled instruction in compensatory techniques for dressing, toilet hygiene, and assessment of need for orthotic device

Second, the categories could be reduced to three (toileting, dressing, and orthotic device assessment) or two (ADLs and orthotic device assessment), and the statements about donning shoes can be combined.

Third, different assist levels are listed for upper body dressing, which is confusing. It would be helpful to know what parts of the task needed what kind of assistance. Also, more information about the type of toilet transfer would be useful. Did the client transfer from a w/c? Was a sliding board, walker, or grab bar used?

Fourth, the UE and LE wording is not inclusive enough because the client is dressing the upper and lower body rather than just the extremities. Specific types of clothing are not indicated (i.e., elastic waist paints, turtleneck sweater). The note also does not indicate where the client got dressed. Was the client sitting on the toilet, edge of the bed, in a w/c, or in a chair?

Finally, under hand status, there is no functional component, and "index finger greatest amount" is not very informative.

Worksheet 13-5: Differentiating Between Observations and Assessments

1. O Client is unable to don Ⓛ LE prosthesis for functional mobility.
2. A Inability to don Ⓛ LE prosthesis Ⓘ prevents client from performing safe functional mobility around the house to live alone.
3. A Decreased tolerance to auditory stimuli limits the student's ability to attend to classroom tasks.
4. O Student required three verbal cues to stay on task due to decreased tolerance to auditory stimuli.
5. O Client was unable to incorporate relaxation and stress reduction techniques, requiring several verbal prompts to complete task.
6. A Inability to incorporate relaxation and stress reduction techniques when interacting with sales clerk limits client's ability to manage shopping tasks Ⓘ after discharge.

Reword the following observations to make them **assessments**.

1. Client required 5 verbal cues to attend to and sequence task of balancing checkbook due to memory deficits.

Decreased memory limits client's ability to perform IADLs such as financial management tasks.

—or—

Memory deficits interfere with client's ability to perform IADLs such as financial management tasks, and limit her ability to return to an Ⓘ living situation.

—or—

Deficits in memory limit the client's ability to do many IADLs, for example, balancing her checkbook.

—or—

Deficits in memory lead to difficulty with IADLs such as financial management tasks necessary for household management.

2. Client needed moderate assistance to complete grooming and laundry tasks due to Ⓛ neglect, impulsive behavior, and decreased attention to task.

    Decreased safety awareness, poor attention, and perceptual deficits limit client's ability to complete homemaking tasks and self-care activities Ⓘ.

    —or—

    Decreased safety awareness and inattention to Ⓛ side interfere with client's ability to complete homemaking tasks and decrease her ability to complete activities of daily living Ⓘ successfully.

    —or—

    Decreased safety awareness and cognitive/perceptual deficits prevent client from performing homemaking and ADLs Ⓘ and safely.

3. After the use of behavior modification techniques, child demonstrated ability to remain seated at his desk for the remainder of the treatment session.

    In assessing this statement you could take a positive or a negative approach:

    Positive:

    Child's ability to remain seated at desk with the aid of behavior modification techniques indicates good potential for improving problem behaviors in school.

    —or—

    Child's positive response to behavior modification techniques shows good potential to meet classroom behavior goals.

    Negative:

    The need for behavior modification techniques to remain seated at desk limit child's ability to succeed with academic tasks.

    —or—

    Child's need for behavior modification in order to remain seated limits his ability to concentrate effectively in classroom situations.

Worksheet 13-6: Problems, Progress, and Rehab Potential

Problems:

After reading through this note, several problems stood out for this OTA:

- *Dynamic sitting balance*
- *Weight shifting*
- *Posture*
- *Transfers*

  These four areas are related to safety and functional mobility. Other apparent problems include:

- *Decreased AROM in Ⓡ UE (mod Ⓐ to reach)*
- *Cognition*

  On thinking a little further, the OTA decided that the "cognition" problem might really be one of the following because the client does seem to understand the goal of the activity:

- *Short-term memory*
- *Motor planning*
- *Problem solving*
- *Initiation*

  Finally, the OTA decides that the problem with initiation is probably some combination of problem-solving and motor planning deficit.

Progress/Rehab Potential

Ability to understand the treatment goal

The OTA then groups the problems according to the impact they have on the client's occupational performance. The OTA decides that the first three cause difficulty with functional mobility and are of particular concern because they create safety issues. The motor planning and initiation problem is a concern in the area of self-care, as is the problem with decreased AROM of the right UE. The need for continual instruction, whether it is a problem with short-term memory or with ability to problem solve, is likely to require a lot of attention from a caregiver at home. The client does, however, understand why he is doing the given task. As long as the goals are not set too high, the client should be able to make good progress in rehabilitation. The OTA's assessment and plan read as follows:

A: *Deficits in postural control, dynamic sitting balance, and weight shifting raise safety concerns when transferring. ↓ AROM and motor planning ability negatively impact ability to perform self-care tasks. A need for continual instruction to prevent unsafe performance of ADL tasks requires a high level of caregiver assistance. Client's ability to understand treatment goal indicates good rehab potential for the goals established. Client would benefit from continued skilled instruction in activities to ↑ balance, safe functional mobility, and facilitate Ⓘ in ADL tasks.*

P: *Continue OT daily for 3 weeks for skilled instruction in self-care tasks and safe transfers. Next session, instruct client in w/c ↔ toilet transfer using grab bar to facilitate forward weight shifting in w/c.*

Another OTA might assess the session a little differently. For example:

A: *Problems include deficits in motor planning, movement initiation, cognition, and muscle weakness in Ⓡ UE, which ↓ safety in ADL tasks and functional mobility. Activity tolerance for Ⓡ UE reaching tasks has improved since yesterday from < 1 minute to > 3 minutes without a rest break. Client would benefit from skilled OT to increase balance, functional mobility, and grasp/release activities with involved UE in order to ↑ Ⓘ in self-care activities.*

P: *Continue OT twice daily for half-hour sessions to work on Ⓡ UE movement and cognitive retraining in order to complete grooming activities with min Ⓐ. Next session will focus on facilitating Ⓡ hand grasp for grooming, such as squeezing toothpaste tube and holding hairbrush.*

—*or*—

A: *Decreased functional use of the Ⓡ UE, decreased sitting balance, and difficulty with sequencing and problem solving limit ability to perform ADLs. Increased shoulder flexion and improved motor planning since initial evaluation, and increased understanding of treatment activities indicate good rehab potential. Client would benefit from continued skilled OT for exercises to increase functional AROM, grasp, and weight shifting to improve dynamic sitting balance. Client would also benefit from evaluation of both cognitive status and ability to initiate activity in order to increase Ⓘ in ADL tasks.*

P: *Continue OT twice daily for 30-minute sessions for 2 weeks to increase dynamic sitting balance in preparation for ADLs. Client will be able to reach for grooming items placed slightly beyond arm's reach with CGA within 1 week.*

Worksheet 13-7: The "Almost" Note

Here we have a note that seems good on the surface, but it demonstrates some problems in critical thinking and organization. The most outstanding problem with this note is that the OTA is mixing the "O" data and the "A" data.

First, it would have helped the "S" if the OTA had asked pertinent questions, such as what the client's pain levels were.

Second, the note should indicate active client participation rather than the client just being "seen" in therapy. There is nothing in the "O" to show that skilled occupational therapy is being provided. The list of observations of assist levels fails to provide the richness of the skill used in treatment. The OTA erroneously puts some of that information in the "A" section, rather than assessing the data. In the "A" the OTA tells us:

Deficits noted in Ⓡ UE coordination, Ⓑ UE strength, and dynamic standing balance. Client Ⓘ in dressing EOB, but is min Ⓐ in dressing when standing with a walker. Ⓛ UE AROM is WFL but Ⓡ UE has deficits noted in shoulder flexion. Client is SBA in bed mobility when rolling to unaffected side and min Ⓐ in sit → stand 2° ↓ UE strength. Client is SBA for transfer to unaffected side in pivot transfer bed → w/c and min Ⓐ w/c → toilet. Client would benefit from skilled OT to continue UE strengthening and coordination exercises and to ↑ dynamic standing balance using walker, in order to ↑ Ⓘ in ADLs.

Even if this information were moved into the "O," there is nothing to tell us what part of the task the assistance was for. The OTA uses a nonstandard abbreviation "VCs." The OTA means verbal cues, but since VC is a standard health term meaning *vital capacity*, it is inappropriate in its usage here and is not on the approved list in this manual. Also, the OTA should be more specific than simply stating, "*↓ range in shoulder flexion.*" For example, is shoulder flexion 90 degrees or 150 degrees? Does the ROM deficit limit ability to dress or use walker?

Third, the coordination deficits mentioned in the "A" section come out of the blue. There is no mention of coordination in the opening statement "*… for work on dressing and functional mobility,*" nor is it mentioned as a problem in the "O." Thus, the statement that coordination deficits are one of the problems noted and the statement that the client would benefit from coordination exercises are unsubstantiated. Remember not to introduce any new information in the "A" section of your note. Information regarding transfers and bed mobility is redundant because it is simply stated twice without any additional assessment or clinical judgment. Also, do not state that the client *is* an assist level but, instead, *needs* the assist level. The assist levels noted for dressing are also a bit confusing.

There is no real assessment of the meaning of the data found in the "S" and the "O." There is a short list of problem areas, but no assessment of their impact on the ability to engage in meaningful occupation, and no assessment of the rehab potential shown by the client's willingness to "do whatever it takes to get out of the hospital."

The best thing for this OTA to do is to rewrite the "O" section, providing a more comprehensive picture of the intervention session. Then, the OTA needs to assess the data based on skilled observations and clinical reasoning. There needs to be an indication of how the observed data impacts the occupational performance of the client before the statements about what the client would benefit from.

Depending on the assessment the OTA makes, the plan to work on balance may be appropriate, or it may be only one of the things to be addressed. The note does not indicate if the client's deficits are due to cognitive problems, such as memory deficits, poor problem solving, or decreased safety awareness. Does the client have limited endurance or poor motor planning? Those might be additional areas that need to be addressed in the plan. Also, the client may benefit from further occupational therapy to work on safe transfers, and further retraining in dressing or other ADLs.

Chapter 14

Worksheet 14-1: Initial Evaluation Report

Background Data

Criteria	How Does the Evaluation Comply With the Criteria?
Are all of the following present: name, date of birth, gender? Are all applicable diagnoses and health information listed along with applicable case number?	*Name, date of birth, and gender are all indicated.* *Dx: Ⓡ CVA; R/O OBS* *2° Dx: Type 2 diabetes* *Hx: Left CTR 2005, diabetic history*
Is it clear who referred the client to occupational therapy, on what date, and what services were requested?	*Dr. Heelue referred her for evaluation and treatment on 5/3/2022.*
Is the funding source listed for this client?	*Medicare*
Is anticipated length of stay indicated for this client?	*2 weeks*
Why is the client seeking occupational therapy services?	*She wants to be independent and return home.*
Are there any secondary problems, preexisting conditions, contraindications, or precautions that will impact therapy?	*Diabetes*

Occupational History and Profile

Is there an occupational history/profile? Is it adequate?	*There is a brief occupational profile. More information can be obtained during intervention.*
Which areas of occupation are currently successful and which are problematic?	*No successful areas noted. ADL and IADL tasks are problematic.*
What factors hinder the client's performance in areas of occupation? What factors support performance in areas of occupation?	***Hinder:*** *↓ problem-solving ability, slow cognitive responses ↓ ability to initiate and sequence tasks. Some client factors not WNL.* ***Support:*** *A nearby daughter who is willing to visit daily and assist with transportation, intact sensation, motor planning and perception WFL, able to stand and transfer with CGA, one-story home, sedentary hobbies, motivation to go home.*
What are the client's priorities? What does the client hope to gain from occupational therapy?	*To be Ⓘ and go back to her own home*
What areas of occupation will be targeted for intervention? Do these match the client's priorities?	*ADLs and IADLs, which do match the client's priorities*
What are the targeted outcomes?	*Discharge to home* *Modified Ⓘ and safety in ADL activities*

Results of the Assessment

What types of assessments were used?	*Mini-Mental State, ADL evaluation, manual muscle test, sensation, observation, interview, AROM*
What were the results of the assessments?	*Results are clearly noted on the evaluation form and in the "A."*
What client factors, performance skills, patterns, contextual aspects, and activity demands are identified as needing attention?	***Client factors:*** *↓ AROM and strength in the Ⓛ UE, ↓ activity tolerance, ↓ problem solving, sequencing, and memory* ***Context:*** *lives alone and daughter unable to provide supervision; needs cues for orientation.* ***Activity demands:*** *Needs cues to initiate and sequence activities and to problem solve.*
What factors (strengths, supports) facilitate the client's occupational performance?	*Supportive daughter, client motivated to be Ⓘ*
Are there other areas that need to be assessed that are not listed?	*Does client use hearing aid, glasses, or mobility devices? Does client have pain, edema, or changes in muscle tone? Additional considerations for occupational profile (e.g., spirituality, virtual contexts, educational level, habits and routines)? Stair rails present at home? Set-up of bathroom (tub or shower stall)? Ability to perform grooming tasks presently?*
Is occupational therapy appropriate for this client? Why or why not?	*Yes—client has good rehab potential to return home and requires occupational therapy to improve ADL function and safety.*

Worksheet 14-2: Intervention Plan

Criteria	How Does the Intervention Plan Comply With the Criteria?
Are the intervention goals and objectives measurable and realistic?	*Yes*
Are the goals and objectives directly related to the client's occupational role performance?	*Yes*
Are specific occupational therapy interventions identified?	*Yes*
Are the interventions listed appropriate to work toward the established goals?	*Yes*
What is the anticipated frequency/duration/intensity of services?	*45-minute sessions 5X wk for 2 weeks*
What is the discontinuation criteria or expected outcomes?	*Ability to live at home safely without supervision*
What is the anticipated discharge location?	*Home*
What is the anticipated plan for follow-up care?	*Meeting with daughter*
Where will service be provided?	*Healthy Hospital as inpatient*
Will these services meet payer requirements?	*Yes, reasonable and medically necessary*
Are there areas of concern that are not addressed in the goals/intervention plan specifically?	*Bathing, specific grooming tasks that may be problematic and snack/light meal preparation do not have goals but the underlying performance skills/factors are being addressed in other areas.*

Worksheet 14-3: Choosing Activities—More Practice

How could you work on these goals simultaneously? What would you choose as intervention activities?

1. *Student will be able to open all containers and wrappers Ⓘ for his lunch at school.*
2. *In order to perform bimanual classroom tasks, student will use Ⓛ hand spontaneously as a functional assist 5/5 opportunities.*
3. *Student will attend to classroom tasks for 10-minute periods with only one verbal cue for redirection.*

You can work with the child at lunchtime in the cafeteria or in another room to teach adaptive techniques and facilitate performance skills. You could have the child try to open all of the lunch items such as lunch box, brown bag, milk carton, sandwich wrapper, straw wrapper, plastic containers, snack bags, and so forth while teaching compensatory techniques, proper positioning, etc. You will note if the child is incorporating use of both hands spontaneously for these tasks and how well the Ⓛ hand is being used as a functional assist for setting up lunch items. You will document skilled occupational therapy happening and also note the number of minutes for attention to task and if child needs to be redirected to task.

—or—

You might also have the child perform another task that involves opening containers, such as a craft project where materials are in snack bags or small jars/containers. Again, you would note the skilled occupational therapy being provided, Ⓛ hand use, and attention span.

Chapter 15

Worksheet 15-1: Evaluating Goal Statements

1. By the time of expected discharge in 1 week, client will be able to dress himself with min Ⓐ for balance using a sock aid and reacher while seated in wheelchair.

   This goal has all the necessary COAST components to be useful.

2. Client will tolerate 15 minutes of treatment daily.

   This goal lacks a function and a time frame. In addition, the behavior (tolerating treatment) is not useful because it is not something a client needs to do after discharge. This would be better stated as "tolerate 15 minutes of grooming/hygiene activity."

3. Client will demonstrate increased coping skills in order to live at home with her granddaughter within 2 weeks.

   This goal lacks specificity, and it needs a condition. "Coping skills" is far too broad. The coping skill(s) in question need to be specified.

4. Resident will demonstrate 15 minutes of activity tolerance without rest breaks using Ⓑ UE in order to complete self-care tasks before breakfast each morning.

   This goal lacks a time frame and needs to be turned around to put function first. For example: Resident will be able to complete grooming and dressing in <15 minutes without rest breaks before breakfast each morning within 2 weeks.

5. In order to be able to toilet self after discharge, client will demonstrate ability to perform a sliding board transfer w/c → mat within the next week.

   This goal has all the necessary COAST components to be useful but would be even better if the assist level of the transfer were noted (e.g., modified Ⓘ).

6. OTA will teach lower body dressing using a reacher, dressing stick, and sock aid within 2 intervention sessions.

   This goal lacks a proper client action and assist level, and should focus on what the client, not the OT or OTA, will do.

7. In order to return to living independently, client will demonstrate ability to balance his checkbook.

   This goal lacks a time frame and would be even better if the assist level for balancing his checkbook were specified (e.g., ability to balance his checkbook Ⓘ).

Worksheet 15-2: Writing Goals That Are Client-Centered, Occupation-Based, and Measurable

1. *Without knowing the client, it is impossible to know what the goal would really be. Here are some suggestions.*

   Within three intervention sessions, client will prepare a sandwich and canned soup with supervision and maintain task attention > 10 minutes without redirection.

   —or—

   Client will demonstrate 10-minute attention span for simple cold meal preparation, requiring no more than 3 verbal cues for redirection by the end of the 3rd treatment session.

2. *By anticipated discharge in 1 week, client will cook a packaged microwave meal with min Ⓐ to follow three-step written directions.*

   —or—

   Client will demonstrate ability to follow a three-step recipe Ⓘ within 1 week.

3. *Client will be able to don shirt with modified Ⓘ using the over-the-head method and a buttonhook within two treatment sessions.*

   —or—

   Client will be able to dress upper body with modified Ⓘ using one-handed techniques and adaptive equipment by 7/27/22.

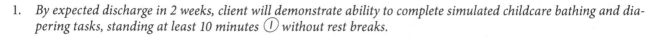

Worksheet 15-3: Writing Goals That Are Client-Centered, Occupation-Based, and Measurable—More Practice

1. *By expected discharge in 2 weeks, client will demonstrate ability to complete simulated childcare bathing and diapering tasks, standing at least 10 minutes Ⓘ without rest breaks.*

   —or—

   Client will complete seated work-simulation tasks (filing and data entry) for 30 minutes without rest breaks within 1 week.

2. *Client will make change from $5.00 correctly 3/3 tries by 9/10/22.*

   —or—

   Client will select ads from the newspaper for an apartment that rents for less than 1/3 of his regular monthly income with minimal verbal cues within the next month.

3. *Within 1 week, client will spontaneously complete showering, dressing, and grooming prior to attending morning groups 3/3 days.*

   —or—

   Within the next 2 days, client will verbalize an interest in participating in at least one future activity without prompting.

Worksheet 15-4: Writing Goals—Developmental Disability

Without knowing the client, it is impossible to know what the goals should really be. Here are some suggestions for functional goals:

1. **Instrumental ADL—meal preparation:** *Client will be able to wash and peel vegetables to make a salad with min verbal cues within 4 weeks.*

   —or—

   Client will prepare a two-step frozen breakfast item with supervision using toaster oven or microwave safely within 3 weeks.

2. **Instrumental ADL—household chore:** *Client will be able to follow the chore schedule for changing bedsheets with one verbal reminder within 4 weeks.*

   —or—

   Client will demonstrate ability to set the table for six place settings using a visual cue (diagram) within 1 week.

3. **Instrumental ADL—shopping:** *Client will locate five items in supermarket using grocery list with 1 verbal cue for each item within 4 weeks.*

   —or—

   Client will be able to locate correct size clothing when shopping within 2 weeks.

4. **Instrumental ADL—money management/functional math skill:** *When shopping, client will use correct denominations to pay cashier Ⓘ for items up to $10.00 within 6 weeks.*

   —or—

   In order to improve shopping skills, client will select and place correct coins in vending machine Ⓘ by 8/31/22.

5. **Communication/interaction skills:** *Client will demonstrate improved social skills by cooperatively playing a simple board game with peers for 20 minutes within 3 weeks.*

   —or—

   Client will demonstrate improved social interaction skills by spontaneously allowing roommate to choose TV program without an altercation within 3 weeks.

6. **Prevocational skills:** *To improve prevocational skills, client will demonstrate ability to correctly punch a time clock 5/5 opportunities within 2 weeks.*

   —or—

   In order to ↑ skills required for employment, client will select appropriate attire for job interview with min verbal cues within 2 weeks.

7. **Temporal organization/time management:** *In order to improve time management skills for ADLs, client will set alarm clock with one verbal cue within 4 weeks.*

—*or*—

In order to improve time management skills for morning self-care, client will follow daily schedule Ⓘ within 1 week.

Worksheet 15-5: Goal Writing—ADL Performance Skills and Factors

Goals will depend on a client's specific circumstances. However, the following are some suggestions for the ADL of brushing teeth:

1. **Fine-motor skills:** *Client will demonstrate improved dexterity for grooming by demonstrating ability to open and close toothpaste cap Ⓘ within 2 weeks.*

—*or*—

Within 3 intervention sessions, client will be able to use a cylindrical grasp to hold toothbrush with affected hand when applying toothpaste.

2. **Hand strength:** *Client will demonstrate improved hand strength for brushing teeth by holding 5-ounce cup of water with affected hand and bringing it to mouth Ⓘ within 1 week.*

—*or*—

Child will demonstrate improved Ⓡ hand strength for grooming by squeezing toothpaste onto toothbrush with min Ⓐ within 1 week.

3. **Standing balance:** *When brushing teeth, child will demonstrate improved dynamic standing balance from poor to fair standing at sink with contact guard assist within 2 months.*

4. **Unilateral inattention:** *Client will demonstrate improved Ⓛ side attention for grooming by locating all items needed for tooth brushing with min verbal cues by 5/10/22.*

5. **Elbow range of motion:** *In order to bring toothbrush to mouth, resident will increase Ⓡ elbow flexion by 30° by 3/19/22.*

6. **Problem solving:** *By 4/2/22, client will demonstrate improved problem-solving skills for grooming by verbalizing several alternatives when there are no more paper cups available for rinsing teeth.*

7. **Spatial relations:** *Child will demonstrate improved spatial relations for grooming by applying toothpaste in a straight line on brush without spilling within 1 wk.*

Chapter 16

Worksheet 16-1: Contact Notes

Criteria	How Does Your Note Comply With the Criteria?
Does the note state the client's full name and identifying number?	*Client's first name, last name, health number, gender, and date of birth are listed.*
Is information relating to the client's diagnosis and precautions/contraindications specified?	*COPD: Maintain O_2 levels at 95% to 100%*
Are the date (and time, if needed) of the contact indicated?	*Date and time of session are listed*
Is the note identified as occupational therapy?	*Yes*
Is the type of note indicated?	*Contact note*
Does the note state the type of contact and purpose of the encounter?	*Instruction in ADL tasks and increase activity tolerance*
Is there a summary of the interventions implemented or information communicated during the contact (e.g., modification of the task or environment, assistive/adaptive devices fabricated or used, education, training, or consultation provided, outcome measures used), and indication of client's present performance level?	*Description of ADL training for bed mobility and self-care along with assessment and reporting of oxygen levels and functional performance during tasks. Instruction in proper breathing techniques provided.*
Is the client's attendance and participation in the contact (or the reason service was missed) indicated?	*Active client participation noted*
Does the note indicate names/positions of persons involved?	*Client and occupational therapy practitioner*
Are all abbreviations and terminology standard and acceptable for the setting?	*Yes*
Are all errors noted and corrected properly?	*No errors identified in this note*
Is the note signed (and cosigned if needed)?	*Signatures of OTA and OT are in place*
Are professional credentials indicated next to the signature?	*Professional credentials and licensure are noted*
Are intervention/procedure codes indicated if needed?	*Not listed in this note (may not be needed)*
Does the note reflect skilled occupational therapy happening?	*Yes. OTA assesses level of self-care function and endurance. OTA uses clinical reasoning to note effects of oxygen levels on activity tolerance and how that impacts ADLs. OTA determines that further instruction in energy conservation, breathing techniques, and positioning is needed to improve ADL abilities.*

Worksheet 16-2: Progress Note

Criteria	How Does Your Note Comply With the Criteria?
Does the note state the client's full name and identifying number?	*Client's first name, last name, health record number, gender, and date of birth are listed.*
Is the date of the progress note specified?	*Yes*
Is the note identified as occupational therapy?	*Yes*
Is the type of note indicated?	*Progress note*
Has new data been obtained and presented?	*Client's attendance, participation, mood, behavior, appearance/grooming, and communication are all noted.*
Is information relating to the client's condition and precautions/contraindications specified?	*Note relates information pertinent to client's diagnosis of depression. No specific precautions/contraindications identified. If client were at risk for suicide, for example, this should be noted.*
Does the note state pertinent client updates, problems, or changes to the intervention plan?	*Goals that have not yet been met are modified or discontinued*
Does the note indicate the frequency of services and how long services have been provided?	*Client attended six out of eight OT groups this week. Start of care date indicated.*
Does the note indicate what areas of occupation are being addressed?	*IADLs, time management, leisure, social skills (communication, assertion)*
Is there a summary of techniques and strategies used? Does the note specify occupational adaptations, assistive technology/adaptive devices, orthotics, or other skilled services provided?	*OT communication group, assertion group, IADL group*
Does the note indicate the type of education, training, or consultation that has been provided and to whom?	*Client participated in OT groups addressing communication, assertion, and IADLs and has been educated regarding a structured leisure plan.*
Does the note indicate what progress (or lack thereof) the client is making toward established goals?	*Progress includes improved mood and hygiene/dressing, increased participation, and spontaneous communication in group; several goals were noted to be met.*
Does the note indicate the client's response to occupational therapy services?	*Client making progress in several areas and demonstrates increased participation in groups.*
Does the note reflect the client's occupational performance?	*Self-care and social/communication skills are noted.*
Are any outcomes measures identified? Are they appropriate to the client's condition/situation and relate to function?	*Objective observations of client's behaviors and mood noted. It might be better if specific standardized assessments were used.*
Are recommendations indicated along with rationale? Will therapy be continued, discontinued, or is there need for referral?	*Continue OT groups until expected discharge date in 2 days. Specific plan was established and an individual session will be provided if needed.*
Does the note reflect the client's input to changes or continuation of the intervention plan?	*Client expressed willingness to follow up with developing a structured leisure plan.*
Are all abbreviations and terminology standard and acceptable for the setting?	*Yes*
Are errors noted and corrected properly?	*No errors indicated in this note.*
Is the note signed (and cosigned if needed)?	*Yes*
Are professional credentials indicated next to the signature?	*Yes*

Chapter 17

Worksheet 17-1: Types of Documentation

1. *g. (OASIS)* — Outcome measure required by Medicare and Medicaid for use in home care
2. *f. (IEP)* — Yearly multidisciplinary plan established for a particular student requiring special services
3. *j. (Intervention plan)* — Contains goals and specific treatment approaches relating to desired client outcomes
4. *d. (Discontinuation report)* — Written when occupational therapy services are no longer needed
5. *b. (MDS)* — Interdisciplinary assessment used in a skilled nursing facility to determine a client's problem areas and care plan
6. *h. (Progress report)* — Summarizes course of treatment and progress toward achieving goals during specified intervals
7. *a. (Contact note)* — Written following a treatment session and includes intervention provided, information communicated, and client's response to furnished service
8. *c. (Initial evaluation)* — Consists of an occupational profile and factors affecting engagement in occupation
9. *i. (Reevaluation report)* — A determination of the client's present status as compared to start of care, including progress, problems, and revision of goals
10. *k. (Occupational profile)* — Includes the client's roles, responsibilities, and factors such as values, culture, physical and social environments, age, and educational level
11. *e. (Transition plan)* — Written to provide consistency when a client switches from one setting to another during the treatment continuum
12. *m. (Clinical pathway)* — A blueprint for a client's care preplanned for each day and for each discipline based on a specific diagnosis
13. *o. (POC)* — Part of the therapy report that must be certified by the physician in home health
14. *n. (IRF-PAI)* — Mandated assessment to determine care levels in an inpatient rehabilitation facility
15. *l. (IFSP)* — Established for children under age 3 years and identifies a service coordinator

References

American Occupational Therapy Association. (2018a). Guidelines for documentation of occupational therapy. *American Journal of Occupational Therapy, 72*(Suppl. 2),7212410010. https://doi.org :10.5014/ajot.2018.72S203

American Occupational Therapy Association. (2018b). Physical agents and mechanical modalities. *American Journal of Occupational Therapy, 72*(Suppl. 2), 7212410055. https://doi.org/10.5014/ajot.2018.72S220

American Occupational Therapy Association. (2020a). Guidelines for supervision, roles, and responsibilities during the delivery of occupational therapy services. *American Journal of Occupational Therapy, 74*(Suppl. 3), 7413410020. https://doi.org/10.5014/ajot.2020.74S3004

American Occupational Therapy Association. (2020b). Occupational therapy practice framework: Domain and process (4th ed.). *American Journal of Occupational Therapy, 74*(Suppl. 2), 7412410010. https://doi.org: 10.5014/ajot.2020.74S2001

American Occupational Therapy Association. (2021a). Occupational therapy scope of practice. *American Journal of Occupational Therapy, 75*(Suppl. 3), 7513410020. https://doi.org/10.5014/ajot.2021.75S3005

American Occupational Therapy Association. (2021b). Standards of practice for occupational therapy. *American Journal of Occupational Therapy, 75*(Suppl. 3), 7513410030. https://doi.org/10.5014/ajot.2021.75S3004

American Psychological Association. (2020). *Publication manual of the American Psychological Association* (7th ed.). Author.

Centers for Medicare & Medicaid Services. (2019). *Medicare benefit policy manual* (Pub. 100-02: Ch. 15, Section 220). Retrieved October 11, 2021 from https://www.cms.gov/Regulations-and-Guidance/Guidance/Manuals/Downloads/bp102c15.pdf

Davis, L., & Rosee, M. (2015). *Occupational therapy student to clinician: Making the transition.* SLACK Incorporated.

Harris, J. C. (2013). New terminology for mental retardation in DSM-5 and ICD-11. *Current Opinion in Psychiatry, 26*(3), 260-262. Retrieved from https://www.medscape.com/viewarticle/782769

Morreale, M. J. (2022). *Developing clinical competence: A workbook for the OTA* (2nd ed.). SLACK Incorporated.

Morreale, M. J., & Amini, D. (2016). *The occupational therapist's workbook for ensuring clinical competence.* SLACK Incorporated.

NetLingo. (2021). NetLingo: Every texting abbreviation & online acronym you'll ever need to know. Retrieved October 29, 2021 from https://www.netlingo.com/acronyms.php

Reed, G. M., First, M. B., Kogan, C. S., Hyman, S. E., Gureje, O., Gaebel, W., Maj, M., Stein, D. J., Maercker, A., Tyrer, P., Claudino, A., Garralda, E., Salvador-Carulla, L., Ray, R., Saunders, J. B., Dua, T., Poznyak, V., Medina-Mora, M. E., Pike, K. M., Ayuso-Mateos, J. L., … Saxena, S. (2019). Innovations and changes in the ICD-11 classification of mental, behavioural and neurodevelopmental disorders. *World psychiatry: Official journal of the World Psychiatric Association (WPA), 18*(1), 3-19. https://www.ncbi.nlm.nih.gov/pmc/articles/PMC6313247/

U.S. Department of Education. (2017). July 11, 2017 (82 FR 31910). Retrieved October 13, 2021 from https://sites.ed.gov/idea/idea-files/july-11-2017-82-fr-31910/

Index

A Quick Checklist for Evaluating Your Note

Use the following two summary charts as a quick reference guide to ensure that your note contains all of the essential elements.

	S: Subjective
☐	1. Use something significant the client says about their treatment or condition.
	O: Objective
☐	1. Begin this section with:
☐	○ Indication of active client engagement/participation
☐	○ Length of session
☐	○ Setting
☐	○ Purpose of session
☐	2. Report your observations succinctly and accurately, either chronologically or using categories.
☐	3. Remember to do the following:
☐	○ De-emphasize the treatment media
☐	○ Specify what part of the task required assistance
☐	○ Specify the exact type and amount of assistance needed
☐	○ Use professional language and standard abbreviations
☐	○ Show skilled occupational therapy happening
☐	○ Leave yourself out
☐	○ Focus on the client's response
☐	○ Avoid being judgmental
	A: Assessment
☐	1. Look at the data in your "S" and "O" sentence by sentence, asking yourself what problems, progress, and rehab potential you see.
☐	2. Ask yourself, "So what? Why is this important in the client's life?" For each underlying factor not within functional limits, identify the impact it will have on an area of occupation.
☐	3. End the "A" with *"Client would benefit from…"*
☐	○ Justify continued skilled occupational therapy
☐	○ Set up the plan
☐	4. Be sure the timelines and interventions you are putting in your plan match the skilled OT you indicate your client needs.
	P: Plan
☐	1. Specify the frequency and duration of occupational therapy intervention.
☐	2. Tell what you will be working on during that time to address the client's needs.
☐	3. Relate to a performance skill/area of occupation and client's OT goals.
☐	4. Indicate any other pertinent follow-up needed for the client's present situation.
	Remember to:
☐	Include the client's identifying information and delineate OT department and type of note.
☐	Correct errors properly, do not erase or use correction fluid, and do not leave blank spaces.
☐	Make certain engagement in occupation is integral to the note.
☐	Sign and date your note.

Morreale, M. J. (2023). *The OTA's guide to documentation: Writing SOAP notes* (5th ed.). SLACK Incorporated.

S: Subjective
- ☐ Use something **significant** the client says about their **treatment** or **condition**.
- ☐ If there is nothing significant, ask yourself whether you are using your interview skills to elicit the proper information about how the client sees things.

O: Objective
- ☐ Begin this section with length of session, where the intervention took place, and for what purpose. Make sure you indicate active client participation. For example:
  Client participated in 30-minute OT session in hospital room for instruction in compensatory dressing techniques.
- ☐ Summarize what you observe, either chronologically or using categories.
- ☐ Focus on performance skills and de-emphasize the treatment media. For example:
  Client worked on three-point pinch using pegs.
- ☐ Relate methods/tasks (i.e., ROM, physical agent modalities) to occupational performance.
  Client worked on three-point pinch using pegs in order to manage buttons on clothing.
- ☐ Specify the **part** of the task needing assistance and the exact **type** and **amount** of assistance provided.
  Client required five verbal cues for correct hand placement during w/c ↔ toilet transfers.
- ☐ Indicate that the client **needed** assistance rather than labeling the client as an assist level.
  "Client required min assist..." rather than *"Client is min assist..."*
- ☐ Use standardized terminology to grade and describe interventions and client performance.
- ☐ Show skilled occupational therapy happening—make it clear that you were not just a passive observer. For example, do not just list all of the assist levels and think that is enough.
- ☐ Write from the client's point of view, leaving yourself out.
  "Client was repositioned in w/c..." rather than *"COTA repositioned client in w/c..."*
- ☐ Focus on the client's response rather than on what you did.
  Client able to don socks using sock aid after demonstration.
- ☐ Avoid judging the client. For example:
  Say client *"...didn't complete the activity."* Don't add *"...because he was stubborn."*

A: Assessment
- ☐ Look at the data in your "S" and "O" sentence by sentence, identifying problems, progress, and rehab potential. Ask yourself what each statement means for the client's occupational performance. Consider the following formula:

Underlying Limiting Factor ———▶	Functional Impact ————▶	Ability to Engage in Occupation

For example, if in your "O" you noted that client falls to the left when sitting unsupported, what do you think this means they will be unable to do for themselves? For example:
  Client unable to sit EOB unsupported to don clothing.
- ☐ Make sure you have not introduced any new information.
- ☐ End the "A" with *"Client would benefit from..."*
- ☐ Justify continued skilled occupational therapy.
  Client would benefit from skilled instruction in use of adaptive devices and compensatory techniques for performing IADL tasks one-handed.
- ☐ Set up the plan and match time lines in your plan to the skilled OT you document that your client needs. For example, if you justify skilled OT by saying only, *"Client would benefit from skilled instruction in energy conservation techniques,"* then do not say that you plan to treat client twice a day for 2 weeks. Skilled instruction in energy conservation should generally take only one session or, at most, two sessions.

P: Plan
- ☐ Specify the frequency, duration of treatment, and specific OT interventions that will be implemented.
- ☐ Identify the performance skills and occupations that will be addressed during that time.
  Continue OT 1 hour daily for 2 weeks for upper body strengthening and instruction in adaptive devices needed for safe and Ⓘ transfers to bed, toilet, and tub.

Morreale, M. J. (2023). *The OTA's guide to documentation: Writing SOAP notes* (5th ed.). SLACK Incorporated.

Printed in the United States
by Baker & Taylor Publisher Services